THE TREATMENT OF PSYCHIATRIC DISORDERS

Third Edition, Revised for DSM-IV

William H. Reid, M.D., M.P.H.

and

George Ulysses Balis, M.D.

with

Beverly J. Sutton, M.D.

BRUNNER/MAZEL, Publishers

A member of the Taylor & Francis Group

Library of Congress Cataloging-in-Publication Data
Reid, William H.
    The treatment of psychiatric disorders / William H. Reid and
George Ulysses Balis, with additional chapters by Beverly J. Sutton.
— 3rd ed., rev. for DSM-IV.
      p.   cm.
    Includes bibliographical references and indexes.
    ISBN 0-87630-765-9 (hard cover)
    1. Mental illness—Treatment.   I. Balis, George U.   II. Sutton,
Beverly J.   III. Title.
    [DNLM: 1. Mental Disorders—therapy.   WM 400 R359t 1997]
RC480.R4 1997
616.89'1—DC20
DNLM/DLC
for Library of Congress   96-7478
                                                    CIP

Published by
BRUNNER/MAZEL, INC.
A member of the Taylor & Francis Group
1900 Frost Road, Suite 101
Bristol, PA 19007

Manufactured in the United States of America

10 9 8 7 6 5 4 3 2 1

To Elise, who supported this project one more time,
To Sophia, Theodora, and Chrysanthy
To our colleagues in the public sector,
and to Robert Boorstin, who speaks eloquently of his own experience
and counsels us that we best serve those who need us
when we see them as patients with mental illness,
not as "consumers" with behavioral health problems.

Contents

Part I

NEUROPSYCHIATRIC DISORDERS

George Ulysses Balis, M.D.

Part II

SUBSTANCE-RELATED DISORDERS

George Ulysses Balis, M.D.

Part III

OTHER DISORDERS PRIMARILY SEEN IN ADULTS

William H. Reid, M.D., M.P.H.

Part IV

DISORDERS USUALLY FIRST DIAGNOSED IN INFANCY, CHILDHOOD, OR ADOLESCENCE

Beverly J. Sutton, M.D.

APPENDICES

Preface to
the Third Edition

This is a book for clinicians. It focuses on the needs of their patients. One is some-times tempted to mitigate "pure" or "scientific" treatment preferences with con-siderations of treatment availability, cost, and/or cost containment. Nevertheless, the authors have generally chosen not to compromise either clinicians' stan-dards or patients' needs. We have tried to suggest the *right* thing to do. The rest is up to you.

Introduction

Audience. Although this book is intended primarily for physicians familiar with psychiatry, it is also written for the many other clinicians who need a concise volume that focuses solely on treatment guidelines and that attempts to integrate the biopsychosocial interventions, which are synergistic for our patients.

Style. There are many ways to approach the writing of a book such as this. One is to have a different expert write each section or subsection. Although this often works well for multivolume reference texts, the loss of continuity and the variability among sections in some edited books were considered unacceptable for our purposes. We hope that readers will find this a relatively concise and affordable, but acceptably complete, resource.

Assumptions. The authors assume that the reader is familiar with psychiatric evaluation and with the diagnostic format of the fourth edition of the *Diagnostic and Statistical Manual of Mental Disorders* (DSM-IV). He or she should have working diagnoses in mind before picking up this book. We also assume that basic medical and technical concepts have been (or will be) learned elsewhere.

Comprehensiveness. Several thousand studies, clinical reports, and texts, most published after 1990, were reviewed for this book. Several hundred are referenced herein. We believe that virtually all standard treatments, and a number of esoteric ones, have been included. Some experimental or unproved therapies are mentioned; every effort has been made to identify them as such.

The text recommends, describes, and briefly expands upon therapeutic modalities; nevertheless, *we make no attempt to present a complete discussion of specific treatment techniques.* We do not warrant, for example, that we have provided complete information concerning workup, prescribing, and follow-up for medications. Doses and other detailed information are sometimes given; however, the clinician must also rely on his or her overall training and experience, other available information sources, and understanding of the individual clinical situation before proceeding.

There is no real substitute for psychiatric training and experience in the treatment of most psychiatric disorders. Accordingly, although this book will be useful for general physicians and many nonmedical mental health professionals, it is not intended to take the place of consultation with, or referral to, a psychiatrist. For the most part, the treatment techniques recommended assume a clinical setting in which appropriate monitoring, peripheral care, and follow-up can be arranged.

Links to DSM-IV. It is important for the reader to note that this volume takes the extremely simplistic stance that the disorder to be treated has been accurately diagnosed according to DSM-IV criteria, and, further, that the DSM-IV criteria are clinically adequate. As every clinician knows, initial diagnostic impressions are not cast in stone. A patient's response to treatment may confirm, refute, or add to one's diagnosis. In addition, it is vitally important that the clinician or other reader be aware that the DSM-IV is not the last or only word in our understanding of mental disorders. Diagnosis and treatment are dynamic and multifaceted, and not nearly as concrete as a lay reader might assume.

Legal Settings. There is particular danger of misunderstanding diagnostic and treatment concepts in legal settings. This book, like the DSM-IV, should not be used in the forensic arena without psychiatric consultation.

Practice Guidelines and Standards of Care. This book discusses treatment practices available at the time it was written. Although we provide treatment *guidelines,* they are not intended to establish a standard of care for any specific patient, clinician, or treatment setting. *Standards of care* are best defined for individual clinical situations, by professionals who understand both the particular medical circumstance at hand and the broader clinical context in which it exists.

The clinical standard should not change with financial or administrative constraints. If one's recommended treatment is not available in one's clinical setting, for whatever reason, it should still be considered and discussed with the patient and/or family, if possible, and efforts should be made to procure it for the patient.

Nor does the standard usually differ from one kind of professional to another. In agreeing to treat the patient, the clinician has, in general, represented that he or she has sufficient professional knowledge and competence either to diagnose and treat appropriately or to recognize his or her limitations and refer the patient elsewhere. Similarly, the patient has a right to expect that the clinician will not knowingly exceed his or her competence, and will be honest about what he or she can and cannot provide. The point is not that all clinicians must be perfect, but that in reasonable clinical situations, consistent with the training and expectations of one's profession, the doctor or therapist should strive to recognize the point at which the patient requires care outside his or her own expertise, and seek appropriate consultation or referral.

Mental Illness and Behavioral Health. The modern lexicon of managed care and health-care reform often avoids such terms as psychiatric treatment and mental illness in favor of the relatively new phrase "behavioral health." The reader will find few, if any, references to behavioral health in this book, since it seems meaningless in a context of treatment of psychiatric disorders. Mental illness is often serious illness, is almost never limited to behavior alone, and should not be trivialized by such an implication. Referring to patients as "consumers" and illnesses as "behavioral issues" may remove some stigma, but in the process, it obscures the need for serious diagnosis and treatment and lowers priorities for funding by legislatures and third-party payers.

Pessimism Versus Realism in Treatment. Although psychiatric disorders as a group have about the same rate of cure or amelioration as those in other medical specialties, they are often viewed with more pessimism. The vast majority of patients are treatable, given appropriate diagnosis and resources for treatment.

Therapeutic pessimism is most often seen regarding the management of the personality disorders. It is important, especially for newly trained clinicians, to recall that there are few medical specialties that expect cures for all patients. The relief of mental or physical pain, with or without a "cure," is often the physician's highest calling.

Treating the "Myth of Mental Illness." Psychiatry is perhaps the only clinical field in which aberrant behavior or emotions alone can warrant "diagnosis" and "treatment." Although sociocultural factors are sometimes important in determining whether or not a particular feeling or behavior (or even hallucination) is normal, mental illness is not a myth. The longer one works with patients and sees the interactions and patterns of biological, psychological, and social factors in their pain, the more one understands that mental disorders deserve consideration beyond mere maladaptation or problems in living.

On the other hand, a clinician with the authority to diagnose and treat such disorders must take his or her responsibility very seriously, record diagnoses honestly (not based on reimbursement needs), and avoid confusing social or political behavior *per se* with mental illness. One should be particularly careful when treating children, adolescents, the elderly, and people whose behavior is deemed antisocial.

Finally, astute readers will note that Dr. George Balis is no longer listed as a contributor, but is now coauthor of *The Treatment of Psychiatric Disorders*. Dr. Balis played a major role in preparing the last two editions and is a strong voice for excellence in medical care. It is time to recognize the collaborative nature of our work.

William H. Reid, M.D., M.P.H.

Part I

NEUROPSYCHIATRIC DISORDERS

George Ulysses Balis, M.D.

The format for Part I differs somewhat from that of the other sections. Although an effort has been made to follow the DSM-IV outline of psychiatric disorders exactly, such a format would be unwieldy when addressing the treatment of the disorders that were called organic mental disorders in the revised third edition (DSM-III-R). We have accordingly grouped these disorders in a clinically useful way, much as it was done in the previous edition.

The remaining specific substance-related disorders of substance dependence, substance abuse, intoxication, and withdrawal are presented in **Part II.**

CHAPTER 1

GENERAL PRINCIPLES OF
NEUROPSYCHIATRIC DIAGNOSIS

The term "organic" was eliminated from the DSM-IV. The "correct" term is now the circumlocution "due to a general medical condition," and "substance-related" if the condition involves the use of a substance. This was done in the noble effort to combat the prevailing Cartesian mind-body dualism in the clinician's thinking (Spitzer *et al.*, 1992). In this reform spirit, it might also appear appropriate to correct the biological versus psychological dichotomy, since all psychological phenomena are eminently biological!

All psychiatric disorders are the result of a multifactorial causative process, which expresses the variable contribution of genetic, developmental, neurophysiologic, systemic, psychological, adaptational, social, and environmental influences. From this perspective, the terms "organic" and "due to a general medical condition" simply denote the significant contribution of brain dysfunction or injury to the multifactorial causative process, and alert the clinician to seek specific etiologic treatment when possible. With this in mind, we will use the term "organic" when we feel it offers simplicity and clarity in communication.

Organic mental syndrome and the older organic brain syndrome have also become extinct in the DSM-IV. Nevertheless, the concept of "syndrome" continues to be very useful in clinical thinking and should be used in the diagnostic process. The term "neuropsychiatric" encompasses those mental disorders that are associated with a brain lesion or dysfunction that is due to a general medical condition or a substance.

In addition to lexically bridging the mind-body dichotomy, it is useful to present a unitary paradigm for conceptualizing psychopathology, based on a systems theory framework.

A UNITARY FRAMEWORK FOR CONCEPTUALIZING PSYCHOPATHOLOGY

From a general systems theory perspective, personality may be viewed as a subsystem level within the multilevel organization of an organism or organismic unity (molecular, cellular, organ system) in which personality represents the emergent phenomena that reflect the structure/process organization of the brain (Balis, 1978a). Family and social systems represent suprasystems relative to personality. Personality is, therefore, the "vantage" system for studying psychological and behavioral phenomena, as they relate to internal matter-energy subsystems (brain, body), to the external family and social suprasystems, and to the environment.

Phenomenologically, personality is introspectively experienced as psychological phenomena and inspectively observed as behavior. Psychological phenomena are viewed as constituting emergent phenomena, expressing the integrative processes of the brain, at the highest level, in the form of introspected experiences (e.g., conscious awareness, perceptions, emotions, cognition). Only a small fraction of the brain's functions are represented at the personality level, that is, only those with an emergent expression at that level (e.g., neocortical and paleocortical processes integrating limbic, hypothalamic, and centrencephalic processes into emergent experiential [conscious] phenomena). Viewed as the level of organization of emergent phenomena associated with certain brain functions, personality is not necessarily a uniquely human apparatus.

Behavior is viewed as the adaptive functions of an organism that serve the maintenance of the steady state. Behavior, therefore, serves adaptation. In its Janus head expression, behavior must be understood as a function of a concrete system, the brain, and as a function of an abstract system, the personality. A fundamental aspect of behavior is that it is organized along dimensional continua. The concept of dimensionality implies that behavior has evolved longitudinally (phylogenetically and ontogenetically) and is organized cross sectionally (molecular, cellular, organ system, personality, social levels). A behavioral dimension is, therefore, a conceptual construct that defines the functional continua along which behavior appears to have evolved in the time frames of phylogeny (evolution) and ontogeny (development), and as it has been organized at each level of the organismic unity (e.g., biochemical, organ system, neurophysiologic, personality, social).

Psychopathology represents a dysfunctional (maladaptive) state of personality functioning that is the result of the dysregulation of the steady-state dynamics within the organism, that is, the result of the failure of the adjustment processes (intraorganismic, intrapsychic) and adaptive processes (behavioral) to maintain constancy in the face of physical, psychological, and interpersonal stresses on the system. The dysfunctional state is the result of a complex interaction between the organizational dynamics of the steady state (system stability) and the stresses that impinge on it. Stress is defined as any dynamic factor (internal or external) that produces a deviation (strain) beyond the optimal range of the organism's steady state.

Deficiencies in the mechanisms for maintaining stability may result in unstable or "vulnerable" systems that are prone to becoming decompensated and dysfunctional. This paradigm provides for a multifactorial causative process of psychopathology, taking into consideration (1) the internal state of the organismic system (vulnerability), as defined by genetic, developmental, and other structure-process parameters; and (2) stress factors (biochemical, physiological, psychological, interpersonal, environmental) acting at various levels of system organization and interacting with each other in a nonlinear causative process. Psychopathology is thus seen as the decompensated ranges of behavioral/psychological dimensions (continua) of the functioning personality. It expresses states of dysregulation in the steady state relative to its internal subsystems (e.g., brain, genes), external suprasystems (family, society), and ecosystems. Symptoms, signs, and maladaptive traits constitute the phenomenology of psychopathology. The clustering of characteristic signs and symptoms constitutes a clinical syndrome, while the clustering of traits constitutes a personality pattern. (The DSM-IV is a taxonomic system that categorizes various syndromes and maladaptive personality patterns as disorders, using descriptive [categorical] criteria rather than dimensional cutoff points.)

The shifting scope of psychiatry has often been determined by factors neither scientific nor clinical, a fact that points to the need for a more careful definition of the disciplinary boundaries and conceptual constructs (Balis, 1978b). The psychiatric model is viewed as the medical model *par excellence* (Engel, 1977), in which the person is the vantage point for conceptualizing clinical matters within the unity of a biosystem (Balis, 1978a). This unitary approach rejects ideological polarity in favor of multilevel theoretical perspectives of selective relevance to a particular clinical situation. It requires one to understand complex phenomena at different levels of organization, through a cognitive process, which Yager (1977) has termed the eclectic mental operation (a process of approaching the available information from several points of entry and repatterning the information in an attempt to see alternative possibilities). The clinician must be able to conceptualize behavior by using alternating vantage points (e.g., personality, brain, family, and social) while recognizing the supremacy of personality as the vantage point for understanding the person. This is precisely the *modus operandi* of the medical model.

THE DIAGNOSTIC PROCESS

A comprehensive evaluation is the principal approach to the diagnosis of all mental disorders. The patient must be understood as a person and as an organismic unit, within a historical perspective and current functioning, and within a family, social, cultural, and environmental matrix.

Both historical and observational information form the database for establishing a diagnosis. Such information generally includes a comprehensive psychiatric and general medical history, family and personal history, mental status examination, physical and neurological examination, screening laboratory tests, and, as appropriate, specialized clinical and laboratory procedures.

Clinical Evidence of Organicity

It is important to recognize the fact that organic psychiatric symptoms are the result of different mechanisms, acting alone or in combination, which may include impairment or loss of function (e.g., loss of memory in Korsakoff's syndrome), exaggerated expression of a central nervous system function (e.g., partial complex seizures), disinhibition of primitive functions (e.g., release phenomena, primitive reflexes), and, most important, psychological reaction to the loss of function (e.g., compensatory or restitutive actions), as determined by patterns of defense mechanisms, the premorbid personality, and coping style (Balis, 1978c).

The diagnostic task for defining an organic contribution to the etiology of a psychiatric disturbance involves two basic steps: identifying a specific organic factor on evidence from history, physical examination, and/or laboratory tests; and judging that factor to be etiologically related to the disturbance. The latter usually involves complex clinical judgment.

A thorough history is the best source of information for identifying organic factors, and includes such items as relevant physical disorders, exposure to environmental or occupational noxae, current use of prescription drugs, alcohol and drug abuse, head injuries, learning disabilities, and family history of hereditary disorders. The history of present illness may also provide valuable clues, including episodic or paroxysmal symptoms, altered states of consciousness, forgetfulness and other evidence of cognitive impairment, emotional lability, and/or behaviors that are out of character for the individual.

Observations from physical examination (including neurological and mental status examination) provide more tangible evidence. The clinician must search for and carefully evaluate the presence of any soft neurological signs (e.g., mild dysarthria, aphasia, incoordination) and symptoms of cognitive impairment. Recognition of subtle behavioral changes—such as cognitive deficits made manifest as mild disorganization of thought (e.g., rambling, disjointedness); subtle changes in awareness as shown by a repeated failure to grasp questions or mistaking the unfamiliar for the familiar, disordered attention (e.g., short attention span, distractibility, wavering in orientation), "picking" behavior evidenced as aimless grooming, or fluctuating occurrence of such behaviors—is particularly significant.

MAJOR NEUROPSYCHIATRIC SYNDROMES

Cerebral Dysfunction

The cerebrum (telencephalon) is the principal brain structure that expresses the emergent psychological phenomena at the level of organization of personality. Since the cerebrum is phylogenetically more recent, it is particularly vulnerable to the effect of various noxae and is usually the first part of the brain to undergo disorganization.

Diffuse pathophysiological changes affecting the cerebrum may result in encephalopathies (e.g., toxic, metabolic) associated with confusional states (delirium), as well as other mental syndromes. Confusional states may also occur in cerebral edema, and in brain compression by mass lesions (e.g., subdural hematoma). The breakdown in arousal and attention mechanisms appears to play a key role in delirium. The clinical picture is suggestive of a state of cerebral decompensation (Engel, 1959).

Structural changes affecting the cerebrum may result in dementia, as well as in a variety of other mental syndromes. Dementias are classified anatomically into localized dementias (cortical, subcortical, axial) and global dementias. Cortical dementias (e.g., Alzheimer's disease, Pick's disease) are characterized by major cognitive deficit and are often associated with aphasias and agnosias, while subcortical dementias (e.g., Huntington's disease, Parkinson's disease) are characterized by milder forms of cognitive deficit, apathy, and absence of language disturbances. Axial dementias are exemplified by the Wernicke-Korsakoff syndrome, characterized by striking changes in recent memory, while global dementia is best typified by advanced Alzheimer's disease (Heilman & Valenstein, 1979).

Hemispheric Dysfunction

A number of studies suggest lateralization in brain functions and hemispheric specialization (Heilman & Valenstein, 1979; Tucker, 1981). Available evidence suggests that the dominant (usually left) hemisphere is specialized not only for verbal information processing (language), but also for higher discriminative cognitive processes involving a more analytic and sequential approach. It also plays a more significant role in response initiation and in processing negative emotions (Tucker, 1981). On the other hand, the right (usually nondominant) hemisphere is more holistic and global, with specialization in nonverbal perceptual analysis involving visuospatial skills. It has a special role in mediating emotional behavior, by processing affective stimuli and programming emotional behavior and by playing a critical part in processing emotions. It is also important in attention-arousal activation.

Destructive lesions (e.g., trauma, tumor, cerebral infarction) are associated with loss or impairment in respective hemispheric functions, and with behavior being dominated by the unopposed functions of the contralateral hemisphere. On the other hand, irritative (ictal) lesions are associated with paroxysmal elicitating of ipsilateral hemispheric functions.

Right Hemisphere Dysfunction. Patients with destructive right hemispheric lesions often appear affectively indifferent, have decreased facial expression and flattened affective reactions, and show impaired comprehension of affect, as indicated by difficulty in comprehending emotional faces and in identifying affective intonations in speech, as well as by difficulty in remembering and expressing the affective component of emotionally charged memories (a phenomenon analogous to isolation of affect). These patients may also appear inappropriately euphoric. Patients with irritative right hemispheric lesions (focal epilepsy) often show depressive and manic syndromes (Flor-Henry, 1969).

Left Hemisphere Dysfunction. Patients with anteriorly located destructive left hemisphere lesions show profound depression dominated by negative cognitive representations and dysphoric affect, in addition to perceptual, cognitive, and expressive defects in speech (aphasia, word deafness). Patients with left hemispheric lesions may also show hyperarousal and are prone to experiencing episodes of catastrophic reaction. Patients with irritative (ictal) left (dominant) hemispheric lesions (e.g., left-sided temporal lobe epilepsy) are more likely to display aggressive behavior and schizophreniform psychosis.

Frontal Lobe Dysfunction

The prefrontal cortex (dorsolateral, medial, and orbitofrontal regions) represents the highest level of integration of behavior, regulating the initiation and maintenance of goal-oriented behavior, "gating" and integrating ongoing external perception and internal inputs, problem solving, and judging one's own behavior (insight), collectively referred to as "executive functions."

Injury to the frontal lobes (e.g., from trauma, infarction, tumors, herpes, Pick's disease) produces characteristic personality and emotional changes, including reduction of initiative and lack of drive with an inability to plan one's actions appropriately, which becomes manifest as apathy, abulia, or aspontaneity (comparable to the negative symptoms of schizophrenia). In more severe forms, one sees bradykinesia, mutism with akinesia, or frontal apraxia (especially in bilateral dorsolateral or mesial lesions); shallow or blunted emotions, facetiousness, and inappropriate jocularity or euphoria (*witzelsucht*); loss of esthetic and ethical nuances of behavior (crude manners, social indiscretion, sociopathy); and low threshold of frustration tolerance (often resulting in violent outbursts). Lesions in the orbitofrontal regions are often related to inappropriate sexual behavior and violent acts. Right frontal lesions are more likely to be associated with inappropriate jocularity, whereas left frontal lesions may be associated with depression.

Neurological signs consist of primitive reflexes (e.g., grasp, groping, snout, and sucking reflexes) and incontinence associated with lack of social concern.

Ictal discharges in the prefrontal areas may result in transient alterations in personality similar to those described following prefrontal lobotomy (release of inhibitions and compulsiveness of behavior).

Temporolimbic Dysfunction

The limbic areas play a significant role in emotion, drive regulation, motivation, and autonomic and visceral function. The neocortical areas are involved in auditory projection and association.

Destructive limbic lesions induce emotional changes, such as ragelike attacks and irritability (e.g., with tumors in the septal region) or marked placidity (in bilateral destruction of amygdala and hippocampal gyrus). Left anterior temporal lesions (i.e., strokes) are frequently related to depression. Recent memory deficit is a common symptom following damage to the limbic structures that are involved in the consolidation process that converts very short-term (working) memory to long-term (recent and remote) memory. These include the bilateral mesial temporal regions, hippocampus, mammillary bodies, and fornix. Damage may be associated with alcoholic Korsakoff's disease, tumors, herpes encephalitis, or cerebrovascular accidents involving the posterior cerebral artery (Heilman & Valenstein, 1979). The limbic system—more specifically, the mesolimbic dopaminergic system with its interconnections with other neurotransmitter systems—represents the final common pathway for developing psychosis (delusions, hallucinations) from lesions of diverse structural, chemical, and systemic etiology, as well as positive symptoms of schizophrenia.

Ictal phenomena (partial seizures) are associated with a broad range of episodic or paroxysmal behavioral and psychological phenomena. They include perceptual disturbances, such as hallucinations, and perceptual distortions, such as micropsias, macropsias, derealization and depersonalization, *deja vu* and *jamais vu*, forced thinking, fear and anxiety, depression and mania, explosive aggression, altered states of consciousness, and amnestic episodes.

Postictal phenomena involve transient confusional states (delirium). Interictal phenomena involve one of two types of so-called temporal lobe epileptic personality: viscous or enechetic type, described as perseverative, circumstantial, rigid, dogmatic, obstinate, pedantic, overreligious, and overbearing; and explosive-aggressive type, characterized by irritability, aggressiveness, impulsivity, emotional instability, and a proclivity to sudden mood changes and violent rage reactions (Balis, 1978c).

Parietal Lobe Dysfunction

The parietal lobes are associated with the discriminative modalities of sensation (e.g., position sense, two-point discrimination, stereognosis), language function (dominant lobe), and perception of body image and proximal external space (nondominant lobe).

Destructive lesions of the left (dominant) parietal lobe produce dysgraphia, dyscalculia, left-right disorientation, and finger agnosia (Gerstmann's syndrome). Some patients may neglect the visual space on the right side. Patients with lesions of the right (nondominant) parietal lobe show abnormalities in their concept of body image (e.g., lack of awareness of the left side of the body, lack of awareness of hemiparesis [anosognosia], denial of illness); in their perception of their proximal external space (e.g., neglect of the left visual field and objects, inability to interpret drawings, such as maps, confusion about figure-background relationships); and in their capacity to construct drawings (constructional apraxia).

Occipital Lobe Dysfunction

The occipital lobes contain the principal projection and association areas of visual function. Unilateral destruction of the projection area (e.g., by occlusion of the posterior cerebral artery) will produce a complete homonymous hemianopsia (cortical blindness). Lesions in the association areas produce deficits in visual recognition and reading.

Basal Ganglia Dysfunction

Dysfunction of one or more of the basal ganglia, although commonly thought to be associated with motor (e.g., extrapyramidal) disorders, appears also to involve cognitive, behavioral, and affective symptoms. Parkinson's disease is often associated with depression and anxiety, while Huntington's disease is commonly marked by depression, mania, psychosis, aggressiveness, irritability, promiscuity, and apathy. Progressive supranuclear palsy may be associated with dementia, irritability, depression, and emotional incontinence (involuntary laughing or crying). Sydenham's chorea is often accompanied by emotional lability, irritability, or apathy. Hepatolenticular degeneration (Wilson's disease) may be associated with psychosis, emotional lability, irritability, or apathy.

DIAGNOSTIC PROCEDURES

Screening Laboratory Tests

With some minor variations, routine laboratory tests within the neuropsychiatric workup generally include a serologic test for syphilis and HIV, complete blood count, thyroid function tests (T_3, T_4, TSH), urinalysis, metabolic screen, serum electrolytes, drug screen, computed tomography (CT), electrocardiogram (ECG), and electroencephalogram (EEG). Several recent studies have shown that the routine tests of serum B_{12}, folate, and thyroid function rarely yield positive results and may not be useful for screening. On the other hand, magnetic resonance imaging (MRI) is usually superior to CT as a screening vehicle.

Depending on the information derived from the clinical and laboratory database, appropriate consultations, additional laboratory or radiological tests, and/or neuropsychological instruments may assist in definitive diagnosis.

Minimental State Examination (MMSE)

The MMSE has become a widely used method for assessing the cognitive mental status. Although it has limited specificity with respect to individual clinical syndromes, it is a brief and useful standardized method for grading patients' cognition. It can also be used to follow the course of a syndrome and to monitor response to treatment. Using a cutoff point of 23, the sensitivity and specificity of the MMSE are quite high for assessing delirium or dementia in hospitalized patients.

Neuropsychological Tests

Commonly used psychological tests for the diagnosis of "organicity" include the Bender Gestalt, the Wechsler Memory Scale, intelligence tests (e.g., WAIS-R), and various scales for measuring cognitive impairment. The more expensive neuropsychological test batteries, such as the Halstead-Reitan Neuropsychological Battery, provide specific information about neurological deficits and localization of the disease process (Lezak, 1985).

Structural Brain Imaging

Structural brain imaging techniques, such as CT and MRI, have become standard methods in psychiatric diagnosis. Whereas CT is used in screening, MRI is the test of choice for investigating patients suspected of brain dysfunction, unless the patient cannot tolerate lying in the MRI machine. In CT, contrast is particularly useful in visualizing vascular malformations and brain regions in the presence of a defective blood-brain barrier (Kinkel, 1992a). The use of contrast media is not without hazards and should not be routine. A major advantage of MRI over CT is the relative invisibility of bone or moving blood on MRI. Head MRI is superior to CT in visualizing small lesions, demyelinating disease (e.g., multiple sclerosis), and nonhemorrhagic cerebrovascular disease (e.g., subcortical arteriosclerotic encephalopathy), and in the differential diagnosis of stroke (e.g., small cerebral emboli, transient ischemic attacks, infarctions very early in their evolution).

MRI can aid in the differential diagnosis of psychiatric disorders associated with various degenerative dementias (e.g., brain atrophy, ventricular enlargement), vascular dementias (e.g., cerebral infarcts, hemorrhages, Binswanger's encephalopathy), and various other neurological disorders that are often associated with psychiatric syndromes, such as systemic lupus erythematosus with cerebral involvement, multiple sclerosis, tumors, and hydrocephalus (Kinkel, 1992b). In addition, MRI screening should be considered in a patient's first episode of psychotic disorder (regardless of age) or mood disorder (over age 45), treatment-resistant psychotic or mood disorder, atypical response to standard treatment, and movement disorder of uncertain etiology.

Functional Brain Imaging

Functional brain imaging, as provided by single photon emission computed tomography (SPECT) and positron emission tomography (PET), although still in the experimental stage, offers a number of avenues to aid in the evaluation of neurologic and psychiatric patients. Most SPECT studies have focused on measuring cerebral blood flow (CBF), since brain activity is tightly coupled to blood flow. SPECT has been applied successfully in the area of cerebrovascular disease (e.g., aiding in the prognosis of stroke), epilepsy (e.g., locating a seizure focus), and dementia, where it can provide clinically useful information with regard to diagnosis, prognosis, and management of therapeutic interventions. In Alzheimer's dementia, both SPECT and PET have shown widespread physiologic disturbance that is characteristically pronounced in the temporal and parietal lobes. These methods may prove to have practical applications in evaluating other psychiatric disorders.

Electroencephalography

The use of electroencephalography (EEG) screening is part of the routine assessment of a psychiatric patient. In addition to a resting record (waking and sleep), a standard EEG includes "activated" tracings that are obtained through hyperventilation and photic stimulation. Special electrode placements for diagnosing temporal EEG abnormalities include sphenoidal and esophageal leads. Sleep deprivation before the day of the recording is another useful activating procedure.

The EEG abnormalities may be nonspecific or specific. Nonspecific abnormalities are divided into focal (e.g., focal slowing, asymmetries) and nonfocal (e.g., bilateral slowing of alpha rhythm, increased fast [beta] activity, and generalized delta/theta activity). Specific abnormalities are paroxysmal (spikes, sharp waves, bursts of slow activity) and are associated with epilepsy (ictal). They are also divided into focal abnormalities (as in temporal lobe epilepsy causing simple or complex partial seizures) and generalized (as in grand mal). Generalized spike-wave activity is associated with petit mal (Miller *et al.*, 1992).

The limitations of the EEG include high rates of false-negative and false-positive findings and low specificity of the patterns obtained. Repeated recordings increase the yield of positive findings. These limitations are even more pronounced in psychiatric populations. Although the EEG is a routine screening procedure in psychiatric diagnosis, its yield of positive findings is generally meager (Balis, 1985). There is little correlation between specific psychiatric symptoms and EEG abnormalities or the site and laterality of seizure focus (Balis, 1985).

The usefulness of EEG is largely limited to the differential diagnosis of epilepsy, delirium and other encephalopathies, certain dementias, and suspected ischemia or postictal depression (Lipowski, 1990). The use of EEG in differentiating complex or simple partial seizures from nonictal psychiatric symptoms is of special interest to psychiatry. Viscerosensory and experiential auras are more likely to have a temporal lobe focus (mostly right-sided), whereas somatosensory and elementary visual auras are more likely to have parieto-occipital foci (Palmini & Gloor, 1992). The degree of EEG slowing in delirium correlates with the severity of clouding of consciousness (Engel, 1959); serial tracings may be useful in monitoring the recovery process. The EEG is diagnostic for subacute sclerosing panencephalitis and Creutzfeldt-Jakob disease. Traditional neuroleptic drugs tend to produce mild generalized slowing, while barbiturates and benzodiazepines produce fast (beta) activity.

Polysomnography and Multiple Sleep Latency Testing

Clinical polysomnography combines all-night EEG and polygraphic recordings of eye movements, electromyogram, and respiratory function for the diagnosis of sleep apnea and other sleep disorders, as well as recordings of penile tumescence for differentiating organic from psychogenic impotence. The multiple sleep latency test (MSLT) is a standardized daytime procedure used to detect sleep-onset REM episodes as an objective confirmation of narcolepsy. Polysomnography recently was used to identify a sleep pattern that may be a trait marker indicating vulnerability to depression (Lauer *et al.*, 1995).

CHAPTER 2

GENERAL PRINCIPLES OF
TREATMENT AND MANAGEMENT

In general, upon completion of the diagnostic process, a treatment plan is formulated that realistically addresses the problems that need to be corrected and serves as the basis for applying various treatments and psychosocial interventions. The treatment plan should be reassessed periodically and modified as necessary to meet changing conditions and responses to treatment. Although a biomedical understanding of the underlying disease process is of primary importance, an understanding of the psychosocial aspects of the illness is also of major significance in treatment and management.

The therapeutic approach can often be divided into treatment and psychosocial management. We will refer to approaches that utilize specific medical procedures (e.g., drug therapy, psychotherapy) as treatment. Treatment is further distinguished as etiological and symptomatic, on the basis of whether the goal of the therapeutic method is to eliminate the cause of the disease or merely to remove or improve its symptoms. Nonspecific psychosocial interventions that are part of the therapeutic effort are referred to as management, and are generally supportive in nature.

Etiological treatment, when available, is of overriding significance, since it aims at removing the cause of the disorder, thus preventing further damage and allowing the reparative process to correct the underlying pathology. It is imperative, therefore, that every effort be made to identify and treat the underlying disorder by eliminating its cause and correcting its consequences, whenever possible. When etiological treatment is unavailable or the cause of the disorder is still unknown, one is limited to symptomatic treatment. Table I.2-1 lists general medical conditions associated etiologically with mental disorders. Table I.2-2 lists common drugs that can induce mental disorders.

TABLE I.2-1

General Medical Conditions Associated with Mental Disorders

	1	2	3	4	5	6	7	8
Intracranial infections								
Encephalitis	+	+	+	+	+	+	+	+
Postinfectious encephalitis	+	+	+	+	+	+	+	+
Meningitis	+	+	+	+	+	+		+
HIV encephalopathy	+	+	+	+	+	+		+
Neurosyphilis	+	+	+	+	+	+		+
Lyme borreliosis		+	+	+		+	+	
Creutzfeldt-Jakob disease		+		+				+
Degenerative disorders								
Alzheimer's disease		+		+		+		+
Parkinson's disease		+				+	+	+
Huntington's chorea		+		+		+		+
Pick's disease		+		+				+
Amyotrophic lateral sclerosis		+				+		+
Hepatolenticular degeneration		+						
Progressive supranuclear palsy		+					+	+
Cerebrovascular disorders								
Transient ischemic attacks		+						
Thrombotic/hemorrhagic/embolic	+	+	+	+	+	+	+	+
Multi-infarct	+	+	+	+	+	+	+	+
Subarachnoid hemorrhage	+	+	+					+
Binswanger's encephalopathy		+				+		+
Epilepsy								
Partial complex seizures	+	+	+	+	+	+	+	
Postictal state	+		+	+				
Interictal state		+	+	+		+		+
Other CNS disorders								
Sydenham's chorea						+		
Head trauma	+	+	+	+	+	+	+	+
Neoplasms	+	+	+	+	+	+	+	+
Other space-occupying lesions	+	+	+	+	+	+	+	+
Multiple sclerosis			+			+		+
Normal pressure hydrocephalus		+				+		+
Temporal arteritis				+		+		
Migraine				+		+		
Transient global amnesia			+					
Sjörgen's syndrome						+		

Key: 1 = delirium, 2 = dementia, 3 = amnestic disorder,
4 = psychotic disorder, 5 = catatonic disorder, 6 = mood disorder,
7 = anxiety disorder, 8 = personality change.

TABLE I.2-1 *(continued)*

General Medical Conditions Associated with Mental Disorders

	1	2	3	4	5	6	7	8
Systemic disorders								
Viral/bacterial infections	+			+	+	+		
Subacute bacterial endocarditis	+	+	+	+	+	+	+	+
Systemic lupus erythematosus	+	+	+	+	+	+		+
Hypertensive encephalopathy	+	+						
Porphyria	+	+	+	+				
Neuroleptic malignant syndrome	+				+			
Metabolic Disorders								
Dialysis encephalopathy	+	+						
Dialysis disequilibrium syndrome	+	+						
Uremic encephalopathy	+							
Hepatic encephalopathy	+	+						
Pulmonary insufficiency	+		+				+	
Burn encephalopathy	+							
Diabetic ketoacidosis	+				+			
Electrolytes—acid/base—water								
Hypercalcemia		+	+			+		+
Hypocalcemia							+	
Hyponatremia	+			+	+			
Hypokalemia	+							
Hypophosphatemia	+							
Dehydration	+			+	+			
Metabolic acidosis	+							
Metabolic alkalosis	+							
Blood gases								
Hypoxia	+	+	+	+	+	+	+	+
Hypercapnia	+	+	+					
Endocrinopathies								
Hyperthyroidism	+			+			+	+
Hypothyroidism	+	+	+	+		+		+
Pheochromocytoma						+	+	
Hypercortisolemia (Cushing's)				+	+	+	+	+
Addison's disease				+		+		+
Hyperinsulinism (hypoglycemia)	+		+				+	
Vitamin deficiencies								
Niacin (pellagra)		+	+	+	+	+		+
Thiamine (Korsakoff-Wernicke)	+		+					+
B$_{12}$ and folate (pernicious anemia)	+	+	+	+	+	+		+

Key: 1 = delirium, 2 = dementia, 3 = amnestic disorder,
4 = psychotic disorder, 5 = catatonic disorder, 6 = mood disorder,
7 = anxiety disorder, 8 = personality change.   *(continued)*

TABLE I.2-1 *(continued)*

General Medical Conditions Associated with Mental Disorders

	1	2	3	4	5	6	7	8
Poisons/chemicals								
Lead	+	+	+			+		+
Mercury			+			+		+
Manganese								+
Organophosphates			+	+		+	+	+
Arsenic	+	+	+	+	+			+
Carbon monoxide	+	+	+		+			+
Miscellaneous								
Carcinoid syndrome						+		
Pancreatic cancer						+		
Iron overload		+				+	+	
Sleep deprivation	+			+	+			
Sensory deprivation				+		+	+	

Key: 1 = delirium, 2 = dementia, 3 = amnestic disorder,
4 = psychotic disorder, 5 = catatonic disorder, 6 = mood disorder,
7 = anxiety disorder, 8 = personality change.

TABLE I-2.2

Substances Inducing Mental Disorders

ACTH	2,5,6,7	Anxiolytics	1, 2, 3, 4, 5, 6, 7, 9, 10
Alcohol	1, 2, 3, 4, 5, 6, 7, 9, 10	Asparaginase	5
Alprazolam	1, 2, 3, 4, 5, 6, 7, 9, 10	Atropine	2, 4, 5
		Baclofen	5
Amantadine	5	Barbiturates	1, 2, 3, 4, 5, 6, 7, 9, 10
Aminocaproic acid	5		
Aminophylline	7, 10	Belladonna	2, 4, 5
Amitriptyline	2, 4, 9, 10	Benzodiazepines	1, 2, 3, 4, 5, 6, 7, 9, 10
Amphetamines	1, 2, 5, 6, 7, 8, 9, 10	Benztropine	2, 4
Anabolic steroids	5, 6, 7, 8, 9	Beta-blockers	3, 4, 5, 6, 9
Antihistamines	2, 4, 10	Bethanidine	6
Anticholinergics	2, 3, 4, 5, 7	Biperiden	2, 4, 5
Antiparkinson	2, 3, 4, 5, 7	Bromides	2, 5

Key: 1 = withdrawal, 2 = delirium, 3 = dementia, 4 = amnestic disorder,
5 = psychotic disorder, 6 = mood disorder, 7 = anxiety disorder, 8 = catatonic
disorder, 9 = sexual dysfunction, 10 = sleep disorder.

TABLE I-2.2 *(continued)*

Substances Inducing Mental Disorders

Bromocriptine	5	Fenfluramine	2, 5, 6, 7, 9, 10
Brompheniramine	2, 4, 10	Fluoxetine	9, 10
Caffeine	7, 10	Fluphenazine	2, 4, 6, 9, 10
Cannabis	2, 5, 7	Flurazepam	1, 2, 3, 4, 5, 6, 7, 9, 10
Carbamazepine	10		
Chloral hydrate	1, 2, 3, 4, 5, 6, 7, 9, 10	Glutethimide	1, 2, 3, 4, 5, 6, 7, 9, 10
Chlordiazepoxide	1, 2, 3, 4, 5, 6, 7, 9, 10	Guanethidine	1, 2, 3, 4, 5, 6, 7, 9, 10
Chloroquine	2, 5	Hallucinogens	2, 5, 6, 7
Chlorpheniramine	2, 4, 10	Haloperidol	2, 4, 6, 8, 9, 10
Chlorpromazine	2, 4, 6, 9, 10	Homatropine	2, 4, 5
Chlorprothixene	2, 4, 6, 9, 10	Hydralazine	7, 9
Cimetidine	2, 3, 5, 6, 9	Hydrocarbons	2, 3, 5, 6, 7
Ciprofloxacin	5, 8	Hydroxyzine	2, 4, 9, 10
Clomipramine	2, 4, 9, 10	Hypnotics	1, 2, 3, 4, 5, 6, 7, 9, 10
Clonazepam	1, 2, 3, 4, 5, 6, 7, 9, 10		
		Imipramine	2, 4, 5, 9, 10
Clonidine	3, 6	Indomethacin	5, 6
Closapine	1, 4, 6, 9, 10	Isoniazid	4, 5, 7
Cocaine	1, 2, 5, 6, 7, 9, 10	Levodopa	3, 5, 7
Cortisone	2, 3, 4, 5, 6, 7	Lidocaine	5, 6, 7
Cycloserine	5	Lithium	2, 3, 4, 9
Desipramine	2, 4, 9, 10	Lorazepam	1, 2, 3, 4, 5, 6, 7, 9, 10
Dexedrine	2, 5, 6, 7, 9, 10		
Diazepam	1, 2, 4, 5, 6, 9, 10	Loxitane	2, 4, 6, 9, 10
Diethylpropion	1, 2, 5, 6, 7, 9, 10	Maprotyline	2, 4, 9, 10
Digitalis	2, 3, 4, 5, 6, 7	Meperidine	2, 6
Diphenhydramine	2, 4, 10	Meprobamate	1, 2, 3, 4, 5, 6, 7, 9, 10
Disopyramide	5, 9		
Disulfiram	2, 3, 5	Mesoridazine	2, 4, 6, 8, 9, 10
Dopamine	7	Methaqualone	1, 2, 3, 4, 5, 6, 7, 9, 10
Doxepine	2, 4, 9, 10		
Ephedrine	2, 5, 6, 7, 10	Methyldopa	3, 4, 5, 6, 9
Epinephrine	7	Methylphenidate	1, 2, 5, 6, 7, 10
Estrogens	6	Methyprylon	1, 2, 4, 6, 10
Ethcorvynol	1, 2, 3, 4, 5, 6, 7, 9, 10	Metrizamide	6
		Molindone	2, 4, 6, 9, 10
Ethosuximide	1, 2, 3, 4, 5, 6, 7, 9, 10	Nadolol	4, 5, 6, 9

Key: 1 = withdrawal, 2 = delirium, 3 = dementia, 4 = amnestic disorder, 5 = psychotic disorder, 6 = mood disorder, 7 = anxiety disorder, 8 = catatonic disorder, 9 = sexual dysfunction, 10 = sleep disorder.

(continued)

TABLE I-2.2 *(continued)*

Substances Inducing Mental Disorders

Narcotics	1, 2, 3, 5, 6, 7, 9, 10	Procainamide	5, 6
		Phenmetrazine	2, 5, 6, 7, 9, 10
Neuroleptics	2, 4, 6, 9, 10	Promethazine	2, 4, 8, 10
Nortriptyline	2, 4, 9, 10	Propranolol	3, 4, 5, 6, 9, 10
Opioids	1, 2, 3, 5, 6, 7, 9, 10	Pseudoephedrine	2, 5, 6, 7, 10
		Reserpine	6
Oral hypoglycemics	7	Salicylates	7
Oral contracept.	6	Scopolamine	2, 4, 5
Organophosphates	4, 8	Sedatives	1, 2, 3, 4, 5, 6, 7, 9, 10
Oxazepam	1, 2, 3, 4, 5, 6, 7, 9, 10		
		Sertraline	9, 10
Paroxetine	9, 10	Steroids	2, 3, 5, 6, 7
Pentazocine	5	Sulindac	5
Pentobarbital	1, 2, 3, 4, 5, 6, 7, 9, 10	Temazepam	1, 2, 3, 4, 5, 6, 7, 9, 10
Perphenazine	2, 4, 6, 8, 9, 10	Thiazide diuretics	6, 9
Phencyclidine	2, 5, 6, 7, 8	Thioridazine	2, 4, 6, 9, 10
Phenelzine	4, 5, 9	Thyroxine	7, 10
Phenmetrazine	2, 5, 6, 7, 9, 10	Tranylcypromine	4, 5, 9
Phenobarbital	1, 2, 3, 4, 5, 6, 7, 9, 10	Trifluoperazine	2, 4, 6, 9, 10
		Trihexyphenidyl	2
Phenylephrine	2, 5, 6, 7, 10	Triazolam	2, 3, 4, 9, 10
Phenytoin	3, 10	Valproate	8, , 9, 10

Key: 1 = withdrawal, 2 = delirium, 3 = dementia, 4 = amnestic disorder, 5 = psychotic disorder, 6 = mood disorder, 7 = anxiety disorder, 8 = catatonic disorder, 9 = sexual dysfunction, 10 = sleep disorder.

Symptomatic treatment is primarily directed toward two areas: (1) the removal or control of the physical symptoms of the underlying disorder and the normalization of physiological functioning in all systems affected by the disease process, and (2) the removal or control of psychiatric symptoms, through the use of various treatment modalities, which include pharmacological and psychosocial approaches. Psychiatric treatment is also directed at restoring the patient's psychosocial functioning to the extent that this is possible, and at improving his or her adjustment to residual behavioral impairment and deficits in adaptation.

The following is a brief review of psychopharmacotherapy, as applied to patient populations at a higher risk for developing mental disorders secondary to a general medical condition, such as medically compromised and geriatric patients, as well as of electroconvulsive therapy, psychotherapies, and psychosocial management.

PSYCHOPHARMACOTHERAPY

High-risk (medically compromised) and geriatric patients represent special populations with different patterns of response to psychotropic drugs, which depend on the nature of the underlying medical condition, the aging process, and other factors. We will briefly review the use of psychotropic drugs in high-risk patients and geriatric populations.

CARDIAC DISEASE

Antidepressants

Tricyclic Antidepressants (TCAs). Tricyclic toxicity is of particular concern in treating the cardiac patient. In addition to orthostatic hypotension (alpha-adrenergic blocking effect) and sinus tachycardia (anticholinergic effect), TCAs prolong intraventricular conduction (quinidinelike effect), and probably decrease myocardial contractility. Patients with preexisting conduction disease, particularly bundle-branch block, are at higher risk for developing symptomatic AV block while on TCAs. Since TCA cardiac effects closely resemble those of class I antiarrhythmic drugs, TCAs may also share the risks associated with use of the latter (Glassman, *et al.*, 1993; Roose & Glassman, 1994). Therefore, TCAs are contraindicated in patients with ventricular premature depolarizations (a risk factor for sudden death after myocardial infarction), are generally contraindicated in patients with manifest ischemic heart disease, and are to be used with caution in patients who have asymptomatic arrhythmias and/or ischemic heart disease (Glassman, *et al.*, 1993).

Selective Serotonin Reuptake Inhibitors (SSRIs). Unlike the TCAs, SSRIs are free of quinidinelike effects and do not produce orthostatic hypotension or tachycardia. Although no serious cardiac effects have been reported with their use in cardiac patients, there have been a few case reports of fluoxetine-associated severe sinus node bradycardia and other types of arrhythmias (Jefferson, 1992). It has been suggested that, in patients with underlying coronary disease, SSRIs may have the potential of causing myocardial infarction due to serotonin's vasoconstrictive effect on lesioned coronary arteries (Hills & Lange, 1991). Although SSRIs are a safer alternative to TCAs, one cannot conclude that they carry no cardiovascular risk (Roose & Glassman, 1994).

Bupropion does not appear do have any direct cardiac effect, and does not produce orthostatic hypotension or tachycardia. While not completely devoid of cardiovascular effects, it is generally well tolerated and is considered relatively safe in patients with cardiac disease (Jefferson, 1993). Bupropion may cause a slight increase in blood pressure in some patients.

Venlafaxine's cardiac effect have not been fully studied. The reported absence of effects on intracardiac conduction in preclinical studies suggests that venlafaxine might prove useful for treating depression in cardiac patients. It may induce sustained hypertension in some patients (probably more than 10% at dosages above 300 mg/day), necessitating the regular monitoring of blood pressure.

Nefazodone is associated with a lower risk of orthostatic hypotension, and appears to lack the cardiac side effects seen with TCAs (Dopheide *et al.*, 1995). It may rarely produce bradycardia in some patients. It should not be used in patients with recent myocardial infarction.

Monoamine oxidase inhibitors (MAOIs) produce postural hypotension but do not have direct cardiotoxic effects. Postural hypotension and sedation are the most serious adverse effects that limit the use of MAOIs as first-line antidepressants.

Antipsychotics

High-potency traditional neuroleptics* (e.g., haloperidol, prolixin, trifluoperazine, thiothixene) have a lower incidence of cardiovascular effects (orthostatic hypotension, tachycardia, arrhythmias) than do low-potency neuroleptics. Their hypotensive effect is due to alpha-adrenergic receptor blockade, while the tachycardia is secondary to anticholinergic action on the vagus nerve. Rare cases of serious arrhythmias and sudden death have been reported with the use of thioridazine and chlorpromazine. The cardiovascular effects of intermediate-potency neuroleptics fall between those of the high- and low-potency drugs. In general, high-potency neuroleptics are safer than those of low potency when used in cardiac patients. The novel neuroleptic risperidone has minimal cardiovascular effects, typically resolving after the first week of therapy (Keegan, 1994).

Anxiolytics

Benzodiazepines do not appear to have any significant adverse effect on the cardiovascular system, and are well tolerated, even in patients with advanced cardiovascular disease. Buspirone has no significant cardiac effects.

Mood Stabilizers

Lithium may induce benign and reversible alterations in the T-wave morphology of the ECG, such as flattening and inversion of the T wave. Lithium may induce arrhythmias, especially sinus node dysfunction, although rarely. It should be used with caution in patients with bradycardia or sinus node dysfunction. Neither valproate nor carbamazepine has a significant cardiac effect.

Note: Until the introduction of clozapine and risperidone, almost all neuroleptic drugs shared most side and adverse effects. We have tried to differentiate the newer, "atypical" neuroleptics (e.g., clozapine, risperidone) when approriate; however, the reader should be aware that "neuroleptic" may sometimes imply older, "traditional" antipsychotic drugs.

RENAL DISEASE

Antidepressants

The TCAs, such as amitriptyline, nortriptyline, desipramine, and their hydroxylated metabolites, do not appear to accumulate significantly with renal failure, making dosage adjustments unnecessary. Similarly, the SSRIs fluoxetine and sertraline do not appear to accumulate significantly, although this is less clear for paroxetine. The total daily dose of venlafaxine should be reduced by about 25% in patients with mild to moderate renal impairment, and by 50% in patients undergoing hemodialysis.

Antipsychotics

The major excretion route of all neuroleptics is the liver. Generally, there is no need for adjusting the dosage of neuroleptics in patients with renal failure.

Anxiolytics

Most benzodiazepines are considered safe in patients with renal failure. Since they are primarily metabolized by the liver, there is no need to adjust their dosage. Some of the active metabolites of lorazepam, oxazepam, and temazepam are excreted by the kidney, however.

Mood Stabilizers

Lithium is almost entirely excreted by the kidney. It is contraindicated in the presence of impaired renal function unless one carefully titrates the dosage and monitors plasma levels closely. Lithium-induced polyuria is a common side effect and may result in diabetes insipidus (4 liters or more of urine daily) in 15 to 20% of patients. Polyuria can be managed by a step-wise approach (e.g., reduce serum lithium level, give the drug in a single bedtime dose, use potassium supplementation, and finally, use amiloride or hydrochlorothiazide [Martin, 1993]). The use of thiazides requires a concomitant reduction of the daily lithium dosage, and daily monitoring of serum lithium during the initial titration phase in order to avoid possible lithium toxicity.

HEPATIC DISEASE

Antidepressants

The TCAs, MAOIs, SSRIs, venlafaxine, and nefazodone are extensively metabolized by the liver. All TCAs have been implicated in hepatotoxicity, both cholestatic and hepatocellular, which is not dose related. Cirrhotic patients have longer elimination half-lives and reduced plasma clearance for these drugs, and may experience adverse effects associated with increased free drug concentration or precipitation of portal-systemic encephalopathy. It is recommended that the total daily dose be reduced by 50% in patients with moderate hepatic impairment. SSRIs appear to be preferable to TCAs in treating patients with liver disease, with a dosage reduced by one-half to two thirds (Hale, 1993).

Antipsychotics

All neuroleptics are metabolized by the liver, mostly through sulfoxide formation, glucuronide conjugation, or hydrozylation. Drugs inducing drug metabolizing enzymes (e.g., barbiturates) tend to lower plasma levels of antipsychotics. Neuroleptics produce asymptomatic, subclinical elevations in liver function tests (i.e., enzymes such as alkaline phosphatase, alaline aminotransferase [ALT], or aspartite aminotransferase [AST]) in 25 to 60% of patients, which usually return to normal with continued treatment. Persistent mild ALT elevation does not appear to be clinically significant; however, any known or suspected hepatotoxic medication must be stopped in patients with ALT or AST levels greater than three times the upper limit of normal. Traditional neuroleptics (especially chlorpromazine) and risperidone can produce jaundice in rare cases (almost always cholestatic; rarely hepatocellular). Liver disease delays the metabolism of neuroleptics and necessitates lower doses.

Anxiolytics

The majority of benzodiazepines are metabolized and eliminated by the liver through microsomal oxidation. The short-acting lorazepam, temazepam, and oxazepam are metabolized by glucuronide conjugation, followed by renal excretion. While conjugation changes little with age, oxidation becomes less efficient in the elderly, who thus are more susceptible to the cumulative effects of drugs metabolized by oxidation, and better tolerate those metabolized via conjugation (e.g., oxazepam, lorazepam). Liver disease may affect the microsomal oxidation of benzodiazepines, rendering patients with such disease susceptible to excessive drug effects. In both instances, the starting dose of benzodiazepines should be about half the dose for healthy young adults. There are case reports of benzodiazepine-induced hepatotoxicity, which is mainly cholestatic. Buspirone's elimination half-life does not appear to be significantly affected by age or hepatic disease.

Mood Stabilizers

Lithium does not appear to cause or aggravate liver disease. Both carbamazepine and valproate are eliminated primarily by hepatic biotransformation. Both (especially carbamazepine) stimulate the hepatic microsomal enzyme oxidation system, necessitating careful initial monitoring. Either may cause hepatic toxicity (particularly valproic acid, which poses the higher risk in young children). Valproate may cause hyperammonemia, which is often clinically insignificant.

PRESCRIBING FOR THE ELDERLY

The elderly patient is more prone to toxic effects. He or she may have liver changes that decrease oxidative mechanisms, lowered serum albumin that provides binding sites, and/or a decline in kidney function, any of which increases drug half-life. For a more complete discussion of the treatment of particular disorders, refer to their specific sections or chapters.

Antidepressants

TCAs. The choice of a specific tricyclic depends on a combination of clinical considerations and the altered metabolism of the elderly patient. Several side effects of the TCAs are especially hazardous, because aging increases plasma half-life and steady-state plasma levels (especially for imipramine and amitriptyline). The hypotensive effect of TCAs does not seem to increase with advancing age (Glassman *et al.,* 1993); nevertheless, orthostatic hypotension is a very common side effect and may precipitate falls, strokes, or heart attacks. Nortriptyline produces less hypotension than does imipramine. Anticholinergic activity is especially prominent with amitriptyline, whereas desipramine and, to a lesser extent, nortriptyline have the least anticholinergic action. The non-TCAs trazodone and bupropion have little or none. Elderly patients are particularly vulnerable to (CNS) anticholinergic toxicity. The tricyclics of choice for the elderly appear to be desipramine, nortriptyline, and doxepin. Of the three, desipramine is the least anticholinergic and doxepin the least cardiotoxic.

The so-called second-generation nontricyclic antidepressants (e.g., maprotyline, amoxapine, trazodone) are reported to have fewer anticholinergic and cardiovascular side effects, and, therefore, may present some advantage over the older drugs for elderly patients (although this claim has not been well substantiated).

The following general guidelines apply in prescribing TCAs for the elderly patient.

1. Obtain a pretreatment ECG and repeat the ECG periodically during the course of treatment.
2. Measure seated and standing blood pressure before treatment is started and before each increase in dose. The concurrent administration of volume-depleting diuretics increases the risk of orthostatic hypotension.
3. Use very low starting doses, giving two-thirds of the dose at bedtime to promote sleep. Raise the dose gradually, while monitoring both thera-

peutic response and side effects. TCA plasma levels may also be monitored, primarily to prevent cumulative toxic levels.

4. Tricyclics should not be used in patients with preexisting cardiovascular disease or in those receiving quinidine, procainamide, and drugs interacting with tricyclics (e.g., clonidine, guanethidine, or bethanidine).

SSRIs. Glassman *et al.* (1993) have suggested that the SSRIs' relative efficacy in the treatment of severely depressed patients and in the elderly has not been adequately established. Sertraline has been found superior to nortriptyline in the treatment of depressed geriatric outpatients. Fluoxetine may be more effective and better tolerated than bupropion in a medically ill geriatric population. In general, depressed patients who have relapsed after an initial favorable response to 20 mg/day of fluoxetine do well on a higher dose (e.g., 40 mg/day) (Maurizio *et al.*, 1995). Fluvoxamine may produce cumulative effects in the elderly.

Bupropion is well tolerated by the elderly (Kirksey & Stern, 1984) and high-risk patients, and is particularly recommended for patients with cardiovascular and pulmonary disease and patients with dementia.

Venlafaxine is well tolerated by the elderly. No dose adjustment is necessary.

MAOIs. Phenelzine and tranylcypromine are safe and well tolerated by the elderly (Jenike, 1985). Their major advantage over the tricyclics is a lack of anticholinergic and cardiotoxic effects. Their major drawbacks are orthostatic hypotension and dietary restrictions. Moclobemide does not necessitate the dietary restrictions required for other MAOIs. Selegiline (Deprenyl), a MAO-B inhibitor, has been found to be effective at high doses (60 mg/day) in treatment-resistant older depressive patients (Sunderland *et al.*, 1994). Selegiline has also been found useful in treating depressed patients with Alzheimer's disease or Parkinson's disease. It should be noted that selegiline may be associated with increased tyramine pressor sensitivity at long-term doses above 20 to 30 mg/day.

Mood Stabilizers

In the elderly, valproate and carbamazepine may have an advantage over lithium, since the latter is more likely to produce toxicity.

Psychostimulants

Several studies advocate the use of CNS stimulants, such as methylphenidate (Ritalin), in depressed-looking medically ill patients who are recovering from chronic illness or surgery (Masand, *et al.*, 1991; Rosenberg *et al.*, 1991). Methylphenidate is thought to be specifically useful in treating medically ill cancer patients (McDaniel, *et al.*, 1995), poststroke patients (Lazarus, *et al.*, 1992), patients with closed head injury, and those with the acquired immunodeficiency syndrome (AIDS) (Rabkin, 1993). Clinical efficacy has been reported in postoperative elderly patients who appear to be apathetic, anergic, and withdrawn, as well as in patients with a lack of initiative (abulia) secondary to frontal lobe lesions or dementia, and elderly patients, who, although withdrawn and apathetic, do not express hopelessness (Salzman, 1995). Most of these studies have reported variable therapeutic efficacy and few adverse effects with methylphenidate. It should be used cautiously because of its potential for elevating blood pressure and potential for abuse.

In cases of treatment-resistant depression, the therapeutic effect of antidepressants may be augmented by the addition of various drugs, serving as potentiators. However, there are few controlled studies with the elderly in using this type of polypharmacy. Current augmentation methods include the use of mood stabilizers, triziodothyronine, SSRI-TCA combinations, MAOI-TCA combinations, estrogen, and psychostimulants.

Antipsychotics

Among the traditional neuroleptics, all are equally effective in controlling psychotic symptoms in the elderly. They differ only in their side effects and toxicity. As with the tricyclics, the choice of a specific antipsychotic agent for an elderly patient should be based on considerations of toxicity and altered metabolism. The dose should be smaller for such patients, generally in the range of 0.03 to 0.45 mg/kg of haloperidol equivalent for traditional drugs. Common significant side effects include sedation, orthostatic hypotension, anticholinergic effects, and extrapyramidal symptoms. Impaired thermoregulation and idiosyncratic reactions should also be noted. Although the sedative effects of neuroleptics may be used therapeutically to induce sleep at night, they often produce confusion and disorientation in the elderly. High-potency neuroleptics are generally safer and the drugs of choice for patients in whom autonomic and sedative effects are most hazardous; however, low-potency neuroleptics (e.g., thioridazine) in small doses may be more appropriate for restless and agitated elderly psychotic patients and those who are sensitive to extrapyramidal reactions. The newer "atypical" neuroleptic risperidone, with its favorable side-effects profile, may become the antipsychotic of choice in the future. There is insufficient experience with the use of olanzapine in elderly patients.

Anxiolytics

Benzodiazepines. In choosing a suitable benzodiazepine for the elderly patient, the clinician must consider pharmacokinetics. The long-acting benzodiazepines have undesirable cumulative effects, often causing excessive sedation. The short-acting benzodiazepines (e.g., lorazepam, oxazepam) are usually the best choice for elderly patients and others expected to show cumulative effects (e.g., those with hepatic insufficiency or prolonged use). Sleep disturbance upon drug cessation is dose dependent and may be reduced by tapering the dose. The prescription of benzodiazepines for the elderly is approximately one third to one half of the younger-adult dose. Excessive sedation, apathy, ataxia, incoordination, memory impairment, disorientation, confusion, and dysarthria are common toxic effects. Elderly men show an impaired capacity to oxidize alprazolam. Benzodiazepines may inhibit respiratory drive and are contraindicated in sleep apnea and in patients with asthma and those with chronic obstructive pulmonary disease (COPD) when there is significant respiratory distress. Buspirone is comparatively well tolerated in these conditions. It is often the anxiolytic of choice for treating the elderly and patients with COPD, asthma, and other pulmonary disease as well as for treating demented and brain-injured patients.

Mood Stabilizers

Elderly patients tend to excrete lithium slowly, and, therefore, require smaller doses as compared with younger individuals. Special attention must be paid to conditions that increase lithium toxicity, such as loss of fluids, a low-salt diet, and the use of thiazide diuretics. Lithium-induced tremor can be controlled with small doses of propranolol. Regular monitoring of the serum lithium level and the periodic assessment of thyroid function, serum electrolytes, and serum creatinin, are part of lithium therapy. Carbamazepine may rarely cause blood dyscrasias. Hematology studies should be done before beginning treatment, and continue with white cell counts every four to eight weeks for the first year, and every three to four months thereafter. When prescribing valproate, liver function, biochemistry profiles, and white blood count (WBC) should be monitored, at least over the first several months of valproate treatment (Brown, 1989).

Lithium maintenance plasma levels in elderly patients should be between 0.6 and 0.8 mEq/L. Therapeutic plasma levels of carbamazepine range between 8 and 12 ng/ml. Plasma levels of valproate are usually kept between 50 and 125 µg/ml.

ELECTROCONVULSIVE THERAPY

Electroconvulsive therapy (ECT) is the most effective method for treating major depression. As currently administered, it has an excellent safety profile and few relative contraindications, which include intracranial space-occupying lesions, recent myocardial infarction, and some cardiac arrhythmias. Its main side effects are cognitive, consisting of a transient postictal confusional state and a longer period of temporary memory impairment, particularly when administered bilaterally. It is well tolerated by the elderly and may be administered even to most high-risk patients after carefully weighing the relative risks and benefits. Unilateral ECT applied to the nondominant side, although somewhat less effective, is indicated for patients with dementia and those who develop severe ECT-induced cognitive impairment. The technique is a first-line treatment for depressed patients with high suicidality, persistent food refusal, and psychotic features; patients with catatonia; and patients with a history of intolerance of antidepressants or failure to respond to pharmacotherapy (Mukherjee *et al.*, 1994; American Psychiatric Association, 1990).

Catatonia secondary to a medical disorder (e.g., lupus erythematosus, multiple sclerosis) appears to respond dramatically to ECT (Taylor, 1990). The therapy has also been used in patients with Parkinson's disease (particularly with the "on-off" phenomenon), neuroleptic malignant syndrome, and intractable seizure disorder.

PSYCHOTHERAPIES

Psychotherapeutic interventions encompass a broad range of nonspecific methods that aim at reversing psychopathology through the use of psychological and behavioristic approaches, in which the therapist–patient relationship serves as the fulcrum for change. They include various formal types of psychotherapy (e.g., psychodynamic, brief, interpersonal, behavioral, cognitive-behavioral, family, and group), as well as supportive techniques.

In treating a patient with a neuropsychiatric disorder, the selection of a particular form of psychotherapy is based on a number of considerations, including the setting; the nature of the underlying medical condition; the patient's motivation for treatment, capacity for insight, ability to form a therapeutic alliance, ego strengths, and cognitive capacity; the nature and severity of psychopathology; and the availability of treatment resources and community support. Psychotherapeutic interventions for such patients should be adjusted to meet the patient's needs, while recognizing the limitations produced by the underlying organic condition, (e.g., memory loss, cognitive impairment). The effectiveness of the interventions depends on a number of clinical characteristics.

1. Knowledge of the underlying pathogenic mechanisms responsible for the physiological and psychological disturbances, and the way these disturbances affect the patient's personality.
2. Understanding of the patient's personality in the face of stress, loss of function, and loss of self-esteem.
3. Sensitivity to the patient's needs and empathic caring in meeting those needs.
4. Appropriate use of psychopharmacology in conjunction with psychotherapeutic interventions, and an appreciation of the need for maintaining compliance with treatment.
5. Understanding of the placebo effect (both positive and negative) and its contribution to the therapeutic process, within the physician–patient relationship (Balis, 1982b).

6. Appreciation for working closely with family members and with other professionals involved in the care of the patient.

In general, focal, time-limited psychotherapies (e.g., cognitive-behavioral therapy, expressive psychotherapy) are useful in patients with psychiatric disorders due to or associated with general medical conditions.

COGNITIVE-BEHAVIORAL THERAPY (CBT)

Several studies have documented the suitability and efficacy of adjuvant CBT (both individual and group) in treating patients with chronic illnesses, including back pain (Keefe *et al.*, 1992), cancer (Greer *et al.*, 1992), AIDS (Markowitz *et al.*, 1992), and somatizations (Sharpe *et al.*, 1992).

INTERPERSONAL PSYCHOTHERAPY (IPT)

IPT is often especially useful for patients having interpersonal problems and difficulty adjusting to life situations. It has been found effective in treating depression (Weissman & Markowitz, 1994), including depressed AIDS patients (Markowitz *et al.*, 1992) and geriatric depressed patients (Sloane *et al.*, 1985). Findings are mixed with regard to treating substance abuse (Carroll *et al.*, 1991).

Supportive psychotherapy and psychotherapeutic management are eminently suitable for patients with neuropsychiatric disorders, in contrast to exploratory (insight-oriented) psychotherapy, which usually has little value.

PSYCHOSOCIAL MANAGEMENT

Medicine not only is an applied scientific discipline, but also is an art that involves the skillful application of management principles. Patient management is an important aspect of comprehensive care that meets the current and anticipated needs of the patient and family. Effective management depends on one's ability to utilize available resources within the hospital, the patient's family, and his or her community, and the ability to work cooperatively with other health professionals, independently or a team approach.

Management interventions aim at reducing morbidity, increasing comfort through relief of suffering, enhancing impaired functions, increasing available competence and skills, reducing the need for lost functions through rehabilitation, and generally optimizing the patient's psychosocial milieu. Psychosocial mamnagement may take place within the patient's physical environment, family, and/or social setting.

Depending on the type of clinical syndrome (e.g., delirium, dementia, personality change), different management approaches must be applied in different settings and circumstances. Effective approaches vary according to whether the patient is in an emergency room, medical–surgical ward, intensive care unit, (ICU), private home, physician's office, or nursing home. The patient's need for particular management skills and interventions will usually vary during the clinical course of the syndrome (e.g. acute, convalescent, or chronic phase). It will also vary according to the prognosis (e.g., reversible or irreversible, residual or progressive) and the potential for using rehabilitative and other community services.

The management of cognitive impairment (e.g., delirium, dementia, amnestic disorder) is of particular significance. These patients require continuous efforts toward reducing needs associated with impaired or lost function, while maximizing the utilization of available function and preventing regression, dependency, and other reactive psychopathology. The management of patients with psychiatric syndromes associated with minimal or no cognitive deficit (e.g., psychosis, catatonia, depression, mania, anxiety, personality change, sexual dysfunction, or sleep problem) is similar to that of patients with the corresponding primary disorders. Treatment follow-up and rehabilitation for substance abuse are an indispensable part of the management of substance-related disorders.

Finally, the patient's family, his or her home environment, and the social milieu are, in most instances, a major focus in the effort to attain effective management. Counseling with family members, especially the spouse or primary caretakers, may involve a range of concerns, including advice regarding the care and supervision of the patient, reducing stress and resolving conflict within the family, dealing with unrealistic expectations about current and future function, and assisting family members in effective coping strategies (especially in caring for the chronically demented, psychotic, or impulsive and emotionally unstable person).

CHAPTER 3

DELIRIUM

Delirium presents with clouding of consciousness (impaired awareness), impaired attention, and global cognitive deficit. The syndrome develops as an acute episode over a short period, tends to fluctuate during the course of the day, and usually resolves within days. It is etiologically related to a general medical condition or substance intoxication or withdrawal, with evidence from history, physical examination, and/or laboratory findings. The confusional state is often associated with illusions, hallucinations, fleeting delusions, and bizarre behavior due to the patient's psychotic experiences and failure to comprehend his or her environment. Affect is variable, often expressing fear and anxiety. Behavior may vary greatly, from agitation, excitement, and combativeness to apathy and lethargy.

Most of the medical conditions listed in Table I.2-1 and substances listed in Table I.2-2 may cause delirium, acting alone or in combination. The most common etiologies involve drugs, various systemic disorders, and primary CNS disorders, including infections, head trauma, neoplasms, and cerebrovascular disorders.

GENERAL TREATMENT PRINCIPLES

The treatment and management of the delirious patient are generally based on the following therapeutic principles (Balis, 1970).

1. Identify and treat the causative factors.
2. Understand the pathogenic mechanisms of the disease process that led to development of the delirium.

3. Recognize emergency situations for early intervention (e.g., hypoxia, hypoglycemia) in order to prevent irreversible brain damage (e.g., dementia) or death.
4. Recognize and treat those psychiatric symptoms that must be removed as soon as possible in order to provide relief or prevent accidents or complications (e.g., agitation, combativeness, suicidal behavior).
5. Understand the cognitive state and factors that may influence it in order to optimize supportive measures in patient management (e.g., impaired capacity for information processing as influenced by an unfamiliar or ambiguous environment).

Etiological treatment, when available, is of primary importance. Every effort should be made to identify the underlying causative factor(s) with the aim of instituting specific treatment at the earlier possible time. A detailed history from relatives or friends is most helpful, especially in identifying drug ingestion, alcohol abuse, head trauma, chemical exposure, or already diagnosed disease (e.g., diabetes, epilepsy, drug idiosyncrasies, or heart disease). In deliria occurring during hospitalization, the diagnostic process is aided by focusing on the setting in which the delirium occurred (ICU, recovery room, dialysis unit), the nature of preexisting disease (e.g., pulmonary insufficiency, cardiac failure, hepatic cirrhosis), or the treatment of the primary disorder (e.g., digitalization, hypnotic-sedatives, gastric suction, irradiation).

The etiology of delirium is often multifactorial, especially in the hospitalized patient. Several subthreshold factors acting concurrently may be sufficient to produce the critical physiological derangement that leads to the decompensated state (Engel, 1959). In this regard, every physiological abnormality should be corrected and every possible etiological factor eliminated, especially nonessential medications or those for which a less toxic drug can be substituted.

Once the causative factor is removed, the condition may be self-limited, with rapid recovery. In some instances, the primary cause may have already ceased to operate (e.g., head trauma, burns, seizures, bleeding, radiation) and only the pathogenic sequelae need to be treated (secondary causes). In others, the primary cause is unknown and only the disease processes are identifiable and amenable to treatment.

Delirium as a complication of serious illness often portends life-threatening or ominous outcome. Early recognition and emergency treatment intervention reduce the risk or degree of brain injury, general morbidity, and mortality. Common preventable etiologies include drug intoxication, hypoglycemia, diabetic acidosis, hypoxia, thiamine deficiency, intracranial hemorrhage, subdural hematoma, subarachnoid hemorrhage, withdrawal delirium, acute cerebral edema, and hyperthermia.

MEDICATION

Symptomatic treatment is primarily medicinal. It should be noted, however, that appropriate management approaches may minimize or make unnecessary the use of drugs. Thus, in a simple confusional state without symptoms of agitation, drug treatment may be unnecessary or may even be contraindicated, since the commonly used psychotropic drugs may aggravate the delirium through their CNS depressant, anticholinergic, or hypotensive effects. Even in florid deliria, pharmacological control of symptoms should be tempered by the realization that appropriately supportive management measures may be of equal importance.

Pharmacological control of delirium generally involves the relief of distressing symptoms (fear, anxiety, panic, irritability, illusory and hallucinatory symptoms, delusions) and disruptive behaviors. Drugs recommended for the symptomatic control of delirious symptoms include antipsychotic and anxiolytic medications. The choice of a particular psychotropic is based on several considerations, including etiology of the delirium, side effects of the drug, and previous experience. Thorough familiarity with a drug's pharmacological actions, pharmacokinetics, biometabolism, and side effects is necessary.

Among the traditional neuroleptics, the high-potency ones have been the preferred agents, with haloperidol the drug of choice. Risperidone may become a favored alternative. Clozapine is not recommended.

The benzodiazepines are safe and effective. They are less sedating than the hypnotics, require high doses to produce CNS depression, and have minimal autonomic and cardiovascular effects. They also have anticonvulsant activity that may be useful in treating withdrawal deliria. The short-acting oxazepam and intermediate-acting lorazepam are often the benzodiazepines of choice, especially for patients expected to show cumulative effects. Lorazepam appears to be ineffective and associated with serious side effects in treating the delirium of medically hospitalized AIDS patients (Breitburt *et al.*, 1996).

Psychotropic drugs have no therapeutic effect on the cognitive deficit and, as mentioned earlier, may worsen it. Physostigmine will restore cognitive functions in deliria induced by anticholinergic agents.

The prescribing schedule of any of these drugs should take the fluctuating course of delirium into consideration. If the symptoms have a characteristic schedule (e.g., only at night), it may be advisable to prescribe the drug only prior to symptom onset. The dosage and route of administration depend on symptom severity, response, patient age (the elderly require much lower doses), and other factors. Small, preferably oral, dosages are appropriate for moderate anxiety and restlessness. Higher doses, given parenterally, are required for the control of severe agitation, panic states, or assaultive behavior. Optimal titration requires close monitoring of response and knowledge of factors that may modify drug effects. Common problems associated with a failure to titrate the drug optimally include oversedation or undersedation with ineffective symptom control.

Sedation with Neuroleptics

In mildly to moderately agitated patients, 2 to 10 mg of oral haloperidol twice a day generally suffices. Parenteral administration may be necessary for the uncooperative patient, with the dosage adjusted to about three-fourths of the oral amount. In severely agitated, assaultive, or panicked patients, haloperidol should be given parenterally, intramuscularly (IM) or intravenously (IV), with an initial dose of 2 to 10 mg, which can be repeated several times a day as needed, while observing for adverse effects, until agitation is controlled. Doses should be lower than those for primary mental disorders. The total daily dose required to produce a calming effect may range from 10 to 40 mg (or higher). Once the effect is achieved, haloperidol should be given orally, in twice-a-day doses, and gradually tapered and discontinued within a week or so. The method is similar for risperidone, with an oral dosage range of 0.5 to 6.0 mg, or higher if necessary.

Sedation with Benzodiazepines

When benzodiazepines are used, the choice depends primarily on differences in plasma half-life and hepatic metabolism. In mildly to moderately agitated patients, 25 to 30 mg of *chlordiazepoxide*, 5 to 10 mg of *diazepam*, 15 to 30 mg of *oxazepam*, or 0.5 to 1.0 mg of *lorazepam* given orally every four to six hours as needed is generally sufficient. These doses may be doubled in more severely agitated patients. Parenteral administration of lorazepam may be required for patients with severe agitation, panic, or combativeness, at dosage levels comparable to those for oral administration. In emergency situations, a slow IV injection of lorazepam (2 mg) or diazepam (10 mg) may become necessary.

Hydroxyzine, an antihistamine, and paraldehyde, a hypnotic, may also be used to control anxiety and agitation, in a manner similar to that described for the benzodiazepines. Hydroxyzine may be given orally or parenterally, while paraldehyde is preferably administered rectally.

In addition to the symptomatic control of the psychiatric manifestations of delirium, close attention must be paid to correcting any concomitant physiological derangement, including fever, insomnia, cardiac arrhythmias, seizures, dehydration, nutritional deficits, and urinary retention.

PSYCHOSOCIAL MANAGEMENT

Psychosocial management of the delirious patient in a hospital setting is the cornerstone of the total therapeutic approach. Its effectiveness is based on an understanding of the cognitive state of the patient and the factors that may influence it, as well as on an appreciation of the patient's psychological needs. Its goals are to optimize the patient's environment and the staff's bedside approach as a means of providing support to the patient's cognitive deficit, to provide protection from accidents, and to improve and maintain the patient's physical and mental state through nonspecific supportive measures that provide control and comfort. The key to successful management is quality nursing care.

One should be guided by the awareness that the patient is confused and disoriented, has impaired memory and cannot retain new information, has difficulty processing information, tends to misinterpret events and distort information, cannot tolerate either excessive or diminished sensory input, and may be experiencing frightening perceptual distortions.

The patient with mild delirium of known etiology and good prognosis (e.g., idiosyncratic reaction to a drug, febrile illness) is best cared for at home, in a stable and familiar environment, provided family members can contribute continuous care and supervision. More serious deliria, and especially those of unknown etiology, require immediate hospitalization. The choice of hospital type depends on several considerations, including the etiology of the underlying illness, the degree and sophistication of medical and diagnostic requirements, and the severity of the behavioral disturbance. For instance, patients with delirium caused by serious physical illness (e.g., heart failure) or with alcohol withdrawal delirium must be treated in a general hospital, usually with psychiatric consultation. On the other hand, violent, suicidal, or acutely psychotic delirious patients with no evidence of serious physical illness (i.e., phencyclidine-induced delirium) may be best treated in a psychiatric hospital.

The physical environment should be stable and unambiguous, with elements that enhance familiarity and orientation, maintain low sensory input, and preserve variability through stimulus change. The patient is best cared for in a quiet, simply furnished, and preferably single-bed room, softly lighted at all times, with mild stimulation provided by a radio or television set. A calendar, clock, and some personal articles (e.g., family pictures) should be at the bedside for orientation and familiarity. Continuous supervision by a sitter, preferably a relative who is thoroughly instructed about the requirements of this task, should be provided. The number of nursing and house staff members involved in the care of the patient should be minimized in order to increase the patient's familiarity with personnel. Special attention should be given to the overriding need for constant supervision and protection from accidents, including suicidal and homicidal precautions when indicated. Physical restraints should be avoided whenever possible, and when applied, should be used for only brief periods. Control of agitation and combativeness is best managed by the personal contact of a supervising family member and by the appropriate use of tranquilizing drugs.

The interpersonal aspects of management are primarily determined by the patient's need to be oriented, to comprehend what is happening to him or her, and to be reassured. Accordingly, every interaction with the patient should be consistent with these needs. Staff members should clearly identify themselves, state their role, remind the patient that he or she is in a hospital, and carefully explain what they intend to do. They should provide reassurance and explain everything that the patient might experience as alien, ambiguous, threatening, or frightening.

Upon recovery from the delirious state, the patient may have complete amnesia for the episode or may have spotty or incomplete recollection. If the patient is amnestic, he or she should be helped to understand the nature of the experiential gap and be reassured that his or her memory is now intact. If the patient remembers the psychotic experiences, their nature and benign prognosis should be carefully explained.

SPECIFIC DELIRIA

The DSM-IV classifies deliria into (1) delirium due to a general medical condition (including delirium associated with the Alzheimer's type and vascular dementias), (2) substance-induced delirium, (3) delirium due to multiple etiologies, and (4) delirium not otherwise specified. The first two types are discussed here.

293.00 DELIRIA DUE TO A GENERAL MEDICAL CONDITION

Most of the disorders listed in Table I.2-1 may cause delirium, coded as 293.00. The following may be of particular clinical interest.

Delirium Associated with Metabolic and Other Encephalopathies

Uremic Encephalopathy. Renal failure and its consequent uremia often present with a uremic delirium. The delirium develops slowly and has a markedly fluctuating course, often associated with psychotic symptoms, hyperexcitability, and electroencephalogram (EEG) abnormalities characterized primarily by diffuse slowing with a tendency to paroxysmal bursts of slow waves. The relation between the degree of elevation of urea and creatinine and the severity of neurologic impairment is highly variable. Dialysis may reverse the delirium, as may renal transplantation (Pincus *et al.*, 1992).

Dialysis Encephalopathy. The dialysis equilibrium syndrome, formerly called the reverse urea syndrome, may present with asterixis (flapping tremor), seizures, delirium, and EEG abnormalities, if not treated early. Its cause is unclear; it is thought to be associated with brain edema due to altered osmolarity. It can be prevented by slower dialysis, more frequent and shorter dialysis sessions, or dialysis against a high glucose concentration (Jefferson & Marshall, 1983). Some cases have been attributed to drug-induced encephalopathy (Taclob & Needle, 1976). The syndrome must be differentiated from subdural hematoma that occasionally develops in hemodialyzed patients receiving anticoagulants and from dialysis dementia (see Chapter 4).

Hepatic Encephalopathy. Delirium develops during the second or "precoma" stage of hepatic encephalopathy, and presents, in addition to the confusional state, with asterixis and characteristic EEG abnormalities (paroxysmal bilateral slow waves superimposed on a relatively normal background). Hyper-ammonemia is a consistent feature, although there is a poor correlation between the severity of the encephalopathy and the level of ammonia (Fraser & Arieff, 1985). Hepatic encephalopathy has been associated with increased GABA-like activity, high tryptophan levels, and electrolyte disturbances. Portal-systemic shunting to treat portal hypertension often results in hepatic encephalopathy. Hepatic encephalopathy is also seen in Reye's syndrome and Wilson's disease. Treatment is generally supportive, directed toward correcting the consequences of hepatic insufficiency (Pincus *et al.*, 1992).

Hypertensive Encephalopathy (HTE). The syndrome presents acutely or subacutely with headache and progresses with symptoms of nausea and vomiting, visual impairment, focal or generalized seizures, transient neurological findings, and an altered state of consciousness (delirium), all in the presence of elevated blood pressure (usually exceeding 220 mmHg). The hypertension may be idiopathic (often after sudden discontinuation of antihypertensive treatment) or a complication of existing disease (e.g., renal disease, pheochromocytoma, eclampsia). It is thought to result from cerebral edema secondary to a breakdown of the blood-brain barrier and extravasation of serum. HTE is a medical emergency requiring aggressive antihypertensive treatment, best achieved with IV nitroprusside in an ICU (Robinson & Toole, 1992).

Fluid-Electrolyte and Acid-Base Encephalopathies. These metabolic disorders include metabolic acidosis (e.g., diabetic ketoacidosis, salicylate poisoning) and metabolic alkalosis (e.g., volume chloride depletion secondary to vomiting, gastric drainage, diuretics, hyperadrenocorticism), which may progress to stupor and coma. In addition to treating the underlying condition, symptomatic treatment involves the administration of bicarbonate to correct the acidosis and volume expansion with sodium chloride to correct the alkalosis. Dehydration and hypernatremia (e.g., lithium-induced diabetes insipidus, excessive sweating), volume sodium depletion (e.g., gastric suction, diarrhea, vomiting, adrenal insufficiency, chronic renal failure, osmotic diuretics), hypokalemia (e.g., vomiting, diarrhea, gastrointestinal fistula), and hypophosphatemia (e.g., antacids, alcohol withdrawal, hyperalimentation) may be associated with delirium, which is readily reversed by correcting the respective electrolyte imbalance.

Delirium caused by hyponatremia secondary to psychogenic polydipsia is of special interest to psychiatrists. Other causes include inappropriate ADH secretion (IADH) and drug-induced hyponatremia (e.g., with carbamazepine). Treatment includes fluid restriction and the use of demeclocycline (Illowsky & Kirsh, 1988).

Burn Encephalopathy. Severe skin burns may lead to "burn delirium," which typically presents with lethargy and confusion, neurological symptoms (e.g., nystagmus, ataxia), and diffuse slowing of the EEG. Treatment is directed at correcting metabolic complications and at providing supportive interventions, including aggressive pain management, brief focused psychotherapy, and pharmacological treatment of psychiatric complications, such as depression, anxiety, and insomnia (Stoddard, 1995).

Hypoalbuminemia. Low serum albumin is a risk factor for delirium. Since albumin is the main transport protein for drugs, caution should be exercised when prescribing for hypoalbuminemic patients (Dickson & Fisher, 1993).

Delirium Due to Neurologic Disorders

Wernicke's Encephalopathy. Produced by thiamine deficiency, Wernicke's encephalopathy is usually secondary to chronic alcoholism, and less often to chronic hemodialysis, thyrotoxicosis, pernicious vomiting of pregnancy, and gastric carcinoma. It usually begins abruptly as a "quiet delirium" and is accompanied by the characteristic neurological triad of external ophthalmoplegia, nystagmus, and cerebellar ataxia. The patient most often appears apathetic, listless, confused, and disoriented. Treatment consists of parenteral thiamine (50 mg IM or IV) followed by oral doses of thiamine and good nutrition with multivitamin supplements. The ophthalmoplegia improves within hours and the delirium clears within a few days after treatment with thiamine. The patient usually emerges from the delirium with an amnestic disorder (Korsakoff's).

Encephalitis. Various encephalitides may present with a vast array of neuropsychiatric symptoms, including delirium. Treatment of these disorders is beyond the scope of this book.

Delirium Complicating Dementias

Delirium is a frequent complication of dementia. The etiology of this delirium is not uniform. It is usually drug induced, often through an anticholinergic mechanism (see Table I.2-2). Other etiologies include metabolic disorders (e.g., diabetic acidosis, hypoglycemia), hypoxia resulting from cardiac or pulmonary disease, and other conditions listed in Table 1.2-1. One of the etiologies of delirium complicating vascular dementia is the disease process itself, which may result in delirium during transient ischemic attacks (TIAs) or during the acute phase of an occlusive episode secondary to cerebral thrombosis or emboli.

290.11, 290.30 Dementia of the Alzheimer's Type with Delirium. As with other deliria, treatment of the delirium in Alzheimer's dementia is generally symptomatic and supportive (Lipowski, 1983; Liston, 1982).

For the control of agitation, high-potency neuroleptics are recommended, especially haloperidol in doses of 0.5 to 5 mg by month (P.O.) or IM twice daily. If the patient develops extrapyramidal symptoms, agitation may alternatively be controlled with small doses of risperidone or a benzodiazepine with a short half-life, such as lorazepam, which can be given in doses of 0.1 to 1 mg P.O. or IM every four hours as needed (p.r.n.). If insomnia is present, it may be treated with a short-half-life benzodiazepine hypnotic, such as temazepam 15 to 30 mg at bedtime p.r.n. or triazolam. The clinician should keep in mind that the use of sedative/hypnotics and benzodiazepines, especially those with longer half-lives (e.g., flurazepam, diazepam), may worsen the confusion in delirium. For more information, see Chapters 4 and 12.

290.41 Vascular Dementia with Delirium. The development of delirium in a patient with vascular dementia is a serious complication because of the possibility that the disease process itself may be causing the delirium. A TIA referable to the carotid or vertebrobasilar arterial territories may present with acute confusional symptoms lasting from a few seconds to 12 hours. The diagnosis of TIAs requires careful evaluation before etiological treatment is instituted, in the effort to abort an irreversible cerebrovascular accident. About one third of patients will have no further symptoms, one-third will have recurrent TIA symptoms, and one-third will go on to have a small or catastrophic stroke (Robinson & Toole, 1992). The choice between medical or surgical (i.e., endarterectomy) treatment depends on a number of factors, including whether or not the carotid or vertebral-basilar system is involved, localization of the lesion, elucidation of the precise cause, the frequency and duration of TIAs, and other risk/benefit considerations.

The pharmacological treatment of TIAs includes risk factor modifications (e.g., control of hypertension, reduction of hypercholesterolemia), platelet anticoagulants (e.g., aspirin, dipyridamole, or ticlopidine), and other anticoagulants (e.g., heparin, warfarin). The starting dose of aspirin is 300 mg/day, which may be increased to 1.2 g a day. Dipyridamole (25 to 75 mg three times a day) is commonly used in conjunction with aspirin. Ticlopidine is prescribed at 0.5 mg/day (Robinson & Toole, 1992). Anticoagulants, used on either a short-term or long-term basis, may arrest the advance of a thrombotic stroke in evolution. It is imperative to rule out intracranial hemorrhage before using anticoagulants. In a thrombotic episode in evolution, anticoagulation with heparin IV or continuous drip therapy is instituted for several days, followed by oral warfarin at doses sufficient to maintain prothrombin time at twice the control value (Hass, 1979). The use of cerebral vasodilators, such as papaverine, nicotinic acid, inhalation of 5% carbon dioxide, aminophylline, and acetazolamide, is controversial and of questionable value.

Sundowner Syndrome. Transient confusional episodes in the demented elderly, known as the sundowner syndrome, are deliriumlike cognitive disturbances judged to be functional and referred to as "pseudodelirium" (by analogy with pseudodementia) (Lipowski, 1983). They generally occur in the evening or at night, as a result of diminished sensory input and social isolation and/or exposure to an unfamiliar environment (e.g., the hospital). Treatment consists of better orientation, room lights, and, if symptoms persist, small doses of a high-potency neuroleptic (e.g., haloperidol, 0.5 to 1 mg, or risperidone) one or two hours before sundown. The dosage may be increased gradually as needed. Risperidone has the advantage of lacking extrapyramidal side effects.

SUBSTANCE-INDUCED DELIRIA

Substance-induced deliria are common, and are generally associated with substance-use disorders, suicidal or accidental drug overdose, and idiosyncratic reactions to prescribed or over-the-counter drugs. The pathogenic mechanism depends on the pharmacological action(s) of the drug. Predisposing or facilitating factors include age (the elderly being most susceptible), biological substrate of the host (genetically determined enzyme systems), dosage, route of administration, and hepatic function (Balis, 1982a). The general management of the delirious patient is discussed under "General Treatment Principles."

Nondelirious alcohol-related withdrawal syndromes are discussed in the section on withdrawal in Chapter 14.

Deliria with Onset During Intoxication

(See also specific treatments for intoxications, Chapter 13.) Intoxication deliria are classified into dose-related and idiosyncratic, depending on the underlying pathogenetic mechanism. Dose-related deliria are induced by relatively high blood concentrations of a potentially deliriogenic drug, such as certain psychoactive drugs (e.g., cocaine, amphetamines, phencyclidine) and anticholinergic agents. Idiosyncratic deliria are not dose-related and can occur early in the course of treatment at therapeutic doses. Genetically controlled enzymatic processes in drug metabolism are thought to be responsible for the induction of the delirium. Many prescription drugs may cause idiosyncratic deliria in predisposed individuals (e.g., codeine, diazepam, glutethimide, chloroquine). They clear rapidly, without sequelae.

291.0 Alcohol Delirium with Onset During Intoxication. This must be differentiated from delirium with onset during withdrawal. High blood alcohol levels suggest intoxication, while the presence of autonomic symptoms (e.g., tachycardia) and seizures suggest a withdrawal mechanism. There are no established guidelines for treatment of alcohol intoxication delirium. Note that benzodiazepines or neuroleptics are contraindicated, since they produce added CNS depression which could cause respiratory depression and coma. For more information, see the section on intoxication in Chapter 13.

292.81 Amphetamine (or Related Substance) Delirium. Sympathomimetic drugs with a CNS stimulant action include amphetamine, methylphenidate, ephedrine, pseudoephedrine, and diethylpropion. Amphetamine and cocaine may induce delirium within 24 hours of intake, and almost immediately following IV administration. In addition to confusional symptoms, associated features include tactile and olfactory hallucinations, labile affect, and violent behavior. The patient should be closely monitored for rising blood pressure and temperature and for convulsions. Treatment of psychostimulant delirium is similar to that of cocaine delirium and psychostimulant intoxication, discussed in Chapter 13.

292.81 Cocaine Delirium. This occurs almost immediately following an IV injection or smoking (free-basing), usually within one hour (but not more than 24 hours) of the oral intake of cocaine. In uncomplicated cases, the delirium clears within six hours. The patient requires placement in a quiet room where safety measures (e.g., physical restraints) may be applied to protect the combative individual. Agitation can be controlled with benzodiazepines (e.g., lorazepam, 1 to 2 mg IM or IV every two to four hours p.r.n.) or neuroleptics (e.g., haloperidol, 5 mg IM or 5 to 15 mg P.O. every two to four hours p.r.n.). It should be noted, however, that cocaine abusers may be sensitive to the extrapyramidal side effects of the neuroleptics because of dopamine depletion (Perry, 1987). Risperidone may be a preferred alternative. The patient's vital signs should be monitored very closely for rising temperature, pulse, and blood pressure. Hyperthermia requires vigorous treatment with both hypothermic blankets and ice packs to prevent grand mal seizures. If convulsions do occur, the patient should be treated with slowly administered IV diazepam, 5 to 15 mg, repeated every 45 minutes to prevent progression to status epilepticus. Uncontrollable severe hypertension (systolic blood pressure remaining above 200 mmHg for an hour or more) should be controlled promptly with propranolol (Perry, 1987).

292.81 Phencyclidine (or Related Substance) Delirium. This delirium may develop within 24 hours after intake of phencyclidine (PCP) or may emerge days later after recovery from an overdose. It may last for a week, with a waxing and waning course. Associated features are those of phencyclidine intoxication, including both physiological changes and behavioral disturbances. Treatment is similar to that described in the section on phencyclidine intoxication in Chapter 13. It includes a calm environment, adequate restraints for combative behavior, and diazepam or haloperidol for agitation. If seizures develop, diazepam should be given IV to prevent progression to status epilepticus.

Deliria with Onset During Withdrawal

(See also treatments for specific withdrawal syndromes, Chapter 14.) This is a special class of substance-induced deliria involving a specific pathogenetic mechanism. They occur in individuals who have developed physiological dependence on alcohol (291.00) or sedative-hypnotic-anxiolytic drugs (292.00), and who abruptly discontinue or drastically reduce their use.

291.00 Alcohol Delirium with Onset During Withdrawal.   Also known as delirium tremens (DTs), this is a serious complication seen in up to 5% of alcohol-withdrawal cases and occasionally leading to death from intercurrent complications. Patients must be hospitalized. After a thorough medical evaluation, treatment should follow the protocol below, or a similar one.

1. The patient should be sedated with a benzodiazepine (e.g., temazepam, diazepam, or lorazepam), given orally, and if necessary, parenterally (IM or IV). Diazepam 10 to 40 mg P.O., temazepam 30 to 60 mg P.O., or lorazepam 1 to 3 mg P.O. may be repeated every one or two hours as necessary until symptoms are suppressed, then reduced to a dose of half the total amount used, administered three or four times a day P.O. Benzodiazepines provide an anticonvulsant effect, reducing the risk of withdrawal seizures. Neuroleptics, on the other hand, tend to increase the risk of convulsions. Magnesium sulfate has been used by some in patients with serum magnesium below 2 mEq/L.

2. The patient should be given daily thiamine (initial dose of 100 to 200 mg IM, with subsequent doses given orally) and a multivitamin supplement, to combat malnutrition and prevent acute thiamine deficiency that may lead to Wernicke's encephalopathy or cardiac failure.

3. Parenteral fluid administration should be carefully individualized and titrated according to the hydration status of the patient. Fluid retention and overhydration develop during rising blood alcohol levels, while dehydration follows a period of high, stable blood alcohol levels. Many patients may actually be overhydrated, in which case parenteral fluids are contraindicated. Dehydration is presumed in cases of vomiting, diarrhea, elevated hematocrit, and other objective signs of dehydration. No more than 50% of an initial fluid deficit should be replaced during the first 24 hours, and no more than 6 liters of dextrose-containing fluid should be given in a 24-hour period. Fluids should be given orally if the patient can tolerate oral intake. Any electrolyte imbalance should be corrected.

4. Hypoglycemia may be present in some patients during the withdrawal period. Patients should be given sufficient carbohydrates in oral fluids (e.g., orange juice). Parenteral fluids, if needed, should contain 5% dextrose.

5. Alcohol withdrawal seizures (grand mal) are generally self-limited and have a relatively benign course. There is no evidence that prophylactic phenytoin will prevent withdrawal seizures. Benzodiazepines are effective in lessening the likelihood of seizures and will suffice for the patient who has no history of epilepsy. Prophylactic anticonvulsant therapy is

indicated in patients known to have an underlying seizure disorder or repeated past episodes of withdrawal seizures. If withdrawal seizures occur repeatedly, 5 to 10 mg diazepam by slow IV is recommended. (See the section on withdrawal in Chapter 14.)

Other specific deliria related to drug abuse (e.g., cannabis, hallucinogens, inhalants, opioids, sedatives, hypnotics, or anxiolytics) are discussed in the sections on intoxication (Chapter 13) and withdrawal (Chapter 14).

292.81 Other Substance Delirium

Many other drugs with CNS effects may induce delirium as a result of drug idiosyncrasy in predisposed individuals (genetically determined) or altered drug metabolism (e.g., advanced age, impaired hepatic function, drug interaction), or because of toxic concentrations of the drug (e.g., overdose, cumulative effects, impaired renal excretion). Table I.2-2 lists drugs known to cause delirium. An anticholinergic mechanism is implicated in the majority of drug-induced deliria.

Anticholinergic Delirium. Drugs with anticholinergic activity include many antispasmodics (atropine, homatropine, belladonna alkaloids, scopolamine, etc.), antiparkinson drugs (benztropine, trihexyphenidyl, biperiden, etc.), analgesics (meperidine), tricyclic antidepressants (especially amitriptyline), neuroleptics (low potency, and especially thioridazine), antihistamines (diphenhydramine, promethazine, hydroxyzine, etc.), cimetidine, and others. Tricyclic drug overdose is a common cause of anticholinergic delirium. According to Preskorn and Simpson (1982), tricyclic plasma levels exceeding 450 ng/ml produced delirium in six of seven patients. Delirium may also occur idiosyncratically with blood concentrations within the therapeutic range. The elderly are particularly vulnerable.

The treatment of anticholinergic delirium is similar to that of anticholinergic intoxication (see Chapter 13). Physostigmine salicylate, 1 to 2 mg IV or IM, will clear the delirium within less than 30 minutes. A second dose of 1 to 2 mg physostigmine may be given 15 minutes later, and may be repeated every two to three hours if needed (Granacher *et al.*, 1976). With tricyclic antidepressant delirium, one must monitor the ECG closely and treat cardiotoxic effects as necessary.

Neuroleptic Malignant Syndrome (NMS). This syndrome presents as an unpredictable response to therapeutic doses of neuroleptics, with a prevalence of 0.15% (Keck *et al.*, 1991). It is more likely to occur with high-potency traditional neuroleptics, especially when given parenterally or in conjunction with lithium and other drugs. Dehydration and exhaustion are thought to be predisposing factors. In the author's opinion, NMS often appears to be a state-dependent response to neuroleptics in patients who are excited or agitated. It is advisable to sedate highly excited patients with a benzodiazepine rather than with a neuroleptic. Similar hypermetabolic syndromes are sometimes seen in the abrupt withdrawal from dopamine agonists (levodopa, bromocriptine, amantadine).

The patient presents with catatoniclike symptoms of mutism, bradykinesia, extrapyramidal cogwheel rigidity and often plastic (lead-type) rigidity, autonomic dysregulation evidenced by marked diaphoresis, tachycardia, fluctuating blood pressure, and a hypermetabolic state indicated by pyrexia, elevated serum creatine phosphokinase (CPK), leukocytosis, elevated liver enzymes, and cardiac arrhythmias, and with confusional symptoms of a waxing and waning course, characteristic of delirium. NMS must be differentiated from neuroleptic-induced hyperthermia, a hypermetabolic state that may present with fever, rigidity, and elevated CPK levels. In hyperthermia, however, the skin is dry and the blood pressure is low or normal. There are notable similarities between NMS and post-anesthetic malignant hyperthermia (MH). The latter is due to a peripheral mechanism related to an idiopathic dysfunction in sarcoplasmic calcium-ion metabolism, resulting in a hypermetabolic state of skeletal muscles. Lethal catatonia may also mimic NMS (see "Catatonic Disorder," Chapter 7).

Without definitive treatment, mortality may approach 50%. In nonlethal cases, NMS symptoms typically resolve within 5 to 10 days (longer if depot neuroleptics were used). Complications include rhabdomyolysis with myoglobulinemia and acute renal failure, aspiration pneumonia, and cardiovascular collapse.

The patient is best managed in a general medical ward. Placement in an ICU may become necessary. Treatment is essentially symptomatic and supportive, consisting of early recognition, immediate discontinuation of the neuroleptic, and careful attention to the detection and aggressive management of complications: control of hyperthermia with antipyretics and cooling blankets; correction of dehydration and electrolyte imbalance; treatment of intercurrent infection, such as pneumonia; dialysis for acute renal failure following rhabdomyolysis; ventilator support in case of acute respiratory failure (due to aspiration, infection, or pulmonary emboli); treatment of cardiac arrhythmias; and management of other secondary complications. Since the patient is usually immobile, prophylactic low-dose heparin has been suggested to prevent venous thrombosis and embolic episodes.

Specific Treatment of NMS. Although controlled studies are not available, various treatments have been advocated in case reports. A comprehensive review by Philbrick and Rummans (1994) supports the view that ECT is the most consistently effective treatment for NMS and neuroleptic-induced malignant catatonia. Among 18 of their own cases, 11 of 13 patients who received ECT survived, compared with only one of five who did not receive ECT. Their patients were generally "initially treated conservatively, and ECT was used as their condition deteriorated." Although the safety of ECT relative to other treatments in high-risk patients is well established (Zielinski *et al.,* 1993; Rice *et al.,* 1994), Davis and colleagues (1991) reported lethal cardiac arrhythmias associated with the treatment in NMS.

Commonly used medications include dopamine agonists (e.g., bromocriptine and amantadine), dantrolene, and benzodiazepines (particularly lorazepam). Bromocriptine has been used in amounts ranging from 7.5 to 60 mg/day, in divided doses every eight hours, initially IV (Granato *et al.*, 1983; Mueller *et al*, 1983). Amantadine, 100 mg twice a day, has had some anecdotal success. Dantrolene has been the most frequently tried drug. It is a direct-acting muscle relaxant that effects calcium release from the sarcoplasmic reticulum, and is often effective in malignant hyperthermia. The dosage range for NMS is 0.8 to 2.5 mg/kg every six hours; oral regimens average 100 to 300 mg/day, in divided doses, for two to three days (Granato *et al.*, 1983). Intravenous lorazepam may be a safe and useful drug (Fricchione *et al.*, 1983). Anticholinergic agents have been used in a few patients, but probably have no therapeutic value and may even hinder recovery. Other approaches reported effective in case reports, but without large numbers or controlled studies, include calcium channel blockers, corticosteroids, and "artificial hibernation" (Philbrick & Rummans, 1994).

In post-NMS cases, neuroleptics must be reintroduced very cautiously, preferably with an atypical neuroleptic, such as risperidone. Neuroleptic rechallenge is best undertaken at least two weeks after complete resolution of the syndrome (Rosebush *et al.*, 1992). Although NMS has been reported to resolve without residual symptoms, the writer has noted two cases followed by residual symptoms—evidenced as severe frontal lobe syndrome with catatoniclike symptoms, dementia, severe perseveration, and gait disturbance—that took several years to resolve.

CHAPTER 4

DEMENTIA

Dementia presents with multiple cognitive deficits, including impairment of memory and disturbances in language, praxis, cognition, and executive functioning, that cause significant impairment and are judged to be related to degenerative, vascular, or other general medical conditions or substances.

Dementia must be differentiated from delirium (no clouding of consciousness in dementia), amnestic disorder (deficit limited to memory), and pseudodementia, a form of depression masquerading as dementia. Recent conceptualizations on a continuum between depressive dementia and dementia spectrum of depression emphasize overlapping pathophysiologic mechanisms rather than differential diagnosis (Emery & Oxman, 1992).

GENERAL TREATMENT PRINCIPLES

The following general guidelines apply to the treatment and management of all dementias, with special emphasis on those arising in the senium. Treatment may be etiological (when the cause is known and treatable) and/or symptomatic.

The early diagnosis of reversible dementias is of the utmost importance. In searching for a treatable cause, first consideration should be given to ruling out depressive pseudodementia (see below). A trial of antidepressants may be justified in the absence of demonstrable etiology. The next step is to search for treatable organic causes, especially when an etiological diagnosis remains uncertain. This is particularly important in older patients, who are more likely to be diagnosed as suffering from Alzheimer's or vascular dementia.

Symptomatic treatment is the only therapeutic approach available for patients suffering from irreversible forms of dementia. Since the cognitive deficit is not amenable to any treatment, therapeutic efforts are directed toward improving impaired functions, promoting general health, and treating psychiatric complications when they develop. Demented patients, especially the elderly, must maintain the best possible physical health in order to prevent physiological derangement of their already compromised cerebral function. Every effort should be made to restore or improve impaired functions (e.g., renal, cardiovascular, respiratory, or endocrine), combat symptoms (pain, insomnia, constipation, impaired mobility), improve impaired hearing and vision, and maintain optimal nutrition. It is especially important to prevent drug interactions and toxic effects from prescribed or over-the-counter medications. Elderly patients are particularly susceptible to side effects because of decreased physiological reserves and slower rates of absorption, metabolism, and elimination of many drugs. Demented patients are highly vulnerable to the development of secondary psychiatric disorders, including delirium, depression, and psychosis.

PSYCHOSOCIAL MANAGEMENT

Effective management of the demented patient demands the physician's commitment to continuing care for a chronically ill and, in most instances, progressively deteriorating patient (Reisberg, 1982). The traditional medical model is expanded to include additional roles required for dealing with social and family problems confronting the patient and his or her caretakers. The physician is often called on to coordinate the activities of several caregivers, including family members, social workers, visiting nurses, in-house aides, and other social service personnel. Knowledge of available community resources and how they can be utilized in the total care of the demented patient, as well as of the patient's medical and psychological needs, family resources and interpersonal dynamics, assets and liabilities, prognosis, and anticipated problems, is crucial to treatment planning.

The physician should maintain continuing interaction with family members; inform them about the patient's condition and the nature, course, and prognosis of his or her illness; and involve them in the treatment, if possible. The local chapter of the Alzheimer's Disease and Related Disorders Association (ADRDA) can be an important source of support. The physician should also assist family members with emotional support and with their feelings of shame, guilt, or anger, especially when they must make decisions about institutional placement. Relatives may become highly critical of the physician or nursing home staff as a means of coping with feelings of guilt or helplessness. These reactions can often be resolved through ventilation and moral support.

The doctor-patient relationship should remain a significant focus throughout the course of the illness. This is most important early in progressive dementias and in patients with nonprogressive dementias, such as those that follow an acute brain insult (e.g., head trauma, encephalitis, anoxic episode). The physician should structure each visit with the patient and provide psychological support by attempting to allay fears and to counteract the sense of helplessness, allow the ventilation of feelings, enhance self-esteem, encourage independence, strengthen healthier coping mechanisms, and correct reality distortions when present.

During the early and milder stages of (especially progressive) dementias, important decisions must be made by the patient (with the help of the family when possible) on a number of issues, including his or her competence to drive a car, capability to continue to work and carry on personal business, retirement, testamentary capacity, and degree of supervision at home and elsewhere. Whenever possible, a power of attorney, advance directives, and living wills should be considered while mental competence is still adequate.

Patients with milder residual deficit and nonprogressive dementias can benefit from retraining and rehabilitation. Every effort should be made to maintain ambulation and prevent regression to a wheelchair or bed. Other psychosocial guidelines include encouraging efforts toward maximum feasible independence and self-care; engaging in pleasurable, useful, or productive activities that enhance self-esteem; maintaining preserved skills and abilities, as well as physical fitness; and appropriate supervision to prevent consequences of poor memory (e.g., fire hazards, getting lost, poor nutrition, deterioration of personal hygiene) or impaired social judgment (e.g., poor management of financial matters and personal affairs).

Appropriate manipulation of the patient's physical environment, whether in an institution or at home, is an important means of supporting impaired cognitive function (such as memory and orientation) and impaired sensory perception. Environmental modulation to establish a "prosthetic environment" for the demented patient includes good room lighting; simple, stable, and familiar furnishings; clocks that sound the time and large calendars on the wall; note pads as memory aids; pill-organizer boxes; hearing aids; eyeglasses; dentures; handrails; and a walker. An extra effort should be made to make life as routine and familiar as possible.

Early Alzheimer's patients may benefit from a support group. Concurrent or conjoint support groups for patients and caregivers may have added benefits for both. In progressive dementias, and as the patient's behavior continues to deteriorate, the physician should refer the family to a social work specialist for assistance in arranging interventions, such as visiting nurses, aides, or sitters; a day-care center; or a hospice, or nursing home (Fisher, 1994). For a more comprehensive review of the treatment and management of dementia patients, see Edwards (1993).

TYPES OF DEMENTIA

IRREVERSIBLE DEMENTIAS

These are associated with permanent neuronal damage and may be either progressive or residual (nonprogressive).

Progressive Dementias

These dementias pursue a relentless course toward a vegetative state and death. They include dementia of the Alzheimer's type, vascular dementia, Parkinson's disease, progressive supranuclear palsy, dementia from inoperable brain tumor, HIV encephalopathy, multiple sclerosis, and other demyelinating diseases, and the less common Huntington's chorea, Pick's disease, and Creutzfeldt-Jakob disease.

Residual (Nonprogressive) Dementias

Such dementias include those resulting from cerebral trauma, protracted cerebral hypoxia or hypoglycemia, and other permanent but nonprogressive injuries to the brain (e.g., subarachnoid hemorrhage, ruptured cerebral aneurysm, radiation injury). Among other causes are bacterial endocarditis resulting in embolic cerebral infarcts, intracranial infections, space-occupying lesions (e.g., tumor, subdural hematoma, colloid cyst), and other CNS disorders (e.g., temporal lobe epilepsy), as well as dementias caused by heavy metals and industrial poisons (lead, carbon monoxide), systemic lupus erythematosus, hypertensive encephalopathy, porphyria, Wilson's disease, hypoxia-anoxia, and vitamin deficiencies (e.g., B_1, B_{12}). Early diagnosis and intervention will usually arrest the underlying dementing process. In some instances, early treatment may alleviate some of the dementia.

REVERSIBLE DEMENTIAS

Reversible dementias are syndromes with a treatable underlying organic disorder. They are of great significance prognostically and therapeutically, since treatment, especially when instituted early, may reverse the dementia. Reversible dementias include endocrinopathies (hypothyroidism, Addison's disease), hypercalcemia, metabolic encephalopathies (diabetic acidosis, hepatic and renal failure), electrolyte/water imbalance, and hypoxia due to cardiac or pulmonary disease. Most substance-induced dementias (e.g., from barbiturates or steroids), discussed below, are eminently treatable. Other medical disorders include normal pressure hydrocephalus, carotid artery occlusal, temporal arteritis, cerebral abscess, neurosyphilis, and Lyme disease. Elderly depressed patients with an initially reversible dementia may develop irreversible dementia at a rate of 9 to 25% per year.

SPECIFIC DEMENTIAS

290.10, 290.00 DEMENTIA OF THE ALZHEIMER'S TYPE

Alzheimer's dementia is the most common dementia in the elderly, affecting 7% of the population over 65 years of age and accounting for 25 to 30% of all cases of dementia and 65% of dementias occurring in the senium (Cummings & Benson, 1983). It begins insidiously and progresses slowly, with memory loss followed by progressive intellectual impairment and personality changes, and later aphasia and apraxia. The patient reaches a vegetative state after 8 to 10 years or longer. Compared with patients with vascular (e.g., multi-infarct) dementia, patients with Alzheimer's seem to enjoy relatively good physical health in the early stages.

The etiology remains unknown. Some cases appear familial, especially those with an onset before age 70 (Li *et al.*, 1993). Recent advances in the neurochemistry of Alzheimer's disease have revealed striking neurotransmitter changes and characteristic cellular proteins (AZ-50). Acetylcholine deficit is of particular interest. The ventral forebrain cholinergic neurons projecting to the cerebral cortex and hippocampus are the most consistently and severely damaged. There is evidence that the apolipoprotein E gene may serve as a predictor of the development of Alzheimer's disease in memory-impaired individuals (Peterson *et al.*, 1995).

A number of studies have tested the therapeutic efficacy of available cholinomimetic drugs, including acetylcholine agonists, precursors, and anticholinesterases. Choline and phosphatidyl choline (PhosChol), dietary precursors of acetylcholine, have been found ineffective in improving the cognitive deficit (Thal, *et al.*, 1981). Clinical trials with IV or oral physostigmine have provided conflicting results, one major disadvantage being its very short plasma half-life (about 30 minutes).

Among the long-acting cholinomimetics, tacrine (Cognex), a centrally active anticholinesterase, has been found in long-term trials to produce modest improvement of cognitive impairment in patients with mild to moderate dementia (Summers, *et al.*, 1986; Davis, *et al.*, 1992). A recent study by Knapp and associates (1994) confirmed the efficacy of tacrine in such patients. Tacrine may produce a number of side effects, including gastrointestinal symptoms (nausea, vomiting, diarrhea), dizziness, headache, ataxia, and ALT (SGPT) elevations. There are isolated reports of jaundice associated with hepatocellular necrosis. A recent study on the hepatotoxic effects of tacrine by Watkins and associates (1994) found ALT levels greater than three times the upper limit of normal in

25% of patients, but 88% of those who discontinued tacrine because of elevated ALT levels were able to resume long-term therapy upon rechallenge. Tacrine is prescribed at an initial dose of 10 mg four times daily, maintained for six weeks while monitoring ALT levels weekly, and then titrated upward at six-week intervals to 120 to 160 mg/day. The concurrent use of tacrine with theophylline may result in a twofold increase in the plasma levels of theophylline. Tacrine does not appear to alter the course of the underlying dementing process.

There has been continuous research in cholinergic (Murphy, 1993) and other pharmacological approaches to cognitive enhancement. Phospaditylserine, a naturally occurring phospolipid that alters neuronal membrane fluidity, was found in a small trial to improve mildly impaired Alzheimer's patients (Crook *et al.*, 1992). Acetyl-L-carnitine has been reported to delay cognitive deterioration in demented patients, probably through an antioxidant or membrane-stabilizing action (Sano *et al.*, 1992). Trials with monoamine oxidase-B inhibitors, such as L-deprenyl, in Alzheimer's dementia are based on the drugs' antioxidant, neuroprotective effects (Tariot *et al.*, 1992). Nimodipine was found to have some effect on delaying cognitive deterioration, probably by blocking the increase in intracellular free calcium, which is known to activate various destructive enzymes leading to cell death (Tollefson, 1992). An early interest in the efficacy of the so-called nootropic drugs, such as piracetam and ACTH-4-10, was recently renewed in a study of oxiracetam, which showed statistically significant effects on some measures (Bottini, 1992). Preliminary reports on the use of cycloserine indicate some beneficial effects for a subgroup of demented patients (Mohr *et al.*, 1993). Recent research evidence suggests that ibuprofen may be prophylactic against Alzheimer's dementia.

Numerous other drugs have been used in the treatment of dementia of the Alzheimer's type with questionable results, including CNS stimulants (e.g., pentylenetetrazol, amphetamines, and amphetaminelike drugs), cerebral vasodilators (e.g., papaverine), and anabolic substances. Hydergine, a dehydrogenated ergot alkaloid, in sublingual doses of 1 to 2 mg three times daily, has received some support as a means of improving cognitive function in the early phase of Alzheimer's dementia (Von Loveren-Huyben *et al.*, 1984).

The treatment of the behavioral and psychological complications of dementia (e.g., psychosis, depression) is discussed below.

VASCULAR DEMENTIAS

Vascular Dementia of Acute Onset (Stroke)

This usually results from a succession of cerebrovascular thrombotic, hemorrhagic, or embolic strokes. It develops rapidly and produces major neurological disturbance (e.g., hemiplegia, aphasia). Tissue Plasminogen Activator (TPA), given I.V. within the first three hours from the onset of the stroke, will reverse the thrombotic process. Treatment of stroke is beyond the scope of this book.

Left-sided anterior strokes are likely to become complicated with depression (see "Complications of Dementia" in this chapter).

Multiple Infarct Dementia

The second most common of the progressive dementias arising in the senium, it is thought to be caused by widespread multiple cerebral infarctions (small strokes), secondary to cerebral arteriosclerosis. It is characterized by a stepwise deteriorating course, focal neurologic signs and symptoms, and evidence of significant cerebrovascular disease. Comorbidity with hypertension and arteriosclerotic heart disease is very common. The differentiation between the Alzheimer's and multi-infarct types of dementia may remain equivocal even after considering clinical criteria, neuropsychological tests, and imaging data. The noninvasive transcranial Doppler sonography aids in differential diagnosis (Ries, *et al.,* 1993). In addition to a positive family history, other predisposing factors that can be addressed in the treatment plan include hypertension, high serum cholesterol or triglycerides, lipoprotein profile, obesity, and smoking.

There is no known effective method for reversing or arresting the course of vascular dementia. Several studies have confirmed the potential usefulness of antiplatelet agglutinating drugs, such as aspirin, ticlopidine, and dipyrimadole, in reducing the risk of infarction in patients with transient ischemic attacks (Robinson & Toole, 1992). Pentoxifylline, which decreases blood viscosity, has been found to slow the progression of vascular dementia, especially in patients who have had at least one stroke (Black *et al.,* 1990). Various other drugs, such as vasodilators (hydergine, papaverine) and lipotropic enzymes, have been proposed for altering the course of vascular disease. No reported controlled studies clearly prove the value of any of these agents. (See "Vascular Dementia with Delirium," Chapter 3).

Dementias Dues to Cerebrovascular Embolism

Associated with subacute bacterial endocarditis and cardiac arrhythmias, these are usually preventable by treating the underlying condition.

Subcortical Vascular Dementia

Binswanger's encephalopathy is associated with foci of ischemic destruction in the deep white matter of the cerebral hemispheres, often in persons with hypertension. The presence of diffuse white matter demyelination can be best demonstrated with MRI, (e.g., evidence of periventricular hypodensities). The disease is often associated with depression, which appears to respond to treatment with antidepressants.

Other vascular dementias include those caused by subarachnoid hemorrhage, subdural hematoma, and carotid artery stenosis. Discussion of these disorders is beyond the scope of this book.

GENERALLY IRREVERSIBLE/UNTREATABLE DEMENTIAS DUE TO OTHER GENERAL MEDICAL CONDITIONS

The DSM-IV has given some prominence to certain dementias by providing codes for them on Axis I as well. They are generally untreatable and, with the exception of dementia due to head injury, are associated with progressive and eventually fatal illness.

294.9; 043.1 on Axis III Dementia Due to HIV Disease

Dementia due to human immunodeficiency virus disease (AIDS dementia complex and HIV encephalopathy) must be differentiated from secondary (opportunistic) CNS infections (e.g., toxoplasmosis, cryptococcosis, herpes encephalitis, mycobacterium tuberculosis), as well as from other causes, such as anergic depression and drug toxicity. It presents with memory impairment, poor concentration, difficulty with problem solving, apathy, social withdrawal, and (often) neurological signs (e.g., hyperreflexia, positive frontal release sign, tremor, ataxia) (Miller *et al.*, 1990). It may progress rapidly and lead to global dementia. Major depression with psychotic features is a common neuropsychiatric complication. The course of the encephalopathy parallels the course of the underlying immunodeficiency.

The treatment of AIDS with antiviral agents (e.g., azidothymidine) may improve or slow the progression of the HIV dementia. The successful treatment of secondary infections may result in cognitive improvement. Depression in patients with early dementia complex may respond to antidepressants or psychostimulants (Ostrow *et al.*, 1988).

294.1; 905.0 on Axis III Dementia Due to Head Trauma

Closed or open head injury may result in dementias of varying severity, depending on the seriousness of the brain injury. Efforts at rehabilitation may bring significant improvement in various areas of functioning (e.g., speech, self-care). Specialized head injury treatment programs may be very useful when available.

294.1; 332.0 on Axis III Dementia Due to Parkinson's Disease

This subcortical dementia, developing in patients with advanced Parkinson's disease, has no distinguishing clinical features. The dementia is usually mild and slowly progressing. Antiparkinsonian drugs (e.g., levodopa, anticholinergics) have no effect on the dementia; anticholinergic medications may aggravate it.

294.1; 333.4 on Axis III Dementia Due to Huntington's Disease

A slowly progressing subcortical dementia, it is associated with predominantly frontal lobe involvement, characteristic choreiform movements, and a family history of the disease. The choreiform movements usually precede the dementia. Complications with depression and psychosis are common and may precede the onset of neurological signs. Depressive and psychotic symptoms usually respond to pharmacological treatment.

290.10; 331.1 on Axis III Dementia Due to Pick's Disease

A middle-life, slowly progressing dementia, it is marked principally by personality changes characteristic of the frontal lobe syndrome (e.g., apathy, fatuous euphoria, emotional blunting, disinhibition, and deterioration in social functioning), which often precede impairment in memory and intellect. Therapeutic interventions are limited to the psychosocial management of personality change related to disinhibition and poor social judgment. (See also "Personality Change," Chapter 10.)

290.10; 046.1 on Axis III Dementia Due to Creutzfeldt-Jakob Disease

This fairly rapidly progressing and devastating dementia is caused by a presumably viral spongioform encephalopathy. It is associated with multiple neurological symptoms, both pyramidal and extrapyramidal, which usually accompany or follow (but in some cases precede) the dementia, and with characteristic (triphasic) EEG abnormalities. There is no available treatment.

294.1 GENERALLY REVERSIBLE/TREATABLE DEMENTIAS DUE TO GENERAL MEDICAL CONDITIONS

Neurosyphilis (General Paresis of the Insane)

Although rare, neurosyphilis continues to be encountered in clinical practice. A positive serology dictates examination of the cerebrospinal fluid (CSF). If earlier syphilis was not adequately treated or there are abnormal CSF findings (e.g., elevated cell count and protein in the CSF), a full course of penicillin should be administered. Besides dementia, neurosyphilis may present with delirium, psychotic disorder, mood disorder, and personality change associated with a prominent frontal lobe syndrome. Treatment of these syndromes is discussed in their respective chapters.

Late Lyme Borreliosis

In its late stages, Lyme disease may present with parenchymatous and meningovascular lesions comparable to those seen in tertiary syphilis. In addition to depression, mania, and psychosis, Lyme disease has been associated with impairment in cognitive function (Krupp *et al.*, 1991). Early treatment of the infection with antibiotics may prevent these late sequelae.

Lewy Bodies' Disease

The disease presents with fluctuating cognitive impairment that involves both episodic confusion and lucid intervals, often associated with hallucinations and extrapyramidal symptoms. Patients with Lewy bodies' disease are unusually sensitive to the effects of neuroleptics, a finding that may serve as a diagnostic marker (Byrne *et al.*, 1992).

Hepatolenticular Degeneration (Wilson's Disease)

This rare inborn error of copper metabolism produces a mild dementia by the deposition of copper in brain tissues. It affects patients below the age of 30, and presents with the classic triad of liver disease, neurological dysfunction (tremor, incoordination, dysarthria), and Kayser-Fleischer corneal rings. There are anecdotal case reports of personality changes, emotional lability, anxiety, psychosis, and depression. The copper chelating agent D-penicillamine is the treatment of choice.

Pellagra (Niacin Deficiency)

A multiple deficiency illness, niacin deficiency is the most prominent. In addition to dementia, psychiatric syndromes may include catatonia, mood disorders, or psychosis. Treatment consists of niacin, multivitamins, and a balanced diet.

Vitamin B_{12} Deficiency (Including Other Folic Acid Deficiency and Pernicious Anemia)

The disease presents insidiously, with symptoms of pernicious anemia and neuropsychiatric features (which may present without lowered hemoglobin or other physical signs). Neurologic changes may include peripheral neuropathy, myelopathy (subacute combined degeneration), and/or encephalopathy. Besides the cognitive changes characteristic of dementia or amnestic disorder, the disease may present with schizophrenialike psychosis, personality change (e.g., apathy, emotional lability), and depression. Folate deficiency is seen, particularly in geriatric patients and epileptics on anticonvulsant therapy. Early replacement therapy with B_{12} (given IM) or folate, respectively, will reverse the symptoms. In more advanced cases, residual dementia will persist.

Epilepsy

Uncontrollable seizures, especially those associated with temporal lobe epilepsy, may cause gradual intellectual deterioration and dementia. Adequate control of seizures will slow or prevent the development of dementia.

Normal Pressure Hydrocephalus

Communicating hydrocephalus with normal CSF pressure causes a dementia characteristically accompanied by gait and sphincter disturbances. As the disorder progresses, the clinical picture is dominated by symptoms of frontal lobe syndrome (e.g., abulia, apathy, mutism, bradykinesia, snout and grasp reflexes, incontinence), which are the result of the expansion of the anterior horns of the lateral ventricles. The disorder is often complicated with depression. Surgical treatment by shunting in carefully selected cases improves the dementia in at least 50% of patients, especially when performed early in the development of the dementia.

Space-Occupying Lesions

Tumors located in the frontal and temporal lobes are the most likely to present with dementia, as well as with other psychiatric conditions. The treatment of these disorders is beyond the scope of this book.

Dialysis Dementia

Developing in some patients on long-term dialysis, it presents with progressive dementia associated with dysarthria, mutism, myoclonus, asterixis, and seizures, and is often accompanied by psychotic symptoms and distinctive EEG changes. The syndrome is thought to be due to a diffuse toxic metabolic disorder of unknown pathogenesis, and is generally irreversible, leading to coma and death. Evidence linking this syndrome to aluminum intoxication is not entirely conclusive (Pincus *et al.*, 1992). Aluminum chelation therapy with deferoxamine has been used to treat the presumed aluminum overload.

Cardiogenic Dementia

This usually hypoxic dementia is secondary to cardiac disorders that compromise cerebral blood flow (e.g., arrhythmias, congestive heart failure, bradycardia, complete heart block). Early treatment of the underlying condition will reverse the dementia, with mild to moderate forms of hypoxic dementia slowly improving over six months or longer. Dementia may also result from repeated embolic episodes secondary to subacute bacterial endocarditis. Antibiotic treatment will prevent its development or progression.

Myxedema Dementia

Caused by severe, untreated hypothyroidism, it can be reversed by replacement treatment with thyroxin.

SUBSTANCE-INDUCED PERSISTING DEMENTIAS

291.2 Alcohol Persisting Dementia

Alcohol-related dementia is presumed to be caused by prolonged, heavy alcohol abuse. Its etiology is still controversial. It must be differentiated from subacute Wernicke-Korsakoff, traumatic, and hepatic encephalopathy. It is associated with more than 10 years of drinking and is nonprogressive if the patient remains alcohol-free. There is evidence for cortical atrophy, which may subside following prolonged abstinence (Francis & Franklin, 1987). There is no established specific treatment. Abstinence, thiamine, and good nutrition are recommended.

292.82 Inhalant Persisting Dementia

Largely irreversible, its clinical aspects are discussed in the section on intoxication, Chapter 13.

292.82 Sedative, Hypnotic, or Anxiolytic Persisting Dementia

The dementia is often seen in elderly patients treated with this class of drugs (especially short- and intermediate-acting benzodiazepines), which can induce it even at therapeutic doses. It is an eminently reversible dementia, which rapidly subsides after tapering and eventually discontinuing the drug.

Other Substance-Related Persisting Dementias

Numerous other drugs may cause reversible dementia following long-term use or chronic intoxication. Among those most commonly implicated are lithium, cyclic antidepressants, β-blockers, methyldopa (especially combined with haloperidol), clonidine, phenytoin, anticholinergic compounds, disulfiram, oral hypoglycemics, anti-inflammatory agents, cimetidine, digitalis, quinidine, levodopa, diuretics, and narcotics. Steroids can produce cognitive decline mimicking early Alzheimer's disease (Varney *et al.*, 1984). These dementias clear following discontinuation or reduction of medication.

DEMENTIA DUE TO MULTIPLE ETIOLOGIES

Dementias with multiple etiologies may involve concurrent Alzheimer's type and vascular dementias, and, most commonly, other noxious factors complicating the two (e.g., drugs [especially in polypharmacy] and physiologic disturbances secondary to other medical disorders). Treatment of these conditions may improve the dementia.

COMPLICATIONS OF DEMENTIA

The DSM-IV provides separate codes for the major psychiatric complications of dementias, including delirium, delusions, hallucinations, depressed mood, perceptual disturbance, behavioral disturbance, and communication disturbance.

290.11, 290.30, 290.41 Delirium

This is the most common psychiatric complication of dementia, especially vascular dementia. For treatment, see "Delirium," Chapter 3.

290.13, 290.21, 290.43 Depressed Mood

A common complication of dementia, its prevalence rate is about 50%. Treatment may include various antidepressant medications, supportive psychotherapy, ECT, and, in early stages of the dementia, psychotherapy. In milder forms, supportive psychotherapy is useful in assisting the patient to grieve and accept cognitive losses and their consequences and to maintain self-esteem. Psychotherapeutic management is directed toward enhancing environmental-social support throughout the course of dementia.

When clinical depression is present, antidepressant medication or ECT is recommended. Although TCAs (e.g., desipramine, nortriptyline) have been the standard drugs in the past, the SSRIs (e.g., fluoxetine, sertraline, pyroxetine, fluvoxamine), bupropion, and venlafaxine, are becoming the preferred antidepressants because of their low potential for side effects (see "Psychophramacotherapy," Chapter 2). The reported improvement of both depression and cognition with the serotonergic citalopram (Nyth *et al.*, 1992) suggests that SSRIs may have cognition-enhancing effects (Schneider, 1993). Monoamine oxidase inhibitors (MAOIs), such as phenelzine and tranylcypromine, have been shown to be effective and well tolerated by the elderly (Jenike, 1985). Their major advantage over the tricyclics is their lack of anticholinergic and cardiotoxic effects. Their major drawbacks are orthostatic hypotension and dietary restrictions. The new MAOI moclobemide does not require dietary restrictions. (See also "Mood Disorders," Chapter 8.)

ECT is indicated for patients who fail to respond to an adequate course of antidepressants, and for the many demented patients who cannot tolerate the adverse effects of these drugs (see "ECT," Chapter 2).

290.xx Delusions, Hallucinations, and Perceptual Disturbance

Psychotic symptoms are usually amenable to neuroleptics. The choice of specific agent should be based on efficacy, side effects, and toxicity, considering altered metabolism in the elderly. High-potency neuroleptics produce the fewest adverse effects and are the neuroleptics of choice. Risperidone is effective in many cases, but has not yet been well studied. There is no experience with olanzapine. (See "Psychopharmacotherapy," Chapter 2.)

Elderly demented patients are particularly susceptible to orthostatic hypotension, as well as to central anticholinergic toxicity (confusion, delirium) and extrapyramidal effects. Neuroleptic treatment should begin with small amounts given in divided doses (e.g., risperidone, 0.5 to 6.0 mg/day; haloperidol, 0.5 to 2.0 mg/day; thioridazine, 25 to 75 mg/day). Blood levels of haloperidol appear to show a linear relationship to clinical response and extrapyramidal effects, with a therapeutic range of 0.5 to 4 ng/ml (Devanand *et al.*, 1992). Monitoring blood levels of haloperidol is recommended, particularly in maintenance treatment. Risperidone may become a first-line drug for controlling psychosis in the demented patient. (See also "Psychotic Disorders," Chapter 6)

290.16, 290.24, 290.46 Behavioral Disturbances

Very common in the demented elderly, behavioral disturbances are principally the result of the underlying brain damage, and are most common in those with prominent frontal lobe damage. The consequent personality change often represents an exaggeration of the individual's premorbid personality traits. Other factors include drug effects (often polypharmacy) on an already compromised brain, unfamiliarity with the environment (e.g., sundowning), failure in task performance (e.g., catastrophic reaction), concomitant physical or mental illness, and interpersonal dynamics in the family or residential setting.

Behavior modification techniques and environmental manipulation are useful in the effort to control such disturbances as aggression, agitation, and sexual disinhibition. Behavioral approaches for agitation include charting behaviors, manipulating the environment, and using sound reduction rooms, music therapy, hearing aids or augmentation, and a transitional object that provides sensory stimulation (Hay, 1995). Phototherapy utilizing an antidepressant-spectrum light source may have a beneficial effect on both sundowning and agitation (Satlin *et al.*, 1992).

The pharmacological management of behavioral disturbances primarily includes neuroleptics and benzodiazepines; among other drugs used are carbamazepine, valproate, and serotonergic medications. Neuroleptics usually have only a limited effect on agitation, hyperactivity, assaultiveness, and irritability. The target symptoms most responsive to neuroleptics include suspiciousness, hallucinatory behavior, excitement, hostility, and uncooperativeness. Steele *et al.* (1986) found both haloperidol (1, 2, and 5 mg/day) and thioridazine (25, 50, and 75 mg/day) effective for managing behavioral symptoms in Alzheimer's dementia. Risperidone may be a better first choice, although it has not been well studied for this indication. Brief or p.r.n. prescribing of short-acting benzodiazepines may also be useful in controlling acute behavioral disturbances. One should note that overprescribing is a common mistake, causing excessive sedation and other toxic signs.

Restlessness, wandering, and agitation tend to be more severe in the evening and at night (sundowner syndrome), and are often part of a psychosis. Neuroleptics show a good to excellent therapeutic response in 60 to 70% of elderly agitated patients with a wide variety of organic and emotional disorders. No therapeutic differences among neuroleptics can be inferred at this time; however, preliminary data (Prado *et al.*, 1995) suggest that risperidone may be an effective and well-tolerated alternative to traditional neuroleptics in very elderly demented patients. Recently, trazodone, 25 mg three times a day, was reported to ameliorate agitation, and especially emotional lability, irritability, and restlessness, associated with dementia (Lebert *et al.*, 1994). Agitation and affective lability refractory to neuroleptics may also respond to carbamazepine (Gleason & Schneider, 1990), benzodiazepines, or lithium (Kunik *et al.*, 1994).

Aggressive behavior is highly prevalent among elderly demented patients, many of whom have found their way to nursing homes. Alcohol and medications (e.g., sedative, hypnotic, or anxiolytic agents; steroids; tricyclic antidepressants; anticholinergic drugs) are commonly implicated in acute aggression in the elderly. Elimination of the offending drug is the treatment of choice.

The treatment of other sources of chronic aggression depends on the underlying specific etiology, such as psychosis (neuroleptics), partial complex seizures (carbamazepine), cyclic mood disorders (lithium, valproate), generalized anxiety (buspirone), or neuroleptic-induced akathesia (propranolol). Buspirone is moderately effective in controlling agitation and aggressive outbursts in the dosage range of 20 to 40 mg/day (Sakauye *et al.*, 1993). Using large doses of propranolol to control chronic violence in the elderly demented patient (Yudofsky *et al.*, 1990) is inadvisable.

Irritability and psychosis are also associated with aggressive behavior. Drug management of acute aggression that does not abate with the above treatments may include carefully monitored, low-dose benzodiazepines (e.g., temazepam, lorazepam) or neuroleptics (e.g., haloperidol, risperidone), given P.O. or IM. For additional information, see "Personality Change" (Chapter 10).

Anxiety is a common symptom. Benzodiazepines are the drugs of choice for acute anxiety states when psychosocial approaches fail to control the symptoms. The short-acting oxazepam and lorazepam are preferred, in approximately one-third to one-half of the young adult dose. Excessive sedation, apathy, ataxia, amnesia, incoordination, disorientation, confusion, and dysarthria are common toxic effects (Salzman, 1995). Buspirone is relatively safe and well tolerated by the elderly, and is recommended for long-term therapy. Antihistamines, such as hydroxyzine, produce excessive initial sedation, have short-lived effects, and, at higher doses, may cause delirium. Antidepressants (TCAs, SSRIs, MAOIs, bupropion) often relieve both anxiety and depression. See "Psychopharmacotherapy" (Chapter 2), "Delirium" (Chapter 3), and "Anxiety Disorder" (Chapter 9).

Insomnia is a ubiquitous complaint of elderly and (especially) demented patients. The latter often cannot fall asleep as a result of becoming disoriented and frightened when the lights are turned out. Leaving a light on all night may be helpful. The artificial bright light used for seasonal affective disorders (phototherapy), administered in two-hour evening sessions, has been shown to improve sleep-wake patterns, sundowning, and agitation in demented patients (Satlin *et al.,* 1992). Patients with sleep-onset insomnia may benefit from L-tryptophan, which can be prescribed as a pill (not currently available in the United States) or provided through high-tryptophan foods, such as milk or tuna fish. Melatonin is sometimes recommended as a benign, nondrug sleep inducer; however, there is little mention of it in the medical literature.

If drug treatment becomes necessary, the clinician has a number of options. Antihistamines (e.g., promethazine, 25 to 50 mg, or diphenhydramine, 25 to 50 mg at bedtime) and thioridazine in small doses (e.g., 25 mg at bedtime) are fairly well tolerated, but their hypnotic effect is short-lived. Chloral hydrate, 250 to 500 mg, is one of the least toxic choices. The short-acting benzodiazepines (e.g., triazolam, temazepam) are the most widely prescribed hypnotics and are well tolerated, although they may work for only a few weeks. They may also produce rebound insomnia, daytime rebound anxiety, and anterograde amnesia. The long-acting benzodiazepines (e.g., flurazepam) often produce unwanted daytime drowsiness, ataxia, and confusion. Zolpidem may be of particular benefit to demented patients (Satlin, 1994). Trazodone, although not a hypnotic, appears to be a safe and effective soporific for the elderly at doses of 25 to 50 mg. (See also "Sleep Disorders," Chapter 12).

Sexual disinhibition (e.g., compulsive public masturbation, attempts at coitus in inappropriate circumstances) is rare in the demented patient. If the behavior becomes intolerable, one may try low doses of neuroleptics or benzodiazepines. Medroxyprogesterone acetate (MPA), which is effective in certain paraphilias in nondemented patients, has been found to control intractable sexually disinhibited behavior in carefully selected demented patients as well (Cooper, 1987).

290.17, 290.25, 290.47 Communication Disturbance

Demented patients often show communication problems secondary to aphasia, especially in the advanced stages (third and fourth) of Alzheimer's dementia, and in vascular dementias with lesions in the dominant (usually left) hemisphere. Vartanian *et al.* (1993) found that the intranasal administration of vasopressin (having selective affinity for the left dominant hemisphere) in patients with cerebrovascular lesions produced increased speech activity and decreased perseveration. Speech therapy is recommended for patients with nonprogressive dementias.

CHAPTER 5

AMNESTIC DISORDERS AND
AGE-RELATED MEMORY DECLINE

This syndrome presents with memory impairment (especially recent memory) evidenced by an inability to learn new information. It occurs in a state of clear awareness (differentiating it from delirium) and without any significant loss of the remaining intellectual abilities (differentiating it from dementia).

The amnestic syndrome is produced by a variety of mechanisms, which can be reversible (as in the case of drugs, such as triazolam, interfering with memory consolidation) or irreversible (from bilateral lesions of specific diencephalic or medial temporal lobe structures).

GENERAL TREATMENT PRINCIPLES

Drug-induced reversible amnestic syndromes, such as those associated with the use of anticholinergics or short-acting benzodiazepines, are treatable by eliminating the offending medication. Amnestic syndromes associated with thiamine deficiency (e.g., chronic alcoholism, malnutrition) are reversible if thiamine is given without delay. There is no symptomatic treatment to correct the memory deficit caused by permanent brain damage. Physostigmine has been reported to improve amnestic disorder after herpes simplex encephalitis. The anticholinesterase tacrine may prove helpful for some patients (see "Alzheimer's Dementia," Chapter 4). Memory therapy (teaching the patient to use visual mnemonics) may be helpful for patients with preserved ability to retrieve visual images.

Psychosocial approaches are similar to those described for demented patients. However, compared with demented patients, amnestic patients have a more circumscribed cognitive deficit, maintain relatively intact verbal capacities, and are less vulnerable to developing major psychiatric complications. Although institutional custodial care may be necessary for patients with more severe forms, most can be cared for at home or in a supervised, structured environment. Efforts at the rehabilitation of patients with milder syndromes should always be part of the management plan. Specialized rehabilitation programs in cognitive retraining are especially valuable for those with head trauma (Kwentus *et al.*, 1985; Lezak, 1978).

SPECIFIC AMNESTIC DISORDERS

294.00 AMNESTIC DISORDERS DUE TO A GENERAL MEDICAL CONDITION

General medical conditions commonly associated with amnestic disorders include Korsakoff's syndrome, cerebrovascular disease (e.g., stroke), multiple sclerosis, temporal lobe epilepsy, head trauma, hypoxia, hypoglycemia, starvation (e.g., in anorexia nervosa), malabsorption, carbon monoxide poisoning, heavy metal intoxication, temporal lobectomy, and a variety of other neurologic traumata and disorders. The following is a brief review of the most significant disorders associated with amnestic phenomena.

Thiamine Deficiency

Besides alcoholism, thiamine deficiency may be seen in a number of other conditions, including malabsorption, eating disorders, hemodialysis, and disseminated malignancy. Treatment of the underlying condition and administration of thiamine (e.g., 50 mg daily) will improve the amnestic syndrome. See also "Alcohol Persisting Amnestic Disorder," below.

Transient Global Amnesia

Occurring in middle-aged or elderly individuals, it consists of a sudden loss of recent memory, lasting from minutes to hours, in the absence of other neurological signs. There is a complete inability to retain new information; however, conscious awareness, immediate recall, and the ability to perform highly complex tasks remain intact. Following the attack, the patent is amnestic for the event. Intense emotion is a frequent precipitant of transient global amnesia. A past history of migraine headaches may be obtained in 30% of cases. The syndrome is thought to be due to episodic transient vascular insufficiency of the mesial temporal lobe (Sluping *et al.*, 1980), possibly from stenosis or occlusion of the posterior cerebral artery (Mathew & Meyer, 1974). Prophylactic treatment with antiplatelet drugs may be considered for patients with recurrent attacks. A trial of antimigraine therapy with a β-blocker or calcium channel antagonist would seem appropriate, especially for those with a past history of migraine (Robinson & Toole, 1992).

Migraine, particularly juvenile migraine, may present with amnestic episodes, often resembling transient global amnesia. (Oliveros & Jensen, 1979). Treatment is that for migraine.

Temporal Lobe Epilepsy

This is characterized by brief amnestic episodes that rarely persist for hours, during which the EEG shows ictal dysrhythmia attributed to limbic seizure foci. Uncontrollable seizures may result in permanent memory impairment (e.g., by "mirror image" lesions of the opposite hemisphere). Treatment aims at complete control of seizures with anticonvulsant drugs. In selected intractable cases, temporal lobectomy may be indicated.

Other neurological disorders associated with amnesia include brain trauma or tumor with damage to diencephalic or temporal regions, bilateral hippocampal infarctions, herpes simplex encephalitis, cerebral anoxic states, and carbon monoxide or heavy metal poisoning. The treatment of the these disorders is beyond the scope of this book.

SUBSTANCE-INDUCED PERSISTING AMNESTIC DISORDERS

291.10 Alcohol Persisting Amnestic Disorder

In addition to transient anterograde amnestic episodes associated with acute intoxication (blackouts), chronic alcohol abuse may produce a persisting amnestic disorder known as Korsakoff's syndrome, the result of a thiamine deficiency secondary to nutritional deficit. In the majority of cases, the onset is acute, presenting as a sequela of Wernicke's encephalopathy; a smaller number of patients experience an insidious onset without a preceding acute encephalopathic episode. The reversibility of the Wernicke-Korsakoff syndrome depends on the promptness of instituting specific treatment with thiamine. Thiamine should initially be given parenterally in doses of 50 mg daily for about one week, and then be switched to oral administration, provided the patient is able to resume a normal diet. Treatment should be continued for several months, with a supplement of B-complex vitamins. About 20% of patients can be expected to recover completely, with another 50% improving to some extent. There is no effective treatment for the residual memory deficit. Clonidine, an α-norepinephrine agonist, may improve memory and recall at doses of 0.3 mg twice a day. See also "Wernicke's Encephalopathy," Chapter 3.

292.83 Sedative, Hypnotic, Anxiolytic Persisting Amnestic Disorder

This class of drugs is commonly associated with amnestic syndromes. The benzodiazepines are of particular interest because they are extensively used as anxiolytics and night sedatives. Benzodiazepines show significant differences in amnesia-inducing potency, with the short- and intermediate-acting compounds (lorazepam, triazolam) having greater amnestic effects than longer-acting benzodiazepines. The ultrashort-acting midazolam (Versed) is an anesthetic that acts through its amnestic effects. The amnestic effects of benzodiazepines are particularly prominent in the geriatric population. Discontinuation of the drug leads to complete recovery (see also "Intoxication," Chapter 13). If the substance is being abused, treatment and rehabilitation of drug abuse and rehabilitation should be part of the total management (see "Substance Use Disorders," Chapter 15).

292.83 Other Substance-Induced Persisting Amnestic Disorders

Anticholinergic compounds, such as scopolamine and atropine, produce marked amnestic effects (Mohs & Davis, 1985). The amnestic effects of tricyclic antidepressants, neuroleptics, antihistamines, and antiparkinsonian drugs, have been attributed to their anticholinergic action. Psychotropic drugs are more likely to be implicated in amnestic syndromes occurring in the elderly, especially those with strong anticholinergic effects, such as amitriptyline, clomipramine, and low-potency neuroleptics (e.g., thioridazine, clozapine). Discontinuation of the drug results in rapid recovery.

Exposure to heavy metals and other toxins, especially lead, arsenic, and organophosphates, may cause impaired memory and other psychiatric symptoms. Treatment of lead intoxication with British Anti-Lewsite (BAL), calcium disodium versenate, or oral penicillamine may improve the symptoms if the intoxication is not severe. Treatment of arsenic intoxication with BAL will clear the syndrome.

294.9 Cognitive Disorder Not Otherwise Specified

Patients with hypoparathyroidism may experience a drop in IQ. Response to treatment with supplementary dietary calcium and vitamin D has been variable. Similarly, patients with hypoxemia due to COPD show progressive neuropsychological impairment, as measured by the WAIS-R and the Halstead-Reitan Neuropsychological Battery (Prigatano *et al.*, 1983). Besides improving oxygenation of the brain, there may be cognitive benefits from improving central cholinergic functioning in hypoxemic persons with centrally acting anticholinesterases (e.g., tacrine) or acetylcholine precursors.

780.9 Age-Related Memory Decline

This is classified under "Additional Conditions That May Be a Focus of Clinical Attention." Normal forgetfulness associated with advanced age is often referred to as benign senescent forgetfulness (Kral, 1978). It is usually associated with an impaired ability to recall names and where items have been placed. There are no established clinical criteria differentiating it from amnestic disorder and no guidelines for treating it. Most individuals with age-related memory complaints show mild cognitive decline after two years (Small *et al.*, 1995). Tacrine or donepezil may be tried.

CHAPTER 6

PSYCHOTIC DISORDERS DUE TO A GENERAL MEDICAL CONDITION OR SUBSTANCE

These disorders were described in the DSM-III-R as "organic delusional disorder" and "organic hallucinosis." Diagnosis involves presumption rather than definitive diagnosis. The course and prognosis depend on the underlying etiology. The most common etiology of organic psychotic disorders, particularly among younger persons, is substance abuse. General medical disorders include degenerative and cerebrovascular disorders, epilepsy, brain tumors, endocrinopathies, systemic lupus erythematosus, and a host of other medical conditions.

GENERAL TREATMENT PRINCIPLES

As with other organic mental disorders, the primary focus is on the identification of the underlying specific disorder or specific causative factor in order to be able to institute appropriate etiological treatment. Diagnostically, psychotic symptoms of organic etiology cannot be differentiated on a phenomenological basis from those with a functional etiology. The common belief that visual hallucinations are characteristic of an organic process or that auditory hallucinations are prominent in functional disorders does not always hold true.

Nevertheless, there are certain features of some hallucinations, delusions, and illusions that are characteristic of some disorders related to medical conditions or substances. For example, microptic (Lilliputian) visual hallucinations, episodic olfactory hallucinations (especially foul odors), simple and repetitive hallucinations (e.g., hearing bells or one's name), various illusory perceptual distortions, and, in general, hallucinations that are simple, ego-dystonic, devoid of apparent psychological meaning, and with intact insight and reality testing are more likely to have an organic etiology (Balis, 1978c).

MEDICATION

Symptomatic treatment should aim at controlling delusions, hallucinations, agitation, and the physical symptoms of the underlying disease. In general, the effective control of delusions and hallucinations may be achieved with medications, usually neuroleptics. In some disorders, the symptomatic treatment of psychosis may involve specific drugs, such as anticonvulsants (in partial complex seizures of temporal lobe epilepsy), diazepam (in hallucinogen persisting perception disorder [flashbacks]), or propranolol and chlorpromazine (in porphyric psychosis). Supportive psychotherapy and other psychosocial approaches follow the same general guidelines as in the primary psychoses.

PSYCHOSOCIAL MANAGEMENT

The management of these patients is similar to that of patients with primary psychotic disorders with the caveat that their other CNS deficits may interfere with social adaptation and training. Management approaches must be directed toward both the underlying illness and the reactive psychopathology that may be present. Patients with continuing substance abuse, for example, require special efforts to engage them in a comprehensive rehabilitation program (see "Substance Use Disorders," Chapter 15). Epileptics have special psychological, social, and vocational needs that should be dealt with as part of their total treatment plan. Patients suffering irreversible loss of vision or hearing require social stimulation to counteract sensory deprivation. Anxious, agitated, or frightened patients must be calmed and reassured. Suicidal tendencies or extreme fear or agitation may make hospitalization necessary.

SPECIFIC PSYCHOTIC DISORDERS

The DSM-III-R wordings "organic hallucinosis" and "organic delusional disorder" were dropped from the DSM-IV, although organic hallucinosis was retained in the ICD-10. The DSM-IV lists the former as "psychotic disorder due to a general medical condition, with hallucinations" (293.82). Recurrent hallucinating is the only essential feature, occurring in a state of clear awareness (differentiating it from delirium) and in the absence of formal thought disturbance (differentiating it from schizophrenia). "Organic delusional disorder" was replaced in the DSM-IV by "psychotic disorder due to a general medical condition, with delusions" (293.81). Since most conditions that cause hallucinations may also cause delusions, the two are often combined.

293.81, 293.82 PSYCHOTIC DISORDER DUE TO A GENERAL MEDICAL CONDITION

Disorders that may cause psychosis include temporal lobe epilepsy, space-occupying lesions of the brain, temporal arteritis, migraine, pernicious anemia, hypo- or hyperthyroidism, hypoparathyroidism, Cushing's syndrome, systemic lupus erythematosus, porphyria, head trauma, Huntington's chorea, and CNS infections, including encephalitis, neurosyphilis, Lyme borreliosis, the spectrum of HIV-related organic brain disease, and disorders involving sensory deprivation (e.g., deafness, blindness). Besides specific etiological treatment (e.g., antibiotics in neurosyphilis or Lyme encephalopathy), neuroleptics are often effective. Clozapine may be preferable to older neuroleptics for treating psychosis in patients with Parkinson's disease (Greene *et al.*, 1993) and Huntington's disease (Sajatovic *et al.*, 1991). Risperidone or olanzapine may be a safer alternative for some patients. Psychosis in patients with HIV-related brain disease is often responsive to extremely low doses of high-potency neuroleptics, such as haloperidol (Ostrow *et al.*, 1988).

Epilepsy

Ictal psychosis in temporal lobe epilepsy (e.g., paroxysmally occurring perceptual distortions, hallucinations, and complex partial seizures), and the short-lived psychotic symptoms accompanying the postictal state (postictal delirium), must be differentiated from the chronic interictal complication of temporal lobe epilepsy known as epileptic psychosis. Improving the control of seizures may prove helpful for ictal and postictal psychosis.

Interictal psychosis (epileptic psychosis) develops in less than 10% of epileptic patients, usually many years after the onset of seizures (Balis, 1978; Blumer, 1977). Umbricht and associates (1995) found that a younger age at the onset of seizures and lower verbal and full-scale IQ differentiated patients with chronic psychosis from those with postictal psychosis. On the other hand, bitemporal seizure foci, clustering of seizures, and absence of a history of febrile convulsions were found to predispose to both chronic psychosis and postictal psychosis. Chronic psychosis in temporal lobe epilepsy may involve left hemispheric dysfunction regardless of seizure focus.

Neuroleptics appear to be of little value. Although there have been no related studies of the newer, atypical neuroleptics, Blumer (1995) reported satisfactory results by using a combination of tricyclic antidepressants and an SSRI (fluoxetine or paroxetine). He assumes that psychiatric disorders of epilepsy result from the secondary mechanisms of inhibition, which can be mitigated by the use of proconvulsant antidepressants.

In some patients, psychotic and seizural episodes show a seesaw relationship, with psychosis occurring when the seizures are controlled and the EEG becomes normal, a phenomenon described by Landolt (1956) as forced normalization. The relevance of this phenomenon to the psychosis remains unclear (Schmitz, 1995). Reduction of anticonvulsant drug dosage in these patients, as a means of allowing seizures to occur, or even induction of a grand mal seizure by ECT, has been suggested for the relief of intractable psychosis. Temporal lobectomy of seizure foci may be considered in some intractable cases as well.

Cardiovascular disorders commonly associated with psychotic manifestations (often with delirium or dementia) include arrhythmias causing transient cerebral ischemic attacks, subacute bacterial endocarditis causing multiple small cerebral embolic infarcts, and the sequelae of open heart surgery. Besides treating the underlying medical condition, psychotic symptoms may be controlled with small doses of nonsedating neuroleptics (e.g., haloperidol, 0.5 to 5.0 mg twice a day, or risperidone, 0.25 to 3.0 mg twice a day).

Temporal (Cranial) Arteritis

This may present with visual hallucinations that respond to systemic corticosteroid therapy. Visual hallucinations that are manifestations of migraine phenomena respond to antimigraine treatment (e.g., ergot alkaloids or propranolol).

Porphyria

It may present with a schizophrenialike psychosis or catatonic states (stupor, excitement), which may progress to delirium and dementia. Chlorpromazine is the only neuroleptic suggested in the literature for porphyric psychosis; however, others may be tried. Propranolol has also been reported to be effective in controlling the psychosis. Barbiturates precipitate porphyric attacks, and are absolutely contraindicated.

Systemic Lupus Erythematosus (SLE)

Presenting with psychosis in approximately 20% of the affected patients (Gurland, *et al.*, 1972), SLE may be schizophreniform, associated with cognitive impairment and personality changes (e.g., emotional lability, impaired judgment), or pure catatonia. The psychosis may be associated with depressive and anxiety syndromes (Ganz *et al.*, 1972). It is often difficult to differentiate SLE psychosis from that induced by concurrent treatment with steroids. If psychosis occurs, symptomatic treatment of the underlying condition with steroids should be coupled with the use of neuroleptics to control the psychosis.

HIV-Associated Psychosis

Patients with HIV infection present considerable psychiatric morbidity, including depression, anxiety, and psychosis. Patients with psychosis have high rates of past stimulant and sedative/hypnotic abuse, greater global neuropsychological impairment, and, at follow-up, a significantly higher rate of mortality (Sewell *et al.*, 1994). These patients are sensitive to the anticholinergic and extrapyramidal side effects of neuroleptics, and should be treated with low doses, if possible, or preferably, with risperidone.

ICU Psychosis

The high incidence of psychosis in patients treated in intensive care units is generally attributable to multiple organic factors, acting alone or in combination. Although psychological factors (e.g., anxiety, fear of death, frightening environment, or monotony) may contribute to the psychotic breakdown, the syndrome must be assumed to be of organic etiology until proved otherwise. The anxious and frightened patient needs reassurance and supportive management. Persistent or rising levels of anxiety may call for a short-acting benzodiazepine (e.g., temazepam), unless contraindicated by the underlying physical condition (e.g., respiratory distress). The presence of psychotic symptoms suggests the use of a neuroleptic (e.g., risperidone or haloperidol), with supportive interventions.

SUBSTANCE-INDUCED PSYCHOTIC DISORDERS

291.3, 291.5 Alcohol Psychotic Disorder

(*Note:* Psychoses associated with alcohol delirium and alcohol intoxication are discussed in their respective sections.) When hallucinations are present, they develop shortly (usually within 48 hours) after the cessation or reduction of the heavy ingestion of alcohol in a person who apparently has alcohol dependence. The hallucinations, formerly diagnosed as alcohol hallucinosis, are characteristically vivid auditory phenomena that develop in a clear sensorium. The course is usually limited to an acute phase typically lasting less than one week. In roughly 25% of cases, it is followed by a chronic phase that may last several months.

Treatment of the acute phase is similar to that of alcohol withdrawal (see "Withdrawal," Chapter 13). The detoxification procedure includes benzodiazepines, rest, vitamins, and nutritional supplements. The chronic phase is treated with neuroleptic drugs and supportive psychotherapy in a manner similar to that for schizophreniform disorder.

291.11, 291.12 Amphetamine (or Related Substance) Psychotic Disorder

The treatment of the acute phase is supportive unless the patient is agitated, in which case neuroleptics may be used. Persistent delusions and flashbacks are treated with neuroleptics. Some patients may later experience recurrent flashbacks of delusional ideas, often triggered by small doses of amphetamines.

291.11, 291.12 Cocaine Psychotic Disorder

Rapidly developing persecutory delusions are the predominant feature, occurring shortly after use. Tactile hallucinations are characteristic. Delusions may be transient, binge limited, or last for a week or longer. Since not all subjects abusing cocaine develop paranoia, it has been suggested that those who do may have lower thresholds or increased susceptibility to drug-induced psychosis. Satel and Edell (1991) suggest that cocaine self-administration may represent a quasinaturalistic method for stressing the neurotransmitter system most often linked to the positive symptoms of schizophrenia. Treatment is similar to that of amphetamine psychotic disorder. The cocaine-induced paranoid symptoms are usually transient, and do not require pharmacological management unless they persist. Symptomatic treatment is based on the use of neuroleptics. (See also Chapter 13.)

291.11, 291.12 Hallucinogen Psychotic Disorder

Formerly called hallucinogen hallucinosis (or a "bad trip"), it may be induced by LSD, MDT, MDMA, mescaline, psilocybin, and similar substances. Large doses of cannabis or tetrahydrocannabinol (THC) also may cause hallucinosis. These patients are typically seen in emergency rooms, frequently brought in by friends or the police. The duration of the syndrome varies with the type of hallucinogen, lasting about six hours for LSD, and from under an hour to a day or two for other substances.

The treatment of this psychotic disorder is the same as for the "bad tripper" (Berger & Tinklenberg, 1979). The physician should be familiar with current patterns of street drug abuse and the street names of various illicit drugs, and with their clinical manifestations.

The patient is placed in a safe, quiet room without impeding freedom of movement, and allowing him or her to get up, walk, or rock, which appears to be helpful. One must attempt to identify the nature of the drug taken, the amount involved, and the amount of time that has elapsed since it was ingested. It is also helpful to inquire about previous exposures to hallucinogens and the patient's reaction to them. Illicit drugs are frequently adulterated (cut) with other toxic drugs, such as atropine and strychnine, which may present serious treatment complications, especially if the patient is treated with anticholinergic drugs. The patient usually presents with a fear that he or she is going to lose control or that he or she will "never come down," which is further aggravated by bizarre illusions and hallucinations, depersonalization, distortions of the body image, and delusions. There are two types of treatment approaches in managing the bad tripper: the "talk-down" method and medications.

In talk-down, the basic goal is to provide continuing reassurance and defining of reality through the establishment of verbal contact with the patient. The therapist tries to reassure the patient about the transient nature of the experience and the forthcoming "coming down," provides empathic support, and repetitively defines the reality of the patient's experience, reducing distortions while the patient is encouraged to describe what is happening to him or her. This method requires considerable time and effort that may not be available in an emergency room (Berger & Tinklenberg, 1979).

Medications are recommended when the patient fails to respond to verbal contact, or when there is not sufficient time to talk the patient down. Although effective, neuroleptics are relatively contraindicated, primarily because they may precipitate an anticholinergic delirium if the illicit drug is adulterated with atropine or some other anticholinergic substance. Neuroleptics should be used only with caution in patients who have "snorted" PCP (phencyclidine, angel dust). Benzodiazepines are the drugs of choice (e.g., diazepam 20 to 30 mg P.O., repeated every three to six hours as necessary [Berger & Tinklenberg, 1979] or lorazepam 2 to 3 mg P.O. or IM). Upon recovery from the acute episode, the patient should be discharged to the care of a responsible person and offered referral to a drug rehabilitation program. Overnight hospitalization may be advisable for the patient who fails to respond to the above treatment.

Chronic hallucinatory psychosis in heavy hallucinogen abusers appears to be refractory to traditional neuroleptics, although it may respond to anticonvulsants (Ifabumuyi & Jeffries, 1976). Treatment with benzodiazepines may be justified if anticonvulsants prove ineffective after an adequate trial. There are no reported studies of the use of the newer atypical neuroleptics (e.g., clozapine, risperidone) in this group of patients.

292.89 Hallucinogen Persisting Perception Disorder (HPPD; Posthallucinogen Perception Disorder in DSM-III)

The essential feature of this infrequent but disabling consequence of hallucinogen use is a persistent perceptual disorder that patients sometimes describe as living in a bubble under water or in a purple haze, experiencing trails of light and images following the movement of their hands (traces) (Smith & Seymour, 1994; Creighton *et al.*, 1991). Associated features include anxiety and depression. Recovery may take several months. Recommended treatment includes supportive psychotherapy, antianxiety medication (benzodiazepines) for the control of anticipatory anxiety and panic episodes, and SSRIs for depression (Smith & Seymour, 1994; Giannini, 1994).

Flashbacks are similar phenomena, distinguished from HPPD in that they are episodic rather than chronic, consisting of the reexperiencing of symptoms experienced while intoxicated with a hallucinogen. The symptoms are often triggered by entering a dark environment or by using cannabis. In about half of patients, the symptoms remit within months. Flashbacks are thought to be due to a kindling effect of specific internal or external stimuli on temporolimbic structures whose seizure threshold was lowered by repeated effects of hallucinogens. Benzodiazepines have been reported to be effective in controlling flashbacks

(Berger & Tinklenberg, 1979), as have anticonvulsants, such as phenytoin (Ifabumuyi & Jeffries, 1976).

291.11, 291.12 Cannabis Psychotic Disorder

Treatment is similar to that for the bad tripper (see "Hallucinogen Psychotic Disorder," above).

291.11, 291.12 Phencyclidine (or Related Substance) Psychotic Disorder

The symptoms of PCP psychosis are essentially the same as those in cocaine psychotic disorder and closely resemble schizophrenia. Patients with PCP psychosis often require physical restraints during the intoxication because of the risk of violent or suicidal behavior (Perry, 1987).

Treatment involves overcoming psychiatric manifestations and clearing PCP from the body. There is evidence that PCP is stored in lipids of the brain and other organs, where it may be retained for a long period. Forced urine acidification (pH below 5) for several weeks with urinary acidifiers, such as ammonium chloride (500 mg three or four times daily), cranberry juice, and vitamin C (1,000 mg/day), are effective in clearing PCP from the blood (Berger & Tinklenberg, 1979). Since acidification does not rid the lipids of stored PCP, periodic forced urine acidification may be required, especially in patients who experience flashbacks. These emergent symptoms occur with febrile illnesses, exercise, and emotional distress, and are thought to result from reintoxication from mobilized PCP.

During the acute phase, diazepam, 10 to 30 mg P.O., or lorazepam, 1 to 3 mg P.O. or IM, may be required to control agitation and violent behavior. Smaller, divided daily doses are indicated in the persistent forms. Neuroleptics are effective in controlling psychotic symptoms; however, the low-potency neuroleptics (e g., chlorpromazine, thioridazine) should be avoided because of the risk of potentiating the anticholinergic effects of PCP. Haloperidol is preferred for the control of both psychotic and assaultive behavior (Berger & Tinklenberg, 1979). See also "Intoxication," Chapter 13.

291.11, 291.12 Inhalant Psychotic Disorder; Opioid Psychotic Disorder; Sedative, Hypnotic, or Anxiolytic Psychotic Disorder

The absence of confusional symptoms differentiates these disorders from delirium. They are generally transient and do not require pharmacological treatment unless the patient becomes agitated, anxious, or combative. Supportive management will suffice in most cases. If necessary, a high-potency neuroleptic may be used to control psychotic symptoms or agitation.

Other Substance-Induced Psychotic Disorders

Many prescription drugs (see Table I.2-2) may induce hallucinations (e.g., amantadine, baclofen, bromocriptine, ephedrine, steroids, propranolol, pentazocine, and levodopa). Although often quite unsettling, the syndrome is generally benign and transient, rapidly subsiding after discontinuation of the drug. Mild sedation with a benzodiazepine may become necessary. Prescription drugs may also induce delusions, as a result of excessive dosage or idiosyncratically. The most commonly implicated drugs include asparaginase, bromocriptine, propranolol, levodopa, chloroquine, cimetidine, cycloserine, digitalis, disopyramide, disulfiram, indomethacin, isoniazid, methyldopa, pentazocine, phenelzine, procaineamide, and sulindac. The psychosis is transient, requiring only brief symptomatic treatment after discontinuing the implicated drug.

290.XX PSYCHOTIC DISORDERS ASSOCIATED WITH DEMENTIA

The treatment of these disorders is discussed in Chapter 4.

CHAPTER 7

CATATONIC DISORDERS DUE TO A GENERAL MEDICAL CONDITION OR SUBSTANCE

This is a newly introduced DSM-IV disorder that corresponds to the organic catatonic disorder of ICD-10. It presents with stupor (immobility, mutism, waxy flexibility), excitement, or alternating stupor and excitement, which are judged to be etiologically related to a general medical condition (e.g., neurological, systemic, toxic) or a substance. Associated features include negativism, posturing, and occasionally echolalia or echopraxia.

GENERAL TREATMENT PRINCIPLES

Sedative challenge has been used for the transient resolution of the catatonic syndrome, although the therapeutic response has been inconsistent (Fink *et al.*, 1993). A modern procedure involves the IV administration of 2 mg of lorazepam (Francis *et al.*, 1993). The older method uses a short-acting barbiturate (e.g., 200 to 500 mg of amobarbital) given by slow intravenous (IV) drip over a 20-minute period (Wilson, 1976).

There are no established guidelines for the treatment of "organic" catatonic syndromes. In addition to treatments for the underlying disease, the catatonic syndrome may resolve with the use of a benzodiazepine, such as parenteral and/or oral lorazepam (Rosebush *et al.*, 1992; Francis *et al.*, 1993; Bush *et al.*, 1993), or electroconvulsive therapy (ECT) if lorazepam fails. Successful parenteral challenge with lorazepam or amobarbital predicts a favorable response (Francis *et al.*, 1993).

Several case reports suggest that ECT is highly effective for the catatonic syndrome, often after one or two sessions (Taylor, 1990; Bush *et al.,* 1993), especially for patients with affective disorder (Rohland & Carroll, 1993; Bush *et al.,* 1993).

SPECIFIC CATATONIC DISORDERS

293.89 CATATONIC DISORDER DUE TO A GENERAL MEDICAL CONDITION

The DSM-IV does not provide codes on Axis I for specific catatonic disorders. The medical condition causing the syndrome must be coded on Axis III.

General medical conditions associated with catatonia include both neurological and systemic disorders (Gelenberg & Turkstra, 1993; Bush *et al.,* 1993). Neurologic disorders include encephalitis and other CNS infections, carbon monoxide poisoning, tumors, strokes, and epilepsy (Taylor, 1990). Systemic disorders include postparathyroidectomy psychosis alternating with periods of catatonia, acid-base and electrolyte imbalance, intermittent porphyria, disseminated lupus erythematosus, diabetic ketoacidosis, and typhoid fever. There are no established guidelines for treating catatonia associated with these disorders; ECT appears to be a first-line treatment.

Encephalitis

There are numerous case reports of catatonic episodes occurring during the acute phase of the illness (Wilson, 1976). Catatonic stupor is associated with immobility, mutism, staring, posturing, negativism, and waxy flexibility, and may alternate with excitement. Viral encephalitis may also present with a schizophrenialike syndrome, which may be difficult to differentiate from schizophrenia, especially in afebrile patients.

Attention to the underlying neurologic or systemic disorder is of primary importance; treatment of the catatonia is often difficult until the underlying medical condition is reversed. Treatment may include a trial of lorazepam or neuroleptics, and ECT if necessary.

Malignant Catatonia

Also known as pernicious, fatal, or lethal catatonia, malignant catatonia is associated with severe medical and neurological complications (including hyperthermia), and has a grave prognosis. Its etiology remains unknown, but some cases are probably due to viral encephalitis (Jefferson & Marshall, 1983). ECT is first-line therapy for malignant catatonia and may be life-saving (Mann *et al.,* 1990). There are case studies reporting that ECT not only reversed the catatonic symptoms, but also completely reversed the life-threatening secondary medical and neurological complications (Rummans, 1991).

Periodic Catatonia

This rare catatonic syndrome of unknown etiology was shown by Gjessing (1947; Gjessing & Gjessing, 1961) to be associated with extreme shifts in the metabolic nitrogen balance. Gjessing found that treatment with thyroxin can prevent relapse in such patients. The syndrome appears to respond well to neuroleptics.

995.2 SUBSTANCE-INDUCED CATATONIC DISORDERS

Since there are no specific codes for substance-induced catatonic disorder, one may use code 995.2 for adverse effects of medication NOS, and code 333.92 for neuroleptic malignant syndrome, both listed under the heading "Other Conditions That May Be a Focus of Clinical Attention."

Substance-induced catatonia is associated with numerous drugs (Herman & Lief, 1988), including high-potency traditional neuroleptics (Gelenberg & Mandel, 1977), sodium valproate (Sackellares, 1979), ciprofloxacin (Akhtar & Ahmad, 1993), amphetamines, and phencyclidine (Taylor, 1990). Removal of the offending drug is generally sufficient to reverse the syndrome. Persistent catatonia may require lorazepam or ECT.

333.92 Neuroleptic Malignant Syndrome (NMS)

In addition to systemic disturbances (e.g., clouding of consciousness, pyrexia, tachycardia, elevated blood pressure), NMS may present with mutism, immobility, lead-pipe rigidity, cogwheel rigidity, and symptoms suggestive of catatonia. The treatment of this syndrome is discussed in the section on delirium (Chapter 3) and under "Schizophrenia and Other Psychotic Disorders," Chapter 16.

CHAPTER 8

MOOD DISORDERS DUE TO
A GENERAL MEDICAL CONDITION
OR SUBSTANCE

The diagnosis of the mood disorder as being related to some "organic" factor is presumptive rather than definitive, and is often not certain. Organic mood disorders may involve major depression, bipolar disorder, or dysthymia, and are generally indistinguishable from primary mood disorders.

GENERAL TREATMENT PRINCIPLES

Etiological treatment of the underlying pathology usually does not promptly reverse the affective syndrome, which may persist for weeks or months after recovery from the primary disease. Symptomatic treatment is directed toward the affective syndrome (depression, mania), as well as the physical symptoms of the primary disorder. Treatment of the affective syndrome follows the general guidelines applicable to the primary affective disorders.

For depression, pharmacotherapy often involves tricyclic antidepressants (TCAs) or selective serotonin reuptake inhibitors (SSRIs). The two classes of drug appear equally effective, the latter lacking the adverse effects of the TCAs (e.g., hypotension, cardiotoxicity, anticholinergic action). Bupropion and venlafaxine are also well tolerated. MAOIs may be tried in refractory cases. Augmentation trials (e.g., by adding lithium or triiodothyronine) are indicated in treatment-resistant cases. Electroconvulsive therapy (ECT) is recommended in cases refractory to medications, when suicidal risk is imminent, or when antidepressant drug toxicity is hazardous or intolerable (e.g., in serious cardiac disease). In some cases, treatment may involve drugs of greater specificity (e.g., carbamazepine in temporal lobe epilepsy). Supportive psychotherapy and other psychosocial modalities follow the same guidelines as in primary depressive disorders.

The treatment of secondary mania or hypomania is similar to that for the primary disorders. Acute manic symptoms are brought under control with neuroleptics or benzodiazepines (e.g., lorazepam, clonazepam). Lithium carbonate and other mood stabilizers (carbamazepine, valproate) have all been reported as effective for ongoing treatment, provided they are not contraindicated by the underlying medical condition.

Suicide risk or behavioral deterioration in the depressed patient, or socially disruptive or seriously maladaptive behavior in the manic, may necessitate hospitalization. The general management of primary mood disorders, both inpatient and outpatient, is discussed in later chapters of this text (see "Mood Disorders," Chapter 17).

SPECIFIC MOOD DISORDERS

The DSM-IV lists three broad types of mood disorders of organic etiology: (1) mood disorder due to a general medical condition; (2) depression associated with Alzheimer's and vascular dementias; and (3) substance-induced mood disorder.

293.83 MOOD DISORDERS DUE TO A GENERAL MEDICAL CONDITION

General medical conditions associated with mood disorder include endocrinopathies (e.g., Cushing's syndrome, hypothyroidism), temporal lobe epilepsy, systemic lupus erythematosus, brain tumors, strokes, deficiency disorders (e.g., pernicious anemia), scleroderma, Parkinson's disease, Huntington's chorea and other neurological disorders, carcinoid syndrome, carcinoma of the pancreas, AIDS, postviral syndromes (influenza, infectious mononucleosis, infectious hepatitis, viral pneumonia), temporal arteritis, lead intoxication, and metabolic disorders.

Thyroid Disease

Depression associated with hypothyroidism is treated with thyroid replacement (T_4) and, in refractory cases, antidepressants or ECT. Sometimes replacement therapy precipitates a psychotic or manic episode. Severe hypothyroidism may also present with psychosis (myxedema madness).

Depression associated with so-called subclinical hypothyroidism is characterized by minor degrees of thyroid hypofunction, documented only by elevated thyroid-stimulating hormone (TSH) or exaggerated TSH responses to thyrotropin-releasing hormone (TRH). This syndrome may be present especially in anergic patients who fail to respond to antidepressants (Gold & Pearsall, 1983). The depression seems to respond to thyroid replacement (Cooper *et al.*, 1984).

Hyperthyroidism is usually associated with an anxiety disorder, psychotic disorder, or, rarely, mania (Corn & Checkley, 1983).

Hypercortisolism

Hyperadrenalism (Cushing's syndrome) is very often associated with psychiatric disorders, depression being the most common. Mania and psychosis are also common; the treatment is primarily etiological. Exogenous steroids may induce major depression, mania, or psychosis. Reduction of the steroid dosage is likely to produce remission. Symptomatic treatment with antidepressants (preferably, bupropion) or antimanic drugs, even in the presence of hypercortisolism, can be effective. If psychotic symptoms are present, small doses of a neuroleptic will usually bring the symptoms under control. Lithium prophylaxis (beginning lithium before initiating steroid treatment) is effective in preventing psychiatric complications of steroid treatment.

Hyperparathyroidism-Hypercalcemia

Medication-resistant depression is the most common psychiatric complication of hypercalcemia. When caused by parathyroid adenoma, removal of the tumor causes remission of the depression. Some patients develop transient postparathyroidectomy psychosis.

Poststroke Depression

Studies by Robinson and associates (1984) have shown that major depression and dysthymia affect about 25% of stroke victims. Major depression occurs characteristically in left-sided anterior lesions. Patients with hypercortisolism three months after a stroke are at risk for major depression later in the course and warrant careful follow-up (Astrom *et al.*, 1993). Poststroke depression is associated with global impairment in cognitive function, which occurs only in major depression and only after left-hemisphere injury, lasts for about one year, and is worst during the acute poststroke phase.

Poststroke depression appears to respond well to all antidepressants, including TCAs, MAOIs, and SSRIs (Robinson *et al.*, 1985; Reding *et al.*, 1986). It also responds to ECT (Murray *et al.*, 1986). In uncontrolled trials, Lazarus *et al.* (1992) found methyphenidate to be a safe, rapid, and effective treatment for poststroke depression in elderly patients. Early treatment (by the fourth week poststroke) may improve the patient's neuropsychological rehabilitation.

Parkinson's Disease

Depression has a prevalence of 40 to 47% in patients with Parkinson's disease (Cummings, 1992). The depression may be a reaction to the physical disability or a direct result of underlying biochemical changes. A review by Cummings (1992) found that depression in Parkinson's disease is distinguished from other depressive disorders by greater anxiety and less self-punitive ideation. Risk factors include female gender, early age of onset, greater left-brain involvement, and a past history of depression.

The TCAs and bupropion improve the depression; there is insufficient experience to recommend the SSRIs. Electroconvulsive therapy produces transient improvement (Burke *et al.*, 1988). Treatment with the dopamine precursor 5-HTP has produced conflicting reports. Selegiline, a monoamine oxidase B inhibitor, may slow the degenerative process and may have mild antidepressant properties. Transplantation of fetal tissue into the basal ganglia may ameliorate the motor disability (Lindvall *et al.*, 1989).

Head Trauma

Fedoroff and associates (1992) found that major depression occurs in about one-quarter of patients after traumatic brain injury and is associated with poor premorbid social functioning, a history of previous psychiatric disorder, and injury to certain brain locations (left dorsolateral frontal cortex and left basal ganglia). On the other hand, Starkstein and associates (1991) have provided support for a link between right hemispheric lesions and mania. Treatment of depression includes antidepressants, various psychosocial therapies, and ECT. In cases involving protracted litigation for compensation following head trauma, early legal settlement often facilitates clinical recovery.

Multiple Sclerosis

A number of case reports and controlled studies have found a high prevalence of mood disorders in patients with multiple sclerosis (Schubert & Foliart, 1993). Multiple sclerosis can present with mood disorders before the onset of neurological symptoms (Whitlock & Siskind, 1980), a fact that suggests using MRI as a screening test in depression. Depression in multiple sclerosis usually responds to antidepressants (Schiffer & Wineman, 1990); group therapy, and/or cognitive psychotherapy.

Lyme Borreliosis

Lyme disease has been associated with major psychiatric disorders. Although depression is the most commonly reported, others include mania, psychosis, panic attacks, impaired cognition, irritability, and emotional lability (Roelecke *et al.*, 1992; Fallon *et al.*, 1993). In addition to antibiotic treatment of the borreliosis, symptomatic therapy involves antidepressants, and ECT in refractory cases. Neuroleptics can be helpful in controlling manic and psychotic symptoms. Because Lyme disease has become more common, and early antibiotic therapy is necessary to prevent its neuropsychiatric sequelae, mental health professionals should consider borrelial infection when faced with an atypical psychiatric disorder (Fallon *et al.*, 1993).

Human Immunodeficiency Virus

Mood disorders have been reported in similar proportions of HIV-infected and uninfected homosexual men. Depression associated with the "spectrum" of HIV-related organic brain diseases cannot be adequately differentiated from primary depression. In the asymptomatic stage of HIV infection, major depression does not appear to be secondary to CNS involvement (Perkins *et al.*, 1994). Most antidepressants are effective in such patients. These patients appear sensitive to the anticholinergic activity of TCAs and require the lower doses appropriate for geriatric patients. The SSRIs and bupropion have several advantages over the TCAs in many patients. It has been suggested that depression in AIDS patients responds to small doses of psychostimulants, such as methylphenidate (Ostrow *et al.*, 1988; Rabkin, 1993).

Epilepsy

Blumer (1995) reports that half of the patients with chronic epilepsy experience an intermittent and polysymptomatic interictal dysphoric disorder (IDD), which responds quite favorably to a combination of a tricyclic antidepressant and an SSRI (e.g., paroxetine, fluoxetine).

Other neurological disorders associated with depression include Huntington's chorea, Sydenham's chorea, progressive supranuclear palsy, normal pressure hydrocephalus, and neurosyphilis. Sjörgen's syndrome commonly presents with an atypical depression (Wyszynski & Wyszynski, 1993). Depression may be a prodromal syndrome of lead encephalopathy, which can be successfully treated with chelation (Schottenfeld & Cullen, 1984). Also, ECT may be of some value for depression in Huntington's chorea (Ranen *et al.*, 1993).

Myocardial Infarction

There is a high rate of depression among patients recovering from myocardial infarction (Fielding, 1991). There is also evidence that such depression places patients at an increased risk for cardiac events, including an increased risk for mortality at six months (Frasure-Smith *et al.*, 1993). Treatment of depression may thus influence survival. Tricyclics are contraindicated in such patients (Glassman *et al.*, 1993). The cautious use of SSRIs or bupropion, following cardiological consultation and under close ECG monitoring, is the preferred treatment (see "Psychopharmacotherapy," Chapter 2).

Cancer

Depression is very common among cancer patients, with the highest prevalence among patients with pancreatic (50%), oropharynx (22 to 50%), breast (13 to 27%), and gynecologic (23%) disease (McDaniel *et al.*, 1995). Appreciating the potential immunoprotective and psychological effect of psychosocial interventions in improving both quality of life and survival time in cancer patients, several studies have reported favorable results with various psychotherapeutic modalities, especially group psychotherapy (Spiegel *et al.*, 1989; Fawzy *et al.*, 1995) and focused psychotherapies (e.g., cognitive-behavioral and expressive psychotherapy) (Markowitz *et al.*, 1992; Sharpe *et al.*, 1992). Antidepressants are also beneficial. Methylphenidate has been found useful in medically ill cancer patients (Fernandez *et al.*, 1987; McDaniel *et al.*, 1995). Other psychosocial interventions include education and behavioral training (see Fawzy *et al.*, 1995).

Chronic Fatigue Syndrome

Chronic fatigue syndrome (CFS), whose etiology remains uncertain, presents with chronic unexplained fatigue, dysphoria, and an array of somatic complaints suggestive of depressive and hypochondriacal disorders (Yargic *et al.*, 1993). CFS has been treated with a variety of therapies, generally with little success. Antidepressants have modest results. Those with a potent noradrenergic activity, such as maprotiline and bupropion, have been found to be the most effective (Goodnick, 1993). The anergic nature of CFS suggests that a trial of methylphenidate may be worth considering. A subgroup of CFS patients with neurally mediated (orthostatic) hypotension may benefit from treatment to raise standing blood pressure (e.g., fludrocortisone combined with atenolol or propanolol, and increased anounts of salt and fluids [Bou-Holaigath *et al.*, 1995]).

Carcinoid Syndrome

Cutaneous flushing, often accompanied by abdominal cramping pain, diarrhea, wheezing, dyspnea, and laboratory evidence of increased urinary secretion of 5-hydroxyindolacetic acid (5-HIAA), is commonly associated with depression (probably due to disturbed 5-HT [serotonin] metabolism). There are no established treatment guidelines, although one might consider potential toxicity from SSRI antidepressants and prefer the noradrenergic bupropion.

Chronic Pain

Regardless of its etiology (physical or psychogenic), chronic pain is often associated with dysthymia or major depression (Blumer, 1982; Gupta, 1986). We view depression in chronic pain as an integral part of a universal biological response to enduring an adverse or catastrophic experience (Balis, 1978d). Antidepressant medications (e.g., TCAs, SSRIs, MAOIs) are effective in relieving both pain and depression (Gupta, 1986). The cognitive-behavioral approach does not seem to alter pain levels, although it increases day-to-day functioning (Nicholas *et al.*, 1992).

Skin Disorders

Skin disorders, such as pruritus, often accompanied by excoriations and agitated behavior, may represent masked depression, which responds well to antidepressant medication, psychotherapy, and ECT.

Despondency

Despondency in physical illness, as seen in demoralized medically ill patients, is best understood as adjustment disorder with depressed mood. Although viewed as primarily reactive to being seriously ill, it may have organic underpinnings. Uncontrolled studies suggest that treatment with methylphenidate, 5 to 15 mg twice a day, may be helpful to some patients. The response to methylphenidate is immediate in those who benefit, and improvement may be sustained at the same dose without tolerance or side effects. The persistence of depressive symptoms may justify a trial of antidepressants (e.g., fluoxetine). Brief psychotherapy (e.g., focused, supportive, group) is recommended.

Depressive Pseudodementia

Recent conceptualizations of so-called pseudodementia, depressive dementia, and a dementia spectrum of depression, emphasize overlapping pathophysiological mechanisms rather than differential diagnoses (Emery & Oxman, 1992). Whether or not cognitive changes in geriatric depression predict irreversible dementia is controversial; recent evidence appears to challenge the notion that depressive pseudodementia heralds dementia (Kramer-Ginsberg & Greenwald, 1993). Both antidepressants and ECT are effective.

Manic Syndromes

Many general medical conditions are associated with secondary mania and hypomania. They include stroke (especially right focal thalamic infarction), brain tumor, focal epilepsy (especially complex partial seizures with nondominant localization), and traumatic brain injury (especially temporal basopolar lesions) (Bamrah & Johnson, 1991; Cohen & Niska, 1980; Jampala & Abrams, 1983; Robinson *et al.*, 1988). Several cases of postoperative mania have been reported. Other general medical conditions associated with mania and hypomanic states include open-heart surgery (Isles & Orrell, 1991), hyperthyroidism (Corn & Checkley, 1983), CNS infections (Thienhaus & Khosla, 1984), uremia (Thomas & Neale, 1991), vitamin B_{12} deficiency, and prolonged sleep deprivation (Wehr *et al.*, 1987). In sleep deprivation, induction of deep sleep results in the rapid resolution of symptoms. Onset of mania in late life suggests organic factors (Tohen *et al.*, 1994). Substance-induced mania is discussed on pages 93–95.

Mood stabilizers (e.g., lithium, carbamazepine, valproate) have been found effective for the symptomatic control of organic mania. However, during the acute manic phase, benzodiazepines (e.g., lorazepam, clonazepam) and neuroleptics (e.g., haloperidol, risperidone) are often necessary for controlling agitation and disruptive behavior. Residual organic factors can complicate treatment with lithium, and may cause serious toxicity. Carbamazepine offers an effective, often safer alternative (Evans *et al.*, 1995). Valproic acid is also well tolerated, and may be tried in cases refractory to the other drugs (McElroy *et al.*, 1992). A trial of carbamazepine or valproate, alone or in combination with lithium or nimodipine (Post *et al.*, 1993), is justified when the patient fails to respond to lithium.

For rapid cycling, carbamazepine or valproate or a combination of lithium with valproate is preferred (Sharma *et al.*, 1993). Carbamazepine is the drug of choice for ictal manic episodes associated with temporal lobe epilepsy. Mood stabilizers are also effective for prophylaxis in drug-induced mania. ECT is an effective and safe treatment for acute mania, and is recommended for patients who have responded poorly to, or cannot tolerate, pharmacotherapy (Mukherjee *et al.*, 1994). In bipolar depression, bupropion is the preferred antidepressant (it is less likely to induce mania).

290.14, 290.21, 290.43 DEPRESSION COMPLICATING DEMENTIA

Depression is a common complication of dementias. Bupropion is well tolerated by the elderly and may be used as a first-line antidepressant. The SSRIs (e.g., fluoxetine) are safe, well tolerated, and as effective as the TCAs, and may prove to be equally effective in treating nonpsychotic depression in the demented patient. The syndrome is also responsive to tricyclic antidepressants; however, they may produce intolerable anticholinergic symptoms and orthostatic hypotension. MAOIs (e.g., phenelzine) appear to be effective and well tolerated in the elderly demented patient (Jenike, 1985). Their main side effects are orthostatic hypotension and insomnia. Moclobemide does not require dietary restriction. Venlafaxine and nefazodone are discussed in Chapter 2.

Electroconvulsive therapy is the treatment of choice for patients who cannot tolerate antidepressant drugs or who are refractory to them.

292.XX (Listed on Axis I of DSM-IV) Substance-Induced Mood Disorder

291.8 Alcohol Mood Disorder
292.84 Sedative, Hypnotic, or Anxiolytic Mood Disorder

There is a very high incidence of depression in individuals abusing these cross-tolerant substances, during both intoxication and withdrawal. Depression occurs, particularly during the late phase of an alcohol binge. Depression may occasionally be associated with benzodiazepine treatment.

Patients abusing these substances, especially alcoholics, may need hospitalization for escalating depression and suicide precautions. The depression is often reactive, with strong Axis II underpinnings. It usually clears, without pharmacological treatment, within a week or so. Detoxification, supportive psychotherapy, and milieu therapy during the acute phase should be followed by a postdischarge treatment plan that includes psychosocial approaches and drug rehabilitation.

292.84 Amphetamine (or Related Substance) Mood Disorder
292.84 Cocaine Mood Disorder

Depression associated with psychostimulant drugs (including anorectics and ephedrinelike compounds) is very common, particularly during the withdrawal phase and in younger populations.

The withdrawal syndrome presents with apathy and psychomotor retardation, which may escalate into a suicidal depression. Hospitalization is often necessary for a person threatening suicide. The decision to use antidepressant drugs should be deferred to allow observation for at least one week. The depression usually clears within that time without medication.

Patients developing depression during intoxication should first be detoxified under close supervision, preferably in a hospital setting, and then treated with antidepressants only if symptoms persist. Supportive and milieu therapy during the acute phase should be followed by psychotherapy, antidepressants (if necessary), and rehabilitation.

292.84 Inhalant Mood Disorder

There are no established treatment guidelines for inhalant-induced depression. See "General Treatment Principles" for mood disorders, and respective sections on "Intoxication" (Chapter 13) and "Substance Dependence-Abuse" (Chapter 15).

282.84 Opioid Mood Disorder

Opioids have a euphoriant as well as a depressive effect. Development of an organic mood syndrome is common in patients undergoing slow detoxification from methadone maintenance and is associated with poor outcome (Levinson *et al.*, 1995). For general treatment, see "Substance Dependence-Abuse" in Chapter 15.

292.84 Hallucinogen Mood Disorder
292.84. Phencyclidine (or Related Substance) Mood Disorder

The essential feature of both disorders is a mood syndrome that usually develops shortly after use and persists more than 24 hours after cessation. Depression is most common; suicide may occur. The course is variable, and may range from a brief experience to a long-lasting episode indistinguishable from a primary mood disorder. Major depressive episodes often call for antidepressants or ECT. Manic episodes may require neuroleptics, and if persisting, mood stabilizers. Individual, group, and/or family psychotherapy should be part of the treatment regimen. For more information, see "Substance Dependence-Abuse," Chapter 15.

292.84 OTHER SUBSTANCE-INDUCED MOOD DISORDER

Antihypertensives

Reserpine is the most commonly implicated. Methyldopa, guanethidine, clonidine, bethanidine, thiazide diuretics, and β-blockers (propranolol) have also been reported to cause depression in small numbers of patients. Recent prospective studies, however, have failed to implicate β-blockers in depression. Treatment includes switching to another drug and using antidepressants, or ECT if the depression does not remit.

Other Cardiovascular Drugs

In addition to depression and mania, digitalis intoxication may cause delusions, hallucinations, delirium, and amnestic symptoms. Depression has also been associated with procainamide and lidocaine.

Corticosteroids and ACTH

They have been reported to cause affective syndromes, both depressive and manic. In manic episodes, dose reduction may bring improvement. If the drug cannot be reduced or discontinued, mania can be controlled with neuroleptics or lithium, carbamazepine, or valproate. Lithium may be considered prophylactically (at serum levels of 0.6 to 0.8 mEq/L) in patients with a prior history of corticosteroid-induced mood disorders who require steroid treatment.

In steroid-induced depression, tricyclics may produce delirium. Alternatives include monitoring tricyclic plasma levels, using smaller doses, or switching to an SSRI; ECT is effective for patients who fail to respond to, or cannot tolerate, pharmacotherapy.

Oral Contraceptives

The evidence implicating oral contraceptives in causing depression has not been adequately substantiated, especially with regard to low doses of estrogen (Kay, 1984). If it occurs, the depression appears atypical, rarely having the vegetative symptoms of sleep and appetite disturbance (Patten & Lamarre, 1992). Use of an alternative contraceptive method is recommended.

Antidepressant-Associated Mania (AAM)

All biological antidepressant treatments occasionally involve the induction of a manic syndrome. AAM may represent a clinical entity distinct from spontaneous mania (Stoll *et al.*, 1993). Treatment includes discontinuing the offending drug, and, if necessary, the brief use of lorazepam or haloperidol to control acute symptoms. If symptoms persist, a mood stabilizer should be prescribed and one should consider a bipolar diagnosis. After recovery, an alternative antidepressant may be tried, preferably bupropion.

Other Drugs

Many other agents have been implicated in case reports of mood disorders, including metrizamide, indomethacin, meperidine, alprazolam, cimetidine, and captopril.

CHAPTER 9

ANXIETY DISORDERS DUE TO A GENERAL MEDICAL CONDITION OR SUBSTANCE

The prevalence of anxiety disorders in medically ill patients is higher than in the general population (Cassem, 1990; Wise & Taylor, 1990). Many conditions and substances may cause anxiety. A comprehensive medical and drug history, coupled with a high degree of alertness to organic etiologies, is an essential part of the diagnostic process.

GENERAL TREATMENT PRINCIPLES

The etiological treatment of the underlying medical condition results in full remission in most cases. Symptomatic treatment includes anxiolytics and various adjunctive methods, such as supportive psychotherapy, relaxation techniques, hypnosis, and biofeedback. Since anxiety is a universal emotional experience in response to external threat or intrapsychic conflict, recognition of all contributing factors (e.g., general medical, intrapsychic, interpersonal) leads to a comprehensive treatment plan.

Guidelines for pharmacological treatment have not been adequately established. In addition to the benzodiazepines, other drugs that may be useful include buspirone, tricyclics, and propranolol. The selection of an appropriate anxiolytic depends on the patient's underlying medical condition, target symptoms, and pharmacologic profile (e.g., side effects, speed of onset, half-life, drug-drug interactions). Failure to respond to adequate dosage suggests a primary organic etiology, such as temporal lobe epilepsy or hyperthyroidism (Beyer *et al.*, 1993).

Patients with these disorders may be seen in a variety of clinical situations, including emergency rooms, ICUs, medical-surgical units, nursing homes, and ambulatory settings. They may require various psychosocial interventions appropriate to the setting and the individual patient's needs.

SPECIFIC ANXIETY DISORDERS

The DSM-IV lists anxiety disorders in two separate organic categories: anxiety disorder due to a general medical condition, and substance-induced anxiety disorder.

293.89 ANXIETY DISORDER DUE TO A GENERAL MEDICAL CONDITION

Anxiety disorders may be caused by endocrinopathies (hyperthyroidism, hypoparathyroidism, pheochromocytoma, hypoglycemia, hyperadrenalism), Parkinson's disease, COPD, and other respiratory disorders, temporal lobe epilepsy, Sydenham's chorea, brain tumors, and cardiac disorders.

Hyperthyroidism

Often presenting as an anxiety disorder, vague symptoms of irritability, emotional lability, and personality change may be its only signs. Kathol and Dalahunt (1986) found that 80% of 29 consecutive hyperthyroid patients in a general endocrine clinic met the DSM criteria for generalized anxiety disorder. Over 90% lost all anxiety symptoms with thyroid therapy alone within days or weeks.

Hypoparathyroidism

Hypocalcemia secondary to hypoparathyroidism is often associated with anxiety and panic attacks (Lawlor, 1988). Benzodiazepines have been reported to provide little relief of anxiety symptoms in hypocalcemia. Medical treatment of the hypoparathyroidism results in remission of the anxiety. Other medical conditions (e.g., chronic renal disease) may also cause hypocalcemia.

Hypoglycemia

Reactive hypoglycemia commonly presents with panic attacks or generalized anxiety related to catecholamine release. The alimentary type, resulting from the unusually rapid absorption of glucose, is treated with dietary management. The diabetic type, due to a delay in insulin secretion, is treated with a combination of dietary management and oral hypoglycemic agents. Insulinomas are treated surgically.

Pheochromocytoma

This relatively rare disorder presents with episodes of generalized anxiety or panic attacks, accompanied by palpitations, profuse sweating, and hypertension. It is diagnosed by its clinical manifestations, measurement of catecholamines in the urine, and angiography. Treatment is based on long-term blockade with α-adrenergic blocking agents (phenoxybenzamine) and surgery.

Hypercortisolism (Cushing's syndrome)

It may be caused by either endogenous (e.g., adrenocortical hyperplasia) or exogenous (e.g., iatrogenic) hypercortisolism. Treatment is directed at the underlying etiology (removal of a tumor, discontinuing corticosteroid therapy, etc.).

Parkinson's Disease

In addition to depression, Parkinson's disease is frequently comorbid with symptoms of generalized anxiety (Robertson-Hoffman & Bonapace, 1993), phobias, and panic attacks (Stein *et al.*, 1990). The panic attacks have been attributed to intense autonomic symptoms associated with the on-off periods of dyskinesia and akinesia. Mixed depression and anxiety are common. For treatment, see "Mood Disorder," Chapter 8.

Temporal Lobe Epilepsy

Ictal paroxysmal anxiety, such as fear or panic attacks in temporal lobe epilepsy, is usually refractory to anxiolytic drugs but responds well to anticonvulsant medications. Ambulatory EEG monitoring of patients with atypical panic attacks (e.g., with sensory distortion or focal paresthesia) may show focal paroxysmal EEG changes during the attack (Weilburg *et al.*, 1993). These ictal anxiety symptoms are responsive to anticonvulsants, such as carbamazepine (McNamara & Fogel, 1990).

Other Neurological Disorders

Brain tumors in the vicinity of the third ventricle and in the temporal lobes may present with an anxiety disorder. Early poststroke anxiety disorder is commonly reported, particularly with left cortical lesions (Starkstein *et al.*, 1990). Etiological treatment, when available, results in remission of the anxiety syndrome. Sydenham's chorea is often associated with obsessive-compulsive symptoms (Swedo *et al.*, 1989) that may require symptomatic treatment with a drug such as clomipramine, fluoxetine, or fluvoxamine.

Respiratory Disorders

Hypoxemic respiratory failure, acute respiratory distress syndrome, and COPD often present with generalized anxiety and/or panic attacks (Karajgi *et al.*, 1990). Pulmonary embolism may present with acute anxiety or panic as well; a prompt and accurate diagnosis is of the utmost importance. Benzodiazepines are relatively contraindicated in these conditions because they may suppress respiration. Buspirone is the anxiolytic of choice for chronic disorders.

Cardiac Disease

Symptomatic cardiac disease (e.g., angina, arrhythmias, acute heart failure) is a common source of anxiety related to fears of heart attack and sudden death. The anxiety is often somatically magnified by the concurrent autonomic symptoms of acute cardiac exacerbations (e.g., chest tightness, shortness of breath, light-headedness, cold sweats). Panic attacks have been associated with postmyocardial infarction. The use of benzodiazepines for the symptomatic control of anxiety has been shown to be safe, even in unstable cardiac disease. Lorazepam is often preferred, although it may require careful tapering to avoid withdrawal symptoms that could be dangerous during unstable cardiac conditions.

Mitral Valve Prolapse (MVP)

Barlow's syndrome often presents with anxiety and palpitations, together with intermittent chest pain and characteristic auscultatory and echocardiographic findings. There are many similarities between panic disorder and MVP symptoms, suggesting that the two may be related. Treatment of MVP is generally supportive (e.g., reassurance, education), with specific drug treatment for arrhythmias if indicated. Propranolol is often the most useful agent.

Benign Hyperventilation

This is a common occurrence that often leads to acute anxiety. A simple test, such as having the patient breathe into a paper bag, can confirm the diagnosis, and can educate and reassure the patient. In addition to treating the underlying condition that causes the hyperventilation, acute episodes may respond to rebreathing of CO_2 (paper bag technique) or to a benzodiazepine.

Iron Overload

Conditions associated with iron overload (e.g., hereditary hemochromatosis) may be related to anxiety, depression, and memory loss. Treatment with deferoxamine or a phlebotomy appears to relieve the psychiatric symptoms (Cutler, 1994).

Miscellaneous Causes

Other general medical conditions include head trauma, brucellosis, demyelinating disease, and heavy metal intoxication. One must understand that anxiety is a ubiquitous symptom that has been reported in most neuropsychiatric disorders. A separate diagnosis is justified only when it is prominent.

292.89 SUBSTANCE-INDUCED ANXIETY DISORDER

Substance-induced anxiety disorders are associated with a variety of substances, including psychostimulants (e.g., amphetamine, cocaine, methylphenidate, ephedrine, and pseudoephedrine), hallucinogens, caffeine, SSRI antidepressants, and withdrawal from alcohol and sedative, hypnotic, or anxiolytic drugs. Anxiety may also be associated with a vast array of prescription drugs.

291.8 Alcohol Anxiety Disorder
292.89 Sedative, Hypnotic, or Anxiolytic Anxiety Disorder

Anxiety is often associated with withdrawal from alcohol or sedative, hypnotic, or anxiolytic drugs. Rebound anxiety may occur with short-acting benzodiazepines (e.g., alprazolam, temazepam), and can be eliminated by switching to a longer-acting benzodiazepine (e.g., diazepam, flurazepam).

292.89 Amphetamine (or Related Substance)
292.89 Cocaine
292.84 Caffeine Anxiety Disorders

Psychostimulant drugs and caffeine are the most commonly implicated in anxiety. The therapeutic approach is based on the treatment of substance abuse and underlying psychopathology. See "Intoxication" (Chapter 13) and "Substance Dependence-Abuse" (Chapter 15).

292.89 Cannabis, Hallucinogen, Inhalant, and Phencyclidine (or Related Substance) Anxiety Disorders

Treatment is discussed under "Intoxication" (Chapter 13) and "Substance Dependence-Abuse" (Chapter 15).

292.89 Other Substance-Induced Anxiety Disorders

Many prescription drugs may induce anxiety disorders, including vasopressors (e.g., dopamine, epinephrine), hydralazine, isoniazid, digitalis (toxicity), levodopa, theophylline, lidocaine, salicylates, steroids, thyroxine, and anticholinergics. Treatment usually includes reduction of dosage, discontinuation of the drug, or substitution of another medication. Anxiety may also accompany abrupt withdrawal from a medication.

Neuroleptic-Induced Akathesia

This may lead to anxiety, agitation, and dysphoria. Severe akathesia has been associated with suicidal (and possibly very rare homicidal) behavior. It is dose-related and more likely to be induced by a high-potency traditional neuroleptic, such as compazine (which is used as an antiemetic) (Sachdev & Kruk, 1994). Parenteral administration of an antiparkinsonian agent is helpful, followed by oral anticholinergics or, preferably, benzodiazepines or β-blockers (e.g., propranolol) (Horiguchi & Nishimatsu, 1992).

CHAPTER 10

PERSONALITY CHANGE DUE TO A GENERAL MEDICAL CONDITION OR SUBSTANCE

The DSM-IV has renamed this syndrome "personality change" instead of "disorder." It requires a persistent change from the individual's previous characteristic personality pattern.

There are two principal types of personality change (Cummings, 1995): apathetic, which is associated with dorsolateral and medial frontal dysfunction and is characterized by apathy, diminished motivation, lack of spontaneity, low initiative, decreased concern, and environmental dependence; and disinhibited, which is associated with orbitofrontal involvement and features impulsiveness, disinhibition, tactlessness, undue familiarity, impaired social judgment, a tendency toward lewd behavior, and facetiousness. Additional "organic" personality types include labile, aggressive, and paranoid (see below).

GENERAL TREATMENT PRINCIPLES

Symptomatic treatment is directed toward controlling emotional lability and impulse dyscontrol. Explosive outbursts of anger and episodes of violent behavior that occur with minimal provocation are the most serious symptoms. Pharmacological control of aggression is discussed under "Aggressive Type." In hospitalized violent patients, behavior therapy and firm limit setting are extremely important. There are no established guidelines for treating the apathetic, paranoid, and disinhibited types.

The psychosocial management of the patient with organic personality change is primarily directed toward enhancing behavioral controls and minimizing undesirable conduct. This may be accomplished through direct counseling to help the patient avoid situations that trigger violent outbursts, abstain from alcohol (which may induce dyscontrol episodes), learn ways to prevent social embarrassment, and make decisions about job changes or early retirement (if necessary). Vocational rehabilitation may be indicated.

Family counseling is an essential part of management. Family members need to be advised about the changes in the patient's personality, behavioral dyscontrol, and impaired social judgment (e.g., embarrassing behaviors, shoplifting, sexual indiscretions). The physician should provide emotional support for their work with the patient, as well as for their own needs. Caretakers should be advised about proper patient management and helped to develop coping strategies and to avoid situations that tend to elicit psychopathology.

It is most important that the family understand the interaction of environmental contingencies (e.g., supports and demands of social situations) with the patient's lifelong coping style in the face of organic disinhibition. For instance, excessive obsessiveness and viscosity in the epileptic personality may be compensatory mechanisms for maintaining control in the face of uncontrollable seizures. Catastrophic reactions (crying, rage, or cognitive disorganization) may occur when the brain-injured person is faced with frustrating tasks. Novel or shifting environments and excessive change of stimulus strain the patient's resources. Patients who are violent, sexually abusive, or otherwise unmanageable may have to be removed from the home.

SPECIFIC DISORDERS (ALL CODED 310.1 ON AXIS I)

Common causes of personality change include head trauma, cerebrovascular disorders, and intracranial space-occupying lesions. Other causes include temporal lobe epilepsy, multiple sclerosis, endocrine disorders, chronic poisoning (e.g., mercury, manganese), neurosyphilis, postencephalitic parkinsonism, and Huntington's chorea. Chronic hypercalcemia (e.g., from hyperparathyroidism) may induce persistent personality changes that can be reversed with the correction of the hypercalcemia. Cerebral neoplasms, subarachnoid hemorrhage, and Wilson's disease are other potentially treatable disorders. Symptomatic treatment depends on the target symptoms.

LABILE TYPE

Lability of affect is a common symptom in patients with brain damage secondary to traumatic, degenerative, vascular, and postencephalitic disorders. Affective lability may accompany other personality change, especially the aggressive and disinhibited types. Emotional lability and disinhibition are often associated with frontal lobe lesions secondary to stroke and traumatic brain injury (Oder *et al.*, 1992). Other conditions associated with emotional lability include Sydenham's chorea, Wilson's disease, and temporal lobe epilepsy (interictal personality change). Progressive supranuclear palsy is often accompanied by unprovoked, episodic crying or laughing, described as emotional incontinence.

There are no established guidelines for the symptomatic treatment of emotional lability. Family members should understand the nature of this personality change and be reassured that the displayed emotions are not necessarily evidence of depression. Patients should be protected from exposure to excessive stimulation. There are very few studies of pharmacologic treatment. One may try valproate, carbamazepine, clonazepam, and other psychotropic drugs on an empirical basis.

DISINHIBITED TYPE

The cardinal feature is disinhibition, with impaired impulse control similar to the pseudopsychopathic or impulsive type. The disturbance is often related to the so-called frontal lobe syndrome, and may be caused by a variety of traumatic (most common), degenerative, vascular, and other CNS disorders (Oder *et al.*, 1992).

In the pseudopsychopathic type, treatment should be primarily behavioral and supportive, including family counseling for problems associated with behavioral dyscontrol and impaired social judgment (e.g., shoplifting, sexual indiscretions). Alcohol abuse and other substance abuse contribute greatly to disinhibition and must be eliminated. In milder cases, a psychosocial center may provide the necessary structure for limit setting. Highly structured environments that provide firm limits and behavior modification are recommended for more severe cases.

There are no established guidelines for pharmacological treatment. Benzodiazepines, especially diazepam, may aggravate disinhibited behavior and should be avoided. Carbamazepine, propranolol, pindolol, and other psychotropic drugs may be tried empirically. The potential role of serotonin (5-HT) in impulse regulation and the possible treatment of impulsive behavior with serotonergic drugs would suggest SSRIs, buspirone (Siever *et al.*, 1993), and risperidone. Medroxyprogesterone was reported by Cooper (1987) to be effective in controlling sexually disinhibited behavior in demented patients, without adverse effects.

AGGRESSIVE TYPE

This type was described in the DSM-III-R as explosive personality. Causes include head trauma, epilepsy, cerebral tumors and other space-occupying lesions, cerebrovascular disorders (stroke, vascular dementia), degenerative disorders (Alzheimer's disease), and encephalitis (Elliott, 1984). Neurologic soft signs may be useful markers of nonspecific brain damage, often associated with impulsive aggressive personality change (Monroe *et al.*, 1978; Balis & Monopolis, 1986). Alcohol is a common precipitant of violent behavior.

Treatment is based on carefully differentiating primary from secondary mental disorders associated with violent behavior (Reid & Balis, 1987).

Organic Violence

Carbamazepine and propranolol (alone or in combination) have been found to improve irritability and episodic rage in patients with temporolimbic epilepsy and those with violence associated with closed head injury. Elliott (1984) has used propranolol in doses of up to 320 mg/day to control aggressive episodes. Some authors report that effective treatment with propranolol requires higher doses (up to 20 mg/kg/day) (Yudofsky *et al.*, 1981). Pindolol has been associated with significant therapeutic benefits without sedation and without other side effects that can occur with propranolol (Greendyke & Kanter, 1986). Metoprolol, a β1-adrenoreceptor blocker, has been reported by Mattes (1985) to suppress aggressive episodes in patients who failed to respond to propranolol and carbamazepine.

Neuroleptic drugs, although often used to control acute episodes of violence, are not satisfactory on a maintenance basis. There is some evidence that risperidone may have an advantage over other neuroleptics in the treatment of hostility and violence. Buspirone has been found moderately effective in reducing hostile, aggressive, and irritable behavior in a variety of patients, including those with dementia, head injury (Levine, 1988), and mental retardation (Rattey *et al.*, 1991).

The surgical treatment of intractable temporolimbic seizures may improve aggressive behavior, as well as mood alterations and psychosis (Mark & Ervin, 1970; Ferguson *et al.*, 1993).

Epilepsy and Violence

The relation of violence to epilepsy deserves special mention. Violent behavior in an epileptic may be ictal, postictal, or interictal. While violence during a seizure is rare, it may occasionally be part of a postictal confusional state.

The concept of epileptic personality and its association with interictal violence has been controversial. A number of investigators have challenged the notion of a specific epileptic personality in noninstitutionalized epileptics, and particularly in patients with familial epilepsy. On the other hand, several studies suggest that patients with temporal lobe epilepsy are more likely to show personality changes, described as adhesive and explosive types (which may coexist in the same patient). It appears that patients with a temporal seizure focus—especially in the dominant hemisphere—are at risk for impulse dyscontrol associated with irritability, explosiveness, and rage reactions (Stevens & Herman,

1981). They are also at higher risk for developing chronic psychosis (Balis, 1978c; Umbricht *et al.*, 1995).

Episodic Dyscontrol

"Episodic dyscontrol" describes (Monroe, 1970; Balis, 1979) episodic violence secondary to limbic dysfunction in persons who have no history of epilepsy or other brain disease. The attacks are minimally provoked, often preceded by an aura, associated with postictal depression and amnesia for the episode, and are ego alien and out of character (Monroe, 1970; Balis & McDonald, 1978; Balis, 1979). Patients may have a childhood history of conduct disorder and hyperactivity (Balis & Monopolis, 1986), and may display "soft" neurological signs (Monroe *et al.*, 1978). The syndrome resembles DSM-IV's intermittent explosive disorder. The concept of dyscontrol syndrome (Mark & Ervin, 1970) describes seizurelike outbursts of explosive anger in patients with limbic brain disease (e.g., epilepsy, tumors). Many patients have histories of repeated traffic violations and car accidents, unusual sexual impulsiveness, and idiosyncratic alcohol intoxication.

The pharmacological treatment of patients with episodic dyscontrol is similar to that described for organic violence, and includes anticonvulsants (especially carbamazepine, alone or in combination with propranolol) (Elliott, 1984; Balis, 1979), primidone (Monroe *et al.*, 1978), or clonazepam. Lithium may have a nonspecific therapeutic effect on aggressive behavior, and, alone or in combination with carbamazepine and/or valproate, may also be effective in explosive violence (Tupin *et al.*, 1972; Sheard *et al.*, 1976). Fluoxetine has been found to decrease overt aggressive behaviors and irritability in some patients with personality disorders (Coccaro & Kavoussi, 1995). Progesterone agonists (e.g., medroxy-progesterone) and testosterone antagonists may be indicated in selected cases of sexually motivated organic violence.

Behavioral interventions should be part of a comprehensive treatment for explosive personality types. Thorough behavioral assessment is a prerequisite for an effective program (Mehr & Holi, 1984; Reid & Balis, 1985). Psychosocial approaches, including individual, group, and family therapy, and behavior modification techniques have been reported to be of value for some patients (Mehr & Holi, 1984), encouraging compliance and helping with the transition to a normal life.

APATHETIC TYPE

This type is also known as pseudodepressive, and is characterized by apathy and indifference. It is often part of a frontal lobe syndrome, with impaired capacity to initiate and maintain goal-directed behavior. More severe cases may present with abulia or frontal apraxia.

There are no established guidelines for treatment. Efforts should be directed at providing a stimulating milieu to combat regression (e.g., referral to a day treatment or psychosocial center). Dopamine agonists (i.e., bromocriptine) appear to be an effective treatment for many patients suffering from "organic" apathy. Bromocriptine, at higher doses, is the drug of choice. A trial of methylphenidate or amphetamine may prove helpful for some patients. Severe cases may require custodial care.

Existence of the so-called amotivational syndrome reported with marijuana, LSD, and other (often psychedelic) substances continues to be controversial. Therapeutic approaches for patients with substance abuse are discussed in Chapter 15.

PARANOID TYPE

This type is seen in some patients with closed head trauma, temporal lobe epilepsy, and other neurological diseases.

The personality change may represent an exaggeration or "caricature" of the patient's premorbid personality. The chronic use of psychostimulants, hallucinogens, phencyclidine, or some prescription drugs (e.g., corticosteroids, anabolic-androgenic steroids) may induce a paranoid personality change, which, in more severe cases, can present as a florid psychotic disorder with delusions. The frequent suspiciousness often causes management problems, negativism, and noncompliance. Explosive outbursts may be present and may be related to a misinterpretation of others' behavior, as well as to poor impulse control. Establishing a therapeutic alliance is a pivotal aspect of treatment and management. Neuroleptics may prove effective in some cases.

CHAPTER 11

SEXUAL DYSFUNCTIONS DUE TO
A GENERAL MEDICAL CONDITION
OR SUBSTANCE

The comprehensive evaluation of a patient whose sexual dysfunction is thought to be caused by a physical condition or substance includes a complete medical and psychiatric history (with thorough attention to drugs and alcohol), a complete sexual history, physical examination with emphasis on neurological and vascular evaluations, urologic or gynecological consultation, laboratory screening for diabetes and androgen deficiency in men or estrogen deficiency in women, and, for men, polysomnography for nocturnal penile tumescence (Schover, 1990; Schover & Jensen, 1988).

Screening for endocrine dysfunction (e.g., serum testosterone, estrogen, and prolactin; thyroid function tests) is routine, and if the test is abnormal, it suggests additional endocrinological evaluation. In men, low serum testosterone may cause impaired sexual desire and erectile function. Hyperprolactinemia secondary to pituitary adenoma may also cause impairment in sexual desire and arousal. Decreased sexual desire or function caused by atherosclerotic obstruction of the aorta and/or iliac arteries may justify further vascular evaluation.

GENERAL TREATMENT PRINCIPLES

The expectations of both the patient and partner are important in selecting appropriate therapy. Sexual dysfunctions secondary to a treatable medical condition may only require a simple intervention, such as removal of an offending substance or medication. On the other hand, a more comprehensive approach is indicated when correction of the underlying condition does not restore impaired sexual function. Additional interventions should include sexual counseling and education with the patient and his or her partner, sex therapy, and individual psychotherapy when indicated.

Depending on the extent of permanent disability, treatment might emphasize accepting alternative methods of having sex (e.g., sharing orgasms through manual or oral caressing) or using prostheses, medications (e.g., papaverine), or sexual aids and devices. Schover (1990) suggests that the couple time sex to avoid periods of pain, use positions that are less strenuous, use pillows to support a weak or painful body part, use a vibrator to compensate for decreased genital sensation, wear attractive nightgowns or undergarments to conceal an ostomy appliance, and take a warm bath or pain medication to decrease pain in preparing for sex.

SPECIFIC SEXUAL DYSFUNCTIONS

SEXUAL DYSFUNCTION DUE TO A GENERAL MEDICAL CONDITION

607.84 Male Erectile Disorder

The most common sexual complaint in men, erectile disorder is estimated to have an organic cause in 10 to 30% of cases (Jefferson & Marshall, 1983); however, the majority involve both organic and psychogenic factors. Treatment of male erectile disorder of organic etiology is principally directed to treating the underlying medical condition (vasculogenic, neurogenic) causing the impotence. Comprehensive evaluation of the many components of erectile function, by a multidisciplinary evaluation team, is important for correct diagnosis and treatment planning; Tiefer and Melman (1990) describe a useful evaluation protocol. The National Institutes of Health (NIH) Consensus Statement on Impotence (1992) describes the recommended vascular examination.

Common causes of impotence include peripheral neuropathy (e.g., diabetic vasculitis), vascular disorders (e.g., small-blood-vessel disease, atherosclerotic obstruction of the aorta and iliac arteries), spinal cord lesions, pituitary tumors, endocrine disorders (e.g., thyroid disorders, reduction in plasma testosterone, elevation of prolactin or estradiol), neurological disorders, prostatectomy, and systemic disease. Risk factors that may be amenable to prevention strategies include diabetes mellitus, hypogonadism, hypertension, atherosclerosis, alcoholism, and smoking.

Contributing psychological factors include a lack of self-confidence, performance anxiety, or a conflicted relationship with the partner. The disorder is likely to be psychogenic if normal erection occurs with a different partner or during masturbation or sleep.

Endocrine treatment is appropriate in hypothalamic-pituitary-gonadal dysfunction (e.g., gonadotropic-hypogonadism, hypergonadotropic-hypogonadism, hyperprolactinemia, or hyperthyroidism). In primary testicular failure or hypothalamic-pituitary dysfunction with low serum testosterone levels, treatment with monthly injections of testosterone in oil (200 to 400 mg) may improve the condition. In the case of prolactin-secreting tumors of the anterior pituitary, hyperprolactinemia is treated with bromocriptine, radiation, or surgical removal of the tumor. Treating the testosterone deficit without reducing the overproduction of prolactin will not improve the sexual dysfunction (Tiefer & Melman, 1990). In hyperthyroidism, the treatment of the erectile disorder is that of the thyroid disease. Erectile disorder may also be associated with increased estradiol, which can be caused by adrenal gland neoplasias (treated with adrenalectomy) or chronic alcoholism (treated with abstinence from alcohol and testosterone). The indiscriminant use of androgen therapy in men with normal testosterone levels is unwarranted and may carry health risks, as in unrecognized prostate cancer.

The treatment of intractable erectile disorder includes penile vascular surgery, intracorporeal injections with vasodilator agents, penile prosthetic devices, and vacuum constriction devices (Tiefer & Melman, 1990).

Vascular surgery may be considered. Any disorder that impairs blood flow may be implicated in the etiology of erectile failure, including systemic obstructive vascular disease and disorders that interfere with the penile veno-occlusive mechanism or produce leakage that interferes with maintenance of the erection. In the case of obstructive vascular disease, arterial bypass procedures may improve erectile dysfunction. Microvascular surgical correction of pudendal and penile artery defects or venous leaks and balloon angioplasty of iliac arteries are new techniques of interest. However, the long-term results of penile vascular surgery have been disappointing (Tiefer & Melman, 1990).

Intracorporeal injections with papaverine and other vasodilating agents (phentolamine, prostaglandin E_1, vasoactive intestinal polypeptide) have become very popular for men with irreversible erectile dysfunction (e.g., caused by diabetic neuropathy, prostatectomy, etc.). After determining the proper dosage of papaverine to effect penile rigidity in under four hours, the patient and his partner are instructed on the proper injection technique (Tiefer & Melman, 1990). Adverse effects include priapism, penile infection, and liver damage. Although effective, papaverine injections are not well tolerated, with the majority of users discontinuing the drug within a relatively short time.

Implanted penile prosthetic devices are of two basic types: (1) a pair of semirigid rods that create a permanent erection; and (2) a multicomponent hydraulic device with two cylindrical rods (implanted in the penis), a saline reservoir implanted in the abdomen, a valve to effect tumescence and detumescence (implanted in the scrotum), and connecting tubes. Follow-up studies of prosthesis recipients and their partners indicate satisfaction in most, despite a variety of disappointments. There were no differences in satisfaction between the two techniques. The primary benefit of the prosthesis, according to Tiefer and Melman (1990), seemed to be to repair the patient's wounded masculine self-esteem.

Vacuum constriction devices are used in an old, noninvasive technique that consists of placing the penis in a tube, creating a partial vacuum that produces an erection, and then placing a constricting band at the base of the penis (Witherington, 1988). There have been few reports of serious adverse effects, although minor bruising (and, potentially, more serious blood vessel rupture) may occur.

Other treatments include the use of yohimbine in the treatment of erectile disorder; its efficacy is thought to be comparable to that of placebo (Morales *et al.*, 1988). Experience with vasodilating drugs (e.g., nitroglycerine, pentaerythritol tetranitrate) in treating erectile dysfunction due to atherosclerotic vascular disease is very limited, and generally has been unsatisfactory. Education concerning sexual function, counseling in dysfunctional relationships, and psychotherapy may be important interventions in cases with psychogenic contribution.

608.89 Male Hypoactive Sexual Desire Disorder

Problems of deficient or absent sexual desire are complex and difficult to treat, requiring a multimodal approach to assessment and treatment. General medical conditions associated with a decrease in or loss of sexual desire include chronic illness, such as systemic diseases resulting in debilitated states (e.g., leukemia, uremia), endocrine disturbances (e.g., hypogonadism, orchidectomy), and hyperprolactinemia secondary to pituitary adenoma. Surgical removal of the prolactine-secreting pituitary adenoma and treatment with the dopamine agonist bromocriptine may restore sexual function.

Libido enhancers, such as pharmacological (e.g., yohimbine) and hormonal (e.g., testosterone) agents, for the symptomatic treatment of low sexual desire have generally been disappointing. Treatment of concurrent depression, a common complication of etiological medical conditions, may prove beneficial. In choosing an antidepressant drug, it is advisable to avoid serotonergic antidepressants (especially clomipramine), giving preference to bupropion and nefazodone.

608.89 Male Dyspareunia

Medical conditions that cause pain during intercourse include local inflammation (e.g., prostatitis, cystitis, urethritis), anatomical deformities of the penis (congenital or following trauma), phimosis, penile ulcers, and condylomata. Treatment of the inflammatory disorder will alleviate the dyspareunia.

Orgasmic Dysfunction

A few medical conditions (e.g., stroke, spinal cord injury) may prevent men from reaching orgasm. Any chronic illness may decrease the intensity of orgasmic pleasure.

Excessive Sexual Desire (Satyriasis)

Sexual disinhibition may be secondary to mania, paraphilia, or early dementia. Medroxyprogesterone acetate has been found to control sexually disinhibited behavior in demented patients, generally without serious adverse effects (Cooper, 1987).

625.8 Female Hypoactive Sexual Desire Disorder

Failure of lubrication is a common factor in decreased or absent sexual desire in women. Other somatic factors may involve vaginal infection or estrogen deficiency (e.g., postmenopausal). As in males, renal disease often decreases libido in women, which may further deteriorate with dialysis and fails to improve after transplantation in most cases. Endocrine and systemic disorders, debilitating states, chronic pain, and other chronic illness affecting sexual desire in men may also impair sexual desire in women (Rosen & Leiblum, 1990). Treatment of the underlying general medical condition may improve the sexual disorder.

625.0 Female Dyspareunia

Failure of lubrication can be easily treated with a lubricating cream or jelly. Post-menopausal dyspareunia is often alleviated with estrogen-replacement therapy. A variety of other gynecological and urological disorders may cause dyspareunia (and vaginismus), including vaginal infections (e.g., trichomonas), ulcers, and condylomata; infections of the lower urinary tract, cervix, and fallopian tubes; endometriosis; ovarian cysts; tumors; retroverted uterus; and scar tissue following episiotomy. The specific treatment of the underlying disorders is beyond the scope of this book. If dyspareunia persists after treatment of a medical condition (and often even if it does not), one must consider and treat psychogenic factors.

625.8 Other Female Sexual Dysfunction

Orgasmic dysfunction may be caused by a number of medical conditions, including diabetic neuropathy, end-stage renal failure, abdominal surgeries, multiple sclerosis, hysterectomy, pregnancy, and postpartum conditions.

SEXUAL DYSFUNCTION DUE TO SUBSTANCE ABUSE

Treatment is directed toward the elimination of the abused substance or medication through detoxification, follow-up treatment, and rehabilitation. See "Intoxication" (Chapter 13), "Withdrawal" (Chapter 14), and "Substance Dependence-Abuse" (Chapter 15).

292.8 Alcohol
292.89 Sedative, Hypnotic, or Anxiolytic
292.89 Opioid

Alcohol is well known for causing sexual problems, primarily impaired erectile ability, in men. In the absence of substantial hepatic or gonadal failure in alcoholic men, normal sexual function is restored during sobriety (Schiavi *et al.*, 1995). CNS depressants, such as sedative, hypnotic, or anxiolytic drugs or opiate pain relievers, may impair sexual desire, arousal, and orgasm in both men and women. Discontinuation returns sexual function to normal.

292.89 Amphetamine (or Related Substance) or Cocaine Sexual Dysfunction

Dextroamphetamine and cocaine are often used for their aphrodisiac effect. A decrease in sexual desire and arousal often occurs during substance withdrawal.

292.89 PRESCRIBED MEDICATIONS

Psychotropic Drugs

Tricyclic antidepressants are the most common psychotropics implicated in reversible sexual dysfunction in both men and women, including decrease in sexual desire and arousal, inhibited orgasm, and painful orgasm. The incidence of sexual dysfunction during antidepressant use varies between 20% and 40% (Balon *et al.*, 1993). Clomipramine, a powerful serotonin reuptake inhibitor, produces the highest incidence of anorgasmia. MAOIs may produce anorgasmia and impotence. The SSRIs (fluoxetine, paroxetine, sertraline) can cause anorgasmia and decreased libido in both men and women, as well as ejaculatory failure in men (Segraves, 1993). Bupropion appears to be relatively devoid of adverse effects on sexual function (Gardner & Johnston, 1985; Segraves, 1993). Neuroleptics can impair both sexual desire and arousal in men and women. Thioridazine may cause inhibition of ejaculation and gynecomastia secondary to hyperprolactinemia. Lithium has been reported to cause erectile failure in some patients.

Lowering the dose, waiting for tolerance to develop, or switching to an alternative medication (e.g., bupropion or nefazodone for depressed patients) restores sexual function in most cases (Segraves, 1993; Gitlin, 1994). Yohimbine has been reported to reverse erectile dysfunction and anorgasmia induced by antidepressants, particularly clomipramine and SSRIs. It is administered either as 5.4 mg three times a day or as 2.7 to 10.8 mg two to four hours before coitus (Hollander & McCarley, 1992). Its potential side effects or adverse effects include hypertension, tachycardia, nausea, and insomnia. Tricyclic-induced anorgasmia has been treated successfully with cyproheptadine, a serotonin receptor antagonist, 4 to 12 mg, or bethanechol, 10 to 20 mg one to two hours prior to coitus.

Other medications are common offenders. Guanethidine has been reported to cause inhibition of ejaculation without loss of erectile ability. Methyldopa has been implicated in inhibition of ejaculation, erectile dysfunction, and decreased libido. Erectile dysfunction has been reported with propranolol, thiazides, and disopyramide. Central nervous system (CNS) depressants, β-blockers, drugs interfering with the hypothalamic-pituitary-gonadal axis (cimetidine, spironolactone), and hormone therapy for cancer of the prostate or breast may also cause low sexual desire. Treatment consists of dose reduction, discontinuation of the offending medication (when possible), or switching to an alternative drug.

CHAPTER 12

SLEEP DISORDERS DUE TO A GENERAL MEDICAL CONDITION OR SUBSTANCE

These disorders involve a prominent disturbance in sleep (insomnia, hypersomnia, nightmares, panicky awakening, or sleepwalking). The ICD-10 continues to define these disorders as organic sleep disorders. The clinician must rule out primary sleep disorders, as well as sleep disturbances secondary to a primary psychiatric condition. Referral to a sleep laboratory for polysomnography is necessary for further evaluation of some specific conditions (e.g., narcolepsy, sleep apnea).

GENERAL TREATMENT PRINCIPLES

Etiological treatment, when available, is the principal intervention. Removal of the causative factor (e.g., detoxification from a substance), reversal of the disease process, normalization of an endocrine or metabolic condition, correction of decompensated physiology (e.g., heart failure), or removal of a sleep-impairing symptom (e.g., pain) will improve or correct the sleep disturbance. If the clinician believes the sleep disorder should be treated symptomatically, the following may apply.

PSYCHOSOCIAL MANAGEMENT

Educating the patient about his or her sleep problem is an important part of the treatment. Regular sleep time, mild to moderate physical exercise, and avoidance of psychostimulants (e.g., caffeine-containing beverages) may all be useful. Patients with substance-use disorder should be treated with detoxification (see

"Intoxication," Chapter 13, and "Withdrawal," Chapter 14), and be referred for rehabilitation (Chapter 15).

PHARMACOLOGIC TREATMENTS FOR INSOMNIA

The treatment of chronic insomnia includes pharmacologic, psychological, and environmental approaches. Behavioral, cognitive, and educational techniques; modification of the sleep environment; physical exercise; relaxation exercises; biofeedback (Morin, 1993); and phototherapy may all be helpful. Nevertheless, medications may be indicated for rapid, short-term relief. *It should be noted that sedative drugs are generally contraindicated in breathing-related sleep disorder and sleep apnea of any etiology.*

The choice of hypnotic should be tailored to the needs of the medically compromised patient, taking into consideration: (1) the nature of the underlying medical condition (e.g., risk of compromising respiration); (2) history of, or potential for, substance abuse; (3) age (e.g., the necessity for small doses of short-acting hypnotics in the elderly); (4) drug interactions (e.g., MAOIs potentiating CNS depressants). Clinically relevant aspects of hypnotic drugs include the development of tolerance, plasma half-life, effect on sleep architecture (REM and slow-wave stages), and potential for abuse. One should use the lowest effective dose for the shortest clinically appropriate period, or use the medication intermittently (Dement, 1992). A combination of pharmacological and nonpharmacological therapies may be particularly useful in chronic insomnia (Mendelson, 1990).

Benzodiazepine hypnotics and anxiolytics, although not ideal, are the most commonly prescribed hypnotics (Walsh & Engelhardt, 1992). They are relatively safe, but have a potential for abuse.

Benzodiazepines are divided into long-acting (e.g., flurazepam, quazepam, prazepam, halazepam, and the anxiolytics diazepam and chlordiazepoxide), which tend to produce cumulative effects and daytime drowsiness, and short-acting (e.g., triazolam, temazepam, and the anxiolytics lorazepam and oxazepam), which may produce rebound insomnia, daytime rebound anxiety, and amnestic effects, particularly in the elderly (Jonas *et al.*, 1992). Triazolam was at one time reported to cause behavior disturbances in some patients, although controlled studies do not indicate that it is more likely than other short-acting benzodiazepines to have such effects. Benzodiazepine hypnotics are generally recommended for short-term use because of tolerance and their potential for abuse. There is some evidence that long-term use in selected cases is safe, and may not necessarily result in increased dosages.

Barbiturates, although very effective, are being replaced by the safer benzodiazepines. Their main problems include respiratory depression, a high potential for abuse, lethality of overdose, hangover, and decrease in REM dreaming.

The prompt effect of short-acting barbiturates (pentobarbital, amobarbital) makes them useful in sleep-onset insomnia.

Other hypnotics, such as ethclorvynol, glutethimide, methyprylon, and methaqualone, have no advantages over the barbiturates, and are inferior to the benzodiazepines. Chloral hydrate (500 to 1,000 mg at bedtime) is considered safe and often effective, especially for the elderly and physically ill. Paraldehyde (administered rectally) has the advantage of being eliminated through the lungs, and the disadvantage of being malodorous. Zolpidem is a new hypnotic with a rapid onset of action and a short half-life. It does not appear to produce rebound insomnia, impair psychomotor performance, or significantly affect sleep architecture (Roger & Cocquelin, 1993). Tolerance and dependence may occur with high doses. The closely related zopiclone, available in Europe, has been reported to have no abuse risk or addictive potential. The clinical activity of zopiclone and zolpidem is probably similar to that of the benzodiazepines (Jonas *et al.*, 1992).

Antihistamines are generally safe, but work for only a short time because of the rapid development of tolerance to their sedating effects. They include hydroxyzine, promethazine, and diphenhydramine.

Sedating antidepressants, in addition to improving sleep in patients with depression, may also be useful in treating general insomnia. Trazodone, a sedating triazolopyridine antidepressant, has been successfully used in insomnia secondary to fluoxetine, bupropion, and MAOIs (Jacobsen, 1990; Nierenberg *et al.*, 1994). It has been reported to increase deep sleep (stages 3 and 4) (Jacobsen, 1990). The most common adverse effect of trazodone in nondepressed poor sleepers is residual daytime drowsiness, which generally resolves after a few days of treatment, or can be managed by dose reduction or by taking the drug earlier in the evening. In the writer's experience, trazodone, 25 to 150 mg at bedtime, appears to be safe and effective for treating insomnia in depressed patients and antidepressant-related insomnia. The total antidepressant dose should be carefully monitored.

SPECIFIC SLEEP DISORDERS

SLEEP DISORDER DUE TO A GENERAL MEDICAL CONDITION

Most sleep disorders due to a general medical condition have a readily apparent cause, the correction of which will lead to improved sleep. Chronic pain, or recurrent pain syndromes (e.g, migraine, cluster headaches), paroxysmal nocturnal dyspnea due to heart failure, COPD (cough), and nocturia secondary to prostatic hypertrophy are examples of such conditions.

780.52 Insomnia

General medical conditions associated with insomnia include dementia, hyperthyroidism, hypercortisolism, and toxic conditions. Etiological treatment, when available, will correct the disturbance. The symptomatic treatment of insomnia involves the use of hypnotics and other sedating drugs (see "General Treatment Principles," above).

780.54 Hypersomnia

General medical conditions causing hypersomnia include hypercapnia, neurological disorders (e.g., encephalitis, meningitis, brain tumors, cerebrovascular lesions, degenerative CNS disorders), endocrinopathies, metabolic disorders, postradiation syndrome, and toxic conditions.

There are no established guidelines for the symptomatic treatment of persisting sleepiness associated with medical conditions. Psychostimulants (e.g., methylphenidate, pemoline, caffeine) may be used. When hypersomnia is caused by prescribed drugs (e.g., antidepressants, neuroleptics, anticonvulsants), one may adjust the dosage to a lower level, wait for the development of tolerance to the sedative effect, or switch to a nonsedating medication. One should also look for undesirable drug interactions (e.g., fluoxetine and imipramine). Avoiding a sleep-conducive environment may also be helpful.

Hypercapnia

CO_2 intoxication, usually associated with hypoxia and respiratory acidosis, and caused by respiratory disease (e.g., hypercapnic respiratory failure, COPD, Pickwick's syndrome), may present with sleepiness and lethargy. Treatment is based on the judicious administration of oxygen and gradual lowering of the P_{CO_2} (under close monitoring of blood gases).

Narcolepsy

See sleep disorders in Part III, Chapter 24.

Sleep Apnea

This may be obstructive (due to obesity or abnormal upper respiratory structure) or central (of two types, based on whether symptoms occur predominantly during REM or non-REM sleep). The obstructive type is treated with surgery or assistive devices. Central sleep apnea associated with REM sleep may be treated with drugs that suppress REM stages, such as TCAs or MAOIs.

780.59 Parasomnias

The treatment of parasomnias due to a general medical condition or a substance is principally etiological, directed toward the underlying medical condition.

292.89 SUBSTANCE-INDUCED SLEEP DISORDER

Substance-induced sleep disorders are differentiated according to whether they are related to intoxication (e.g., insomnia associated with the use of psychostimulants, hypersomnia caused by substances of abuse) or withdrawal (e.g., insomnia during withdrawal from alcohol, sedative/hypnotics, or anxiolytics). Treatment is based on detoxification (see "Withdrawal," Chapter 14) and referral for rehabilitation as appropriate (see "Substance Dependence-Abuse," Chapter 15).

Insomnia

This may be caused by a variety of prescription drugs, especially in predisposed individuals. Examples include the SSRI antidepressants, ephedrine, pseudoephedrine, vasopressors, and aminophylline. Treatment consists of lowering the dosage or switching to another drug. A small dose of trazodone (50 to 75 mg at bedtime) is usually sufficient to control the mild insomnia associated with such drugs as the SSRIs.

Hypersomnia

Daytime sleepiness is a common side effect of many drugs (e.g., low-potency neuroleptics; some antidepressants, anticonvulsants, and antihistamines). One should also consider drug interactions, liver disease, hypoalbuminemia, and other factors that may lead to toxic levels of a sedating drug. Treatment consists of adjusting the dosage or switching to a nonsedating drug.

Medications whose long plasma half-lives lead to cumulative effects (e.g., long-acting sedatives/hypnotics, such as phenobarbital or flurazepam, or anxiolytics, such as diazepam) may produce daytime sleepiness, especially in the elderly. Switching to a short-acting hypnotic (e.g., triazolam, temazepam) or anxiolytic (e.g., oxazepam) is helpful; however, short-acting benzodiazepines may produce rebound insomnia and "rebound" anxiety.

Parasomnias

Some psychotropic medications are associated with the occurrence of nightmares. Switching to another drug may correct the problem. Abrupt withdrawal from hypnotics that suppress REM sleep may cause nightmares through REM rebound. One should taper the dosage before discontinuing the drug.

Some SSRIs (e.g., fluoxetine) may induce or exacerbate REM sleep behavior disorder, a disturbance occurring during REM sleep in those uncommon patients whose REM sleep is not accompanied by muscular paralysis. During this phenomenon, one may act out one's dream content. Benzodiazepines, particularly clonazepam, may prove helpful.

References for Part I

Akhtar, S., & Ahmad, H. (1993): Ciprofloxacin-induced catatonia (letter). *Journal of Clinical Psychiatry,* 54:115–116.

American Psychiatric Association Task Force on Electroconvulsive Therapy (1990): *The Practice of Electroconvulsive Therapy.* Washington, D.C.: American Psychiatric Press.

Astrom, M., Olsson, T., & Asplud, K. (1993): Different linkage of depression to hypercortisolism: Early versus late stroke. *Stroke,* 24:52–57.

Balis, G.U. (1970): Delirium and other states of altered consciousness. In *Tice's Practice of Medicine,* Vol. 10. Hagerstown, MD: Harper & Row.

Balis, G.U. (1978a): General systems theory and biosystems: An introduction. In: G.U. Balis, L. Wurmser, & E. McDaniel (Eds.), *Psychiatric Foundations of Medicine, Vol. I: Dimensions of Behavior.* Woburn, MA: Butterworths.

Balis, G.U. (1978b). Conceptual models of disordered behavior. In: G. U. Balis, L. Wurmser, & E. McDaniel (Eds.), *Psychiatric Foundations of Medicine, Vol. 3, Basic Psychopathology.* Woburn, MA: Butterworths.

Balis, G.U. (1978c): Behavior disorders associated with epilepsy. In G.U. Balis, L. Wurmser, & E. McDaniel (Eds.), *Clinical Psychopathology, Psychiatric Foundations of Medicine, vol. 4: Clinical psychopharmacology.* Boston: Butterworths.

Balis, G.U. (1978d): The nature of pain: Psychogenic pain. In G.U. Balis, L. Wurmser, & E. McDaniel (Eds.), *Psychiatric Foundations of Medicine, Vol. 6: Psychiatric Problems in Medical Practice.* Boston: Butterworths.

Balis, G.U. (1979): The effects of drugs in episodic dyscontrol disorders. In S. Fielding & R.C. Effland (Eds.), *New Frontiers in Psychotropic Drug Research.* New York: Futura.

Balis, G.U. (1982a): Criterion value of atypical drug responses in the diagnosis of atypical psychiatric disorders. *Journal of Nervous and Mental Diseases,* 170(12):737–743.

Balis, G.U. (1982b): Therapeutic relationship and the placebo effect. *La Vie Medical au Canada Français,* 2:444–457.

Balis, G.U. (1985): Electroencephalographic correlates of psychopathology. *Proceedings,* Fourth World Congress of Biological Psychiatry, Philadelphia.

Balis, G.U., & McDonald, M. (1978): Episodic dyscontrol: Definitions, descriptions, and measurement. In R.R. Monroe, G.U. Balis, J.D. Barcik (Eds.), *Brain Dysfunction in Aggressive Criminals.* Boston: Lexington Books.

Balis, G.U., & Monopolis, S. (1986): Developmental behavioral antecedents of violence. *Proceedings,* Annual Meeting, American Psychiatric Association.

Balon, R., Yeragani, V.K., Pohl, R., & Ramesh, C. (1993): Sexual dysfunction during antidepressant treatment. *Journal of Clinical Psychiatry,* 54:209–212.

Bamrah, J.S., & Johnson, J. (1991): Bipolar affective disorder following head injury. *British Journal of Psychiatry,* 258:117–119.

Berger, P.A., & Tinklenberg, J.R. (1979): Medical management of the drug abuser. In A.M. Freedman, R.L. Sack, & P.L. Berger (Eds.), *Psychiatry for the Primary Care Physician.* Baltimore: Williams & Wilkins.

Beyer, J., Burke, M., Meglin, D., *et al.* (1993): Organic anxiety disorder: Iatrogenic hyperthyroidism. *Psychosomatics,* 34:181–184.

Black, R.D., Barrcley, L.I., Nolan, K.A., *et al.* (1990): Pentoxifylline in cerebrovascular dementia. *Journal of the American Geriatric Society,* 40:237–244.

Blumer, D. (1977): Treatment of patients with seizure disorders referred because of psychiatric complications. *McLean Hospital Journal,* June.

Blumer, D. (1995): Treatment of interictal psychiatric disorders. *Proceedings,* Annual Meeting, American Psychiatric Association, Miami.

Blumer, D., & Heilbronin, M. (1982): Chronic pain as a variant of depressive disease: The pain-prone disorder. *Journal of Nervous and Mental Diseases,* 170:381–424.

Bou-Holaigal, I., Rowe, P.C., Kay, J., & Calkins, H. (1995): The relationship between neurally mediated hypotension and the chronic fatigue syndrome. *Journal of the American Medical Association,* 274:961–967.

Bottini, G., Vallar, G., Cappa, S., *et al.* (1992): Oxiracetam in dementia: A double-blind, placebo-controlled study. *Acta Neurologica Scandinavica,* 86:237–241.

Breitbart, W., Morotta, R., Platt, M.M., *et al.* (1996): A double-blind trial of haloperidol, chlorpromazine, and lorazepam in the treatment of delirium in hospitalized AIDS patients. *American Journal of Psychiatry,* 153:231–237.

Brown, R. (1989): U.S. experience with valproate in manic depressive illness: A multicenter trial. *Journal of Clinical Psychiatry,* 50 (suppl. 3):13–16.

Burke, W.J., Peterson, J., & Rubin, E.H. (1988): Electroconvulsive therapy in the treatment of combined depression and Parkinson's disease. *Psychosomatics,* 29:341–346.

Bush, A.G., Francis, A.J., Fink, M., *et al.* (1993): Catatonia: Symptomatology, diagnosis and response to treatment. In *1993 New Research Program and Abstracts,* 146th Meeting, American Psychiatric Association, San Francisco, p. 251.

Byrne, E.J., Burns, A., & Waite, J. (1992): Neuroleptic sensitivity in dementia with cortical Lewy bodies. *British Medical Journal,* 305:1158–1159.

Carroll, K.M., Rounsaville, B.J., & Gawin, F.H. (1991): A comparative trial of psychotherapies for ambulatory cocaine abusers: Relapse prevention and interpersonal psychotherapy. *American Journal of Drug and Alcohol Abuse,* 17:229–247.

Cassem, E.H. (1990): Depression and anxiety secondary to medical illness. *Psychiatric Clinics of North America,* 13:597–612.

Coccaro, E.F., & Kavoussi, R.J. (1995): Fluoxetine and aggression in personality disorder. *New Research Program and Abstracts,* 1995 Annual Meeting, American Psychiatric Association, Miami, p. 101.

Cohen, M.R., & Niska, R.W. (1980): Localized right cerebral hemisphere dysfunction and recurrent mania. *American Journal of Psychiatry,* 137:847–848.

Cooper, A.J. (1987): Medroxyprogesterone acetate (MPA) treatment of sexual acting out in men suffering from dementia. *Journal of Clinical Psychiatry,* 48:368–370.

Cooper, D.S., Halpern, R., Wood, L.L., *et al.* (1984): L-Thyroxine therapy in subclinical hypothyroidism: A double-blind placebo-controlled trial. *Annals of Internal Medicine,* 101:18–24.

Corn, T.H., & Checkley, S.A. (1983): A case of recurrent mania with recurrent hyperthyroidism. *British Journal of Psychiatry,* 143:74–76.

Creighton, F., Black, D., & Hyde, C. (1991): Ecstasy psychosis and flashbacks. *British Journal of Psychiatry,* 159:713–715.

Crook, T., Petrie V., Wells C., & Massari, D.C. (1992): Effects of phosphatidylserine in Alzheimer's disease. *Psychopharmacology Bulletin,* 28:61–66.

Cummings, J.L. (1992): Depression and Parkinson's disease. *American Journal of Psychiatry,* 149:443–454.

Cummings, J.L. (1995): Frontotemporal degenerations and behavior. *Proceedings,* 1995 Annual Meeting, American Psychiatric Association, Miami, p. 155.

Cummings, J.L., & Benson, D.F. (1983): *Dementia: A Clinical Approach.* Boston: Butterworths.

Cutler, P. (1994): Iron overload and psychiatric illness. *Canadian Journal of Psychiatry,* 39:8–11.

Davis, J.M., Janicak, P.G., Sakkas, P., *et al.* (1991): Electroconvulsive therapy in treatment of the neuroleptic malignant syndrome. *Convulsive Therapy,* 7(2):111–120.

Davis, K.L., Thal, L.J., Gamzu, E., *et al.* (1992): Tacrine in patients with Alzheimer's disease: A double-blind, placebo-controlled multicenter study. *New England Journal of Medicine,* 327:1253–1259.

Dement, W.C. (1992): The proper use of sleeping pills in the primary care setting. *Journal of Clinical Psychiatry,* 53 (suppl. 12):50–56.

Devanand, D.P., Cooper, T., Scakeim, H.A., *et al.* (1992): Low dose oral haloperidol and blood levels in Alzheimer's disease. A preliminary study. *Psychopharmacology Bulletin,* 28:169–173.

Dickson, L.R., & Fisher, W. (1993): Polypharmacy and hypoalbuminemia in delirium. *Proceedings,* Annual Meeting, American Psychiatric Association, San Francisco.

Dopheide, J.A., Stimmel, G.L., & Yi, D.D. (1995): Focus on nefazodone: A serotonergic drug for major depression. *Hospital Formulary,* 30:205–212.

Edwards, A.J. (1993): *Dementia.* New York: Plenum.

Elliott, F.A. (1984): The episodic dyscontrol syndrome and aggression. *Neurological Clinics,* 2:113–125.

Emery, V.O., & Oxman, T.E. (1992): Update on the dementia spectrum of depression. *American Journal of Psychiatry,* 149:305–317.

Engel, G. (1959): Delirium: A syndrome of cerebral insufficiency. *Journal of Chronic Diseases,* 9(3).

Engel, G.L. (1977): The need for a new medical model: A challenge for biomedicine. *Science,* 196:129–136.

Evans, D.L., Byerly, M.J., & Greer, R.A. (1995): Secondary mania: Diagnosis and treatment. *Journal of Clinical Psychiatry,* 56 (suppl. 3):31–37.

Fawzy, F.I., Fawzy, N.W., Arndt, L.A., *et al.* (1995): Critical review of psychosocial interventions in cancer care. *Archives of General Psychiatry,* 52:100–113.

Fedoroff, J.P., Starkstein, S.E., Forrester, A.W. (1992): Depression in patients with acute traumatic brain injury. *American Journal of Psychiatry,* 149:918–923.

Ferguson, S.M., Rayport, M., & Schell, C.A. (1993): Behavioral outcome of temporal seizure surgery. In *1993 Proceedings,* 146th Annual Meeting, American Psychiatric Association, San Francisco, p. 115.

Fernandez, F., Adams, F., Holmes, V.F., *et al.* (1987): Methylphenidate for depressive disorders in cancer patients, *Psychosomatics,* 28:455–461.

Fielding, R. (1991): Depression and acute myocardial infarction: A review and reinterpretation. *Society of Science and Medicine,* 32:1017–1027.

Fink, M., Bush, G., & Francis, A. (1993): Catatonia: A treatable disorder occasionally recognized. *Directions in Psychiatry,* 13:1–7.

Fisher, J.W. (1994): Legal aspects of the psychosocial management of the demented patient. *Psychiatric Annals,* 24:197–201.

Flor-Henry, P. (1969): Psychosis and temporal lobe epilepsy: A controlled investigation. *Epilepsia,* 10:363.

Francis, A.J., Bush, G., Petrides, G, *et al.* (1993): Treatment of catatonia: A prospective study and quantitative response. In *Proceedings,* Annual Meeting, American Psychiatric Association, San Francisco, p. 185.

Francis, F.J., & Franklin, J.E., Jr. (1987): Alcohol-induced organic mental disorders. In R.E. Hales & S.C. Yudofsky (Eds.), *Textbook of Neuropsychiatry* (pp. 141–156). Washington, D.C.: American Psychiatric Press.

Fraser, C.L., & Arieff, A.I. (1985): Hepatic encephalopathy. *New England Journal of Medicine,* 313:865.

Frazure-Smith, N., Lesperance, F., & Talajik, M. (1993): Depression following myocardial infarction. *Journal of the American Medical Association,* 270:1819–1925.

Fricchione, G.L., Cassem, N.H., *et al.* (1983): Intravenous lorazepam in neuroleptic-induced catatonia. *Journal of Clinical Psychopharmacology,* 3, 334–338.

Ganz, V.F., Gurland, B.J., Demming, E., *et al.* (1972): The study of the psychiatric symptoms of systemic lupus erythematosus: A biometric study. *Psychosomatic Medicine,* 34:207–219.

Gardner, E.A., & Johnston, J.A. (1985): Bupropion: An antidepressant without sexual pathophysiological action. *Journal of Clinical Psychopharmacology,* 5:24–29.

Gelenberg, A.J., & Mandel, M.R. (1977): Catatonic reaction to high potency neuroleptic. *Archives of General Psychiatry,* 34:947–950.

Gelenberg, A.J., & Turkstra, L.S. (1993): Secondary catatonia. In *Proceedings,* Annual Meeting, American Psychiatric Association, San Francisco.

Giannini, J. (1994): Inward the mind's I: Description, diagnosis, and treatment of acute and delayed LSD hallucinations. *Psychiatric Annals,* 24:134–136.

Gitlin, M.J. (1994): Psychotropic medications and their effects on sexual function: Diagnosis, biology, and treatment approaches. *Journal of Clinical Psychiatry,* 55:406–413.

Gjessing, R. (1947): Biological investigations in endogenous psychoses. *Acta Psychiatrica Scandinavica,* 47(suppl.):93–254.

Gjessing, R., & Gjessing, L. (1961): Some main trends in the clinical aspects of periodic catatonia. *Acta Psychiatrica Scandinavica,* 37(I):254–335.

Glassman, A.H., Roose, S.P., & Bigger, J.T. (1993): The safety of tricyclic antidepressants in cardiac patients. *Journal of the American Medical Association,* 269:2673–2675.

Gleason, R.P., & Schneider, L.S. (1990): Carbamazepine treatment of agitation in Alzheimer's outpatients refractory to neuroleptics. *Journal of Clinical Psychiatry,* 51:115–118.

Gold, M., & Pearsall, H. (1983): Hypothyroidism—or is it depression? *Psychosomatics,* 24:646–656.

Goodnick, P.J. (1993): Chronic fatigue syndrome therapy: Mechanism and response. In *New Research Program and Abstracts,* Annual Meeting, American Psychiatric Association, San Francisco, p. 85.

Granacher, R.P., Baldessarini, R.J., & Messner, E. (1976): Physostigmine treatment of delirium induced by anticholinergics. *American Family Physician,* 13:99–103.

Granato, J.E., Stern, B.J., Ringel, A., *et al.* (1983): Neuroleptic malignant syndrome: Successful treatment with dantrolene and bromocriptine. *Annals of Neurology,* 14:89–90.

Greendyke, R.M., & Kanter, D.R. (1986): Therapeutic effects of pindolol on behavior disturbances associated with organic brain disease: A double-blind study. *Journal of Clinical Psychiatry,* 47:423–426.

Greene, P., Cote, L., & Fahn, S. (1993): Treatment of psychosis in Parkinson's disease with clozapine. In H. Narabayashi *et al.* (Eds.), *Advances in Neurology,* vol. 60 (pp. 703–706). New York: Raven.

Greer, S., Moorey, J.D.R., Watson, M., *et al.* (1992): Adjuvant psychological therapy for patients with cancer: A prospective randomized trial. *British Medical Journal,* 304:675–680.

Gupta, M.G. (1986): Is chronic pain a variant of depressive illness? A critical review. *Canadian Journal of Psychiatry,* 31:241–248.

Gurland, B.J., Ganz, V.F., Fleiss, J.L., *et al.* (1972): The study of the psychiatric symptoms of systemic lupus erythematosus. *Psychosomatic Medicine,* 34:199–206.

Hale, A.S. (1993): New antidepressants: Use in high risk patients. *Journal of Clinical Psychiatry,* 54(suppl. 8):61–70.

Hass, W.K. (1979): Acute ischemic cerebrovascular disease. In W.F. Cohn (Ed.), *Current Therapy* (pp. 676–677). Philadelphia: Saunders.

Hay, L. (1995): Treatment of agitation in elderly patients with dementia: Behavioral approaches. *Proceedings,* Annual Meeting, American Psychiatric Association, Miami.

Heilman, M.N., & Valenstein, E. (Eds.) (1979): *Clinical Neuropsychology.* New York: Oxford University Press.

Herman, N., & Lief, J.S. (1988): Drug-induced catatonia. *Canadian Journal of Psychiatry,* 33:633–634.

Hills, D.L., & Lange, R.A. (1991): Serotonin and acute ischemic heart disease. *New England Journal of Medicine,* 324(10):688–690.

Hollander, E., & McCarley, A. (1992): Yohimbine treatment of sexual side effects induced by serotonin reuptake blockers. *Journal of Clinical Psychiatry,* 53:207–209.

Horiguchi, J., & Nishimatsu, O. (1992): Usefulness of antiparkinsonian drugs during neuroleptic treatment and the effect of clonazepam on akathesia and parkinsonism occurring after antiparkinsonian drug withdrawal: A double-blind study, *Japanese Journal of Psychiatry,* 46:733–739.

Ifabumuyi, O.L., & Jeffries, J.J. (1976): Treatment of drug-induced psychosis with diphenylhydantoin. *Canadian Psychiatric Association Journal,* 21:565–569.

Illowsky, B.P. & Kirsh, D.G. (1988): Polydipsia and hyponatremia in psychiatric patients. *American Journal of Psychiatry,* 145:675–683.

Isles, L.J., & Orrell, M.W. (1993): Secondary mania after open-heart surgery. *British Journal of Psychiatry,* 159:280–282.

Jacobsen, F.M. (1990): Low-dose trazodone as a hypnotic in patients treated with MAOIs and other psychotropics: A pilot study. *Journal of Clinical Psychiatry,* 51:298–302.

Jampala, V.C., & Abrams, R. (1983): Mania secondary to left and right hemisphere damage. *American Journal of Psychiatry,* 140:1197–1199.

Jefferson, J.W. (1992): Treatment of depressed patients who have become nontolerant of antidepressant medication because of cardiovascular side effects. *Journal of Clinical Psychiatry Monograph,* 10(1):66–71.

Jefferson, J.W. (1993): Cardiovascular effects of bupropion. *Journal of Clinical Psychiatry Monograph,* 11(1):43–48.

Jefferson, J.W., & Marshall, J.R. (1983): *Neuropsychiatric Features of Medical Disorders.* New York: Plenum.

Jenike, M.A. (1985): Monoamine oxidase inhibitors as treatment for depressed patients with primary degenerative dementia (Alzheimer's disease). *American Journal of Psychiatry,* 142:763–764.

Jonas, J.M., Coleman, R.S., Sheridan, A.Q., & Kalinske, R.W. (1992): Comparative clinical profiles of triazolam versus other shorter-acting hypnotics. *Journal of Clinical Psychiatry,* 53(suppl. 12):19–31.

Karajgi, B., Rifkin, A., Doddi, S., *et al.* (1990): The prevalence of anxiety disorders in patients with chronic obstructive pulmonary disease. *American Journal of Psychiatry,* 147:200–201.

Kathol, R.G., & Dalahunt, J.W. (1986): The relationship of anxiety and depression to symptoms of hyperthyroidism using operational criteria. *General Hospital Psychiatry,* 8:23–28.

Kay, C.R. (1984): The Royal College of General Practitioners' oral contraception study: Some recent observations. *Clinical Obstetrics and Gynecology,* 11:759.

Keck, P.E., Pope, H.G., & McElroy, S.L. (1991): Declining frequency of neuroleptic malignant syndrome in a hospital population. *American Journal of Psychiatry,* 148:880–882.

Keefe, F.J., Dunsmore, J., & Burnett, R. (1992): Behavioural and cognitive-behavioural approaches to chronic pain: Recent advances and future directions, *Journal of Consulting Clinical Psychology,* 60:528–536.

Keegan, D. (1994): Risperidone: Neurochemical, pharmacologic and clinical properties of a new antipsychotic agent, *Canadian Journal of Psychiatry,* 39(suppl. 2):S46–S52.

Kinkel, W. (1992a): Computerized tomography in clinical neurology. In R.J. Joynt (Ed.), *Clinical Neurology,* vol. 1 (pp. 1–115). Philadelphia: Lippincott.

Kinkel, W. (1992b): Nuclear magnetic resonance imaging in clinical neurology. In R.J. Joynt (Ed.), *Clinical Neurology,* vol. 1 (pp. 1–68). Philadelphia: Lippincott.

Kirksey, D., & Stern, W. (1984): Multicenter private practice evaluation of the safety and efficacy of bupropion in depressed geriatric outpatients. *Current Therapeutic Research,* 35:200–210.

Knapp, M.J., Solomon, P.R., & Davis, C.S. (1994): A 30-week randomized controlled trial of high-dose tacrine in patients with Alzheimer's disease. *Journal of the American Medical Association,* 271:985–991.

Kral, V.A. (1978): Benign senescent forgetfulness. In R. Katzman, R.D. Terry, & K.K. Bick (Eds.), *Alzheimer's Disease: Senile Dementia and Related Disorders.* New York: Raven.

Kramer-Ginsberg, E., & Greenwald, B.S. (1993): Depressive pseudodementia: Six to seven year outcome. In *1993 New Research Program and Abstracts,* Annual Meeting, American Psychiatric Association, San Francisco, p. 234.

Krupp, L.B., Masur, D., Schwartz, J., *et al.* (1991): Cognitive functioning in late Lyme borreliosis. *Archives of Neurology,* 48:1125–1129.

Kunik, M.E.,Yudofsky, S.C., Silver, J.M., & Hales, R.E. (1994): Pharmacologic approach to management of agitation associated with dementia. *Journal of Clinical Psychiatry,* 55(suppl. 2):13–17.

Kwentus, J.A., Hart, R.P., Peck, E.T., *et al.* (1985): Psychiatric complications of closed-head trauma. *Psychosomatics,* 26:8–17.

Landolt, H. (1956): Electroencephalographie dans les psychoses epileptiques et les episodes schizophreniques. *Review of Neurology,* 95:595.

Lauer, C.J., Schreiber,W., Holseboer, F., *et al.* (1995): In quest of identifying vulnerability markers for psychiatric disorders by all-night polysomnography, *Archives of General Psychiatry,* 52:145–153.

Lawlor, B.A. (1988): Hypocalcemia, hypoparathyroidism, and organic anxiety syndrome. *Journal of Clinical Psychiatry,* 49:317–318.

Lazarus, L.W.,Winemiller, D.R., Lingam,V.R., *et al.* (1992): Efficacy and side effects of methylphenidate for poststroke depression. *Journal of Clinical Psychiatry,* 53:447–449.

Lebert, F., Pasquier, F., & Petit, H. (1994): Behavioral effects of trazodone in Alzheimer's disease. *Journal of Clinical Psychiatry,* 55(12):536–539.

Levine, A.M. (1988): Buspirone and agitation in head injury. *Brain Injury,* 2:165–187.

Levinson, I. & Galymker, I.I. (1995): Methadone withdrawal psychosis. *Journal of Clinical Psychiatry,* 56:73–76.

Lezak, M. (1985): *Neuropsychological Assessment.* New York: Oxford University Press.

Lezak, M.D. (1978): Living with the characterologically altered brain injured patient. *Journal of Clinical Psychiatry,* 39:592–598.

Li, G., Silverman, J.M., Smith, C.J., *et al.* (1993): Onset and familial risk in Alzheimer's disease. *Proceedings,* Annual Meeting, American Psychiatric Association, San Francisco.

Lindvall, O., Rehncona, S., Brundin, P., *et al.* (1989): Human fetal dopamine neurons grafted into the striatum in two patients with severe Parkinson's disease. *Archives of Neurology,* 46:615–631.

Lipowski, Z.J. (1983): Transient cognitive disorders (delirium, acute confusional states) in the elderly. *American Journal of Psychiatry,* 140:1426–1436.

Lipowski, Z.J. (1990): *Delirium: Acute Confusional States.* New York: Oxford University Press.

Liston, E.H. (1982): Delirium in the aged. *Psychiatric Clinics of North America,* 5:49–66.

Mann, S.C., Caroff, S.N., Bleir, H.R., *et al.* (1990): Electroconvulsive therapy of the lethal catatonia syndrome: Case report and review. *Convulsive Therapy,* 6(3):239–247.

Mark,V.H., & Ervin, F.R. (1970): *Violence and the Brain.* New York: Harper & Row.

Markowitz, J.C., Klerman, G.I., & Perry, S.W. (1992): Interpersonal psychotherapy of depressed HIV-positive outpatients. *Hospital and Community Psychiatry,* 43:885–890.

Martin, A. (1993): Clinical management of lithium-induced polyuria. *Hospital and Community Psychiatry,* 44:427–428.

Masand, P., Pickett, P., & Murray, G.B. (1991): Psychostimulants for secondary depression in medical illness. *Psychosomatics,* 32:203–208.

Mathew, R.J., & Meyer, J.S. (1974): Pathogenesis and natural history of transient global amnesia. *Stroke,* 5:303–311.

Mattes, J.A. (1985): Metoprolol for intermittent explosive disorder. *American Journal of Psychiatry,* 142:1108–1109.

Maurizio, F., Rappe, S.M., Pava, J.A, *et al.* (1995): Relapse in patients on long-term fluoxetine treatment: Response to increased fluoxetine dose. *Journal of Clinical Psychiatry,* 56:52–55.

McDaniel, J.S., Musselman, D.L., Porter, M.R., *et al.* (1995): Depression in patients with cancer: Diagnosis, biology, and treatment. *Archives of General Psychiatry,* 52:89–99.

McEllroy, S.L., Keck, P.E., Jr., Pope, H.G., Jr., *et al.* (1992): Valproate in bipolar disorder: Literature review and treatment guidelines. *Journal of Clinical Psychopharmacology,* 12:42S–52S.

McNamara, M.E., & Fogel, B.S. (1990): Anticonvulsant-responsive panic attacks with temporal lobe EEG abnormalities. *Journal of Neuropsychiatry and Clinical Neuroscience,* 2:193–196.

Mehr, J.J., & Holi, T.C. (1984): Behavioral treatment for aggression in residents of institutions for the emotionally disturbed and the mentally retarded. In S. Saunders, A.M. Anderson, C.A. Hart, *et al.* (Eds.), *Violent Families and Individuals: A Handbook for Practitioners.* Springfield, IL: Charles C Thomas.

Mendelson, W.B. (1990): Insomnia: The patient and the pill. In R.R. Bootzin, J.F. Kihlstron, & D.L. Schacter (Eds.), *Sleep and Cognition* (pp. 139–147). Washington, D.C.: American Psychological Association.

Miller, E.N., Selnes, O.A., & McArthur, J.C. (1990): Neuropsychological performance in HIV-1 infected homosexual men: The multicenter AIDS cohort study (MCAS). *Neurology,* 40:197–203.

Miller, J.W.., Snyder, A.Z., Coben, L.A., *et al.* (1992): Clinical electroencephalography and related techniques. In R.J. Joynt (Ed.), *Clinical Neurology,* Vol. 1, (pp. 1–115). Philadelphia: Lippincott.

Mohr, E., Knott, V., Herting, R., & Mendis, T. (1993): Cycloserine treatment in Alzheimer's disease. In *Neuropsychopharmacology, Supplement/Abstracts* (p.96). First International Congress of Hormones, Brain and Neuropsychopharmacology, Rhodes, Greece. New York: Elsevier.

Molis, R.C., & Davis, K.L. (1985): Interaction of choline and scopalamine in human memory. *Life Sciences,* 37:193–197.

Monroe, R.R. (1970): *Episodic Behavior Disorders.* Cambridge, MA: Harvard University Press.

Monroe, R.R., Balis, G.U., Lion, J., *et al.* (1978): *Brain Dysfunction in Aggressive Criminals.* Boston: Lexington Books.

Morales, A., Condra, M.S., Owen, J.E., *et al.* (1988): Oral and transcutaneous pharmacologic agents in the treatment of impotence. *Urologic Clinics of North America,* 15:87–93.

Morin, C.M. (1993): *Psychological Management of Insomnia.* New York: Guilford.

Mueller, P.S., Vester, J.W., & Fermaglich, J. (1983): Neuroleptic malignant syndrome: Successful treatment with bromocriptine. *Journal of the American Medical Association,* 249:386–388.

Mukherjee, S., Sackeim, H.A., & Schnur, D.B. (1994): Electroconvulsive therapy of acute manic episodes: A review of 50 years' experience. *American Journal of Psychiatry,* 151:169–176.

Murphy, M.F. (1993): Cholinergic approaches to cognitive enhancement. In *Neuropsychopharmacology, Supplement/Abstracts* (pp. 15–16). First International Congress of Hormones, Brain and Neuropsychopharmacology, Rhodes, Greece. New York: Elsevier.

Murray, G.B., Shea, V., & Conn, D.K. (1986): Electroconvulsive therapy for post-stroke depression. *Journal of Clinical Psychiatry,* 47:258–260.

Nicholas, M.K., Wilson, P.H., & Goyen, J. (1992): Comparison of cognitive-behavioral group therapy and an alternative non-psychological treatment for chronic low back pain. *Pain,* 48:339–347.

Nierenberg, A.A., Adler, L.A., Peselow, E., *et al.* (1994): Trazodone for antidepressant-associated insomnia. *American Journal of Psychiatry,* 151:1069–1072.

NIH (1992): Consensus Statement on Impotence, vol 10(4), National Institutes of Health, Office of the Director.

Nyth, A.L., Gottfries, C.G., Lyby, K., *et al.* (1992): A controlled multicenter clinical study of citalopram and placebo in elderly depressed patients with and without concomitant dementia. *Acta Psychiatrica Scandinavica,* 86:138–145.

Oder, W., Goldenberg, G., Spatt, J., *et al.* (1992): Behavioural and psychosocial sequelae of severe closed-head injury and regional blood flow: A SPECT study. *Journal of Neurology, Neurosurgery, Psychiatry,* 55:475–480.

Olivurus, B. de Fine, & Jeusen, T.S. (1979): Transient global amnesia in migraine. *Headache,* 19:335–338.

Ostrow, D., Grant, I., & Atkinson, H. (1988): Assessment and management of the AIDS patient with neuropsychiatric disorders. *Journal of Clinical Psychiatry,* 49(5,suppl):14–22.

Palmini, A., & Gloor, P. (1992): The localizing value of auras in partial seizures: A prospective and retrospective study. *Neurology,* 42:801–808.

Patten, S.B., & Lamarre, C.J. (1992): Can drug-induced depressions be identified by their clinical features? *Canadian Journal of Psychiatry,* 37:213–215.

Perkins, D.O., Stern, R.A., Golden, R.N., *et al.* (1994): Mood disorders in HIV infection: Prevalence and risk factors in a nonepicenter of the AIDS epidemic. *American Journal of Psychiatry,* 151:233–236.

Perry, S. (1987): Substance-induced organic mental disorders. In R.E. Hales & S.C. Yudofsky (Eds.), *Textbook of Neuropsychiatry* (pp. 157–176). Washington, D.C.: American Psychiatric Press.

Peterson, R.C., Smith, G.E., Ivnik, R.J., *et al.* (1995): Apolipoprotein E status as a predictor of the development of Alzheimer's disease in memory-impaired individuals. *Journal of the American Medical Association,* 273:1274–1278.

Philbrick, K.L., & Rummans, T.A. (1994): Malignant catatonia. *Journal of Neuropsychiatry and Clinical Neuroscience,* 6:1–13.

Pincus, J.H., Cohan, S.L., & Glaser, G.H. (1992): Neurologic complications of internal disease. In R.J. Joint (Ed.), *Clinical Neurology*, vol. 4, (pp. 1–76). Philadelphia: Lippincott.

Post, R.M., Pazzaglia, P.J., Ketter, T.A., *et al.* (1993): Carbamazepine and nimodipine in refractory bipolar illness: Efficacy and mechanisms. In *Neuropsychopharmacology, Supplement/Abstracts* (pp. 17–18). First International Congress of Hormones, Brain and Neuropsychopharmacology, Rhodes, Greece. New York: Elsevier.

Prado, N., Kramer-Kinsberg, E., Kremen, N., *et al.* (1995): Risperidone in dementia with behavioral disturbances. *New Research Program and Abstracts*, Annual Meeting, American Psychiatric Association, p. 55.

Preskorn, S.H., & Simpson, S. (1982): Tricyclic-antidepressant-induced delirium and plasma drug concentration. *American Journal of Psychiatry*, 139:822–823.

Prigatano, G.P., Parsons, O.A., Wright, E., *et al.* (1983): Neuropsychologic test performance in mildly hypoxemic patients with chronic obstructive pulmonary disease. *Journal of Consulting Clinical Psychology*, 51:108–116.

Rabkin, J.G. (1993): Psychostimulant medication for depression and lethargy in HIV illness: A pilot study. *Progress Notes, American Society on Clinical Psychopharmacology*, 4:1.

Ranen, N.G., Peyser, C.E., & Folstein, S.E. (1993). ECT treatment for depression in Huntington's disease. In *1993 New Research Program and Abstracts*, 146th Meeting, American Psychiatric Association, San Francisco, pp. 249–250.

Rattey, J., Sovner, R., Parks, A., *et al.* (1991): Buspirone treatment of aggression and anxiety in mentally retarded patients: A multiple-baseline, placebo lead-in study. *Journal of Clinical Psychiatry*, 52:159–162.

Reding, M.J., Orto. L.A., Winter, S.W., *et al.* (1986): Antidepressant therapy after stroke: A double-blind trial. *Archives of Neurology*, 43:763–765.

Reid, W.H., & Balis, G.U. (1987): Evaluation of the violent patient. In R.E. Hales & A.J. Frances (Eds.), *Annual Review of Psychiatry*, Vol. 6, (pp. 491–509). Washington, D.C.: American Psychiatric Association Press.

Reisberg, B. (1982): Office management and treatment of primary degenerative dementia. *Psychiatric Annals*, 12:631–642.

Rice, E.H., Sombrotto, L.B., Markowitz, J.C., & Leon, A.C. (1994): Cardiovascular morbidity in high-risk patients during ECT. *American Journal of Psychiatry*, 151:1637–1641.

Ries, F., Horn, F., Hillekamp, J., *et al.* (1993): Differentiation of multi-infarct and Alzheimer dementia by intracranial hemodynamic parameters. *Stroke*, 24:228–235.

Robertson-Hoffman, D.E., and Bonapace, A.S. (1993): Anxiety and depression in Parkinson's: Comorbidity. In *1993 New Research Program and Abstracts*, Annual Meeting, American Psychiatric Association, San Francisco, p. 71.

Robinson, M.K., and Toole, J.F. (1992): Ischemic cerebrovascular disease. In R.J. Joynt (Ed.), *Clinical Neurology*, Vol. 2, (pp. 1–64). Philadelphia: Lippincott.

Robinson, R.G., Boston, J.D., Startstein, S.E., & Price, T.R. (1988): Comparison of mania and depression after brain injury: Causal factors. *American Journal of Psychiatry*, 145:172–178.

Robinson, R.G., Kubos, K.L., Starr, L.B., *et al.* (1984): Mood disorders in stroke patients: Importance of location of lesions. *Brain*, 107:81–93.

Robinson, R.G., Lipsey, J.R., and Price, T.R. (1995): Diagnosis and clinical management of poststroke depression. *Psychosomatics,* 26:769–778.

Roeleke, U., Barnett, W., Wilder-Smith, E., *et al.* (1992): Centrented neuroborreliosis: Bannworth's syndrome evolving into acute schizophrenia-like psychosis. *Journal of Neurology,* 239:129–131.

Roger, M., & Cocquelin, J.P. (1993): Multicenter, double-blind, controlled comparison of zolpidem and triazolam in elderly patients with insomnia. *Clinical Therapeutics,* 15:127–136.

Rohland, B.M., & Carroll, B.T. (1993): ECT in the treatment of the catatonic syndrome. In *1993 New Research Program and Abstracts,* Annual Meeting, American Psychiatric Association, San Francisco, p. 71.

Roose, S.P., & Glassman, A.H. (1994): Antidepressant choice in the patient with cardiac disease: Lessons from the cardiac arrhythmia suppression trial (CAST) studies. *Journal of Clinical Psychiatry,* 55(suppl A):83–87.

Rosebush, P.I., Hildebrand, A.M., & Mazurek, M.F. (1992): The treatment of catatonia: Benzodiazepines or ECT? *American Journal of Psychiatry,* 149:1279.

Rosen, R.C., & Leiblum, S.R. (1990): Assessment and treatment of desire disorders. In S.R. Leiblum, & R.C. Rosen (Eds.), *Principles and Practice of Sex Therapy,* (pp. 19–50). New York: Guilford.

Rosenberg, P.B., Ahmed, I., & Hurwitz, S. (1991): Methylphenidate in depressed medically ill patients. *Journal of Clinical Psychiatry,* 52:263–267.

Rummans, T.A., & Bassingthwaigthe, M. (1991): Severe medical and neurologic complications associated with near-lethal catatonia treated with ECT. *Convulsive Therapy,* 7(2):121–124.

Sachdev, P., & Kruk, J. (1994): Clinical characteristics and predisposing factors in acute-drug-induced akathesia. *Archives of General Psychiatry,* 51:963–974.

Sackellares, J.C. (1979): Stupor following administration of valproic acid to patient receiving other antiepileptic drugs. *Epilepsia,* 20:697–703.

Sajatovic, M., Verbanac, P., Ramirez, L.F., *et al.* (1991): Clozapine treatment of psychiatric symptoms resistant to neuroleptic treatment in patients with Huntington's chorea *Neurology,* 41:156.

Sakauye, K.M., Camp, C.J., & Ford, P.A. (1993): Effects of buspirone on agitation associated with dementia. *American Journal of Geriatric Psychiatry,* 1:82–83.

Salzman, C. (1995): Update on selected topics pertaining to geriatric psychopharmacology. *Current Affective Illness,* 14:5–13.

Sano, M., Bell, K., Cotte, L., *et al.* (1992): Double-blind parallel design pilot study of acetyl levocarnitine in patients with Alzheimer's disease. *Archives of Neurology,* 49:1137–1141.

Satel, S.L., & Edell, W.S. (1991): Cocaine-induced paranoia and psychosis proneness. *American Journal of Psychiatry,* 148:495–498.

Satlin, A. (1994): Sleep disorders in dementia. *Psychiatric Annals,* 24:186–191.

Satlin, A., Volicer, L., Ross, V., *et al.* (1992): Bright light treatment in behavioral and sleep disturbances in patients with Alzheimer's disease. *American Journal of Psychiatry,* 149:1028–1032.

Schiavi, R.C., Stimmel, B.B., Mandeli, J., *et al.* (1995): Chronic alcoholism and male sexual function. *American Journal of Psychiatry,* 152:1045–1051.

Schiffer, R.B., & Wineman, N.M. (1990): Antidepressant pharmacotherapy of depression associated with multiple sclerosis. *American Journal of Psychiatry,* 147:1493–1497.

Schmitz, B. (1995): Forced normalization: The relevance psychiatry. *Syllabus and Proceedings,* Annual Meeting, American Psychiatric Association, Miami, pp. 93–94.

Schneider, L.S. (1993): Treatment of depression, psychosis, and other conditions in geriatric patients. In H.G. Morgan & D.J. Kupfer (Eds.), *Current Opinion in Psychiatry,* Vol. 4, No. 4, (pp. 562–567). Salem, MA: Current Science Ltd.

Schottenfeld, R.S., & Cullen, M.R. (1984): Organic affective illness associated with lead intoxication. *American Journal of Psychiatry,* 141:1423–1426.

Schover, L.R. (1990): Sexual problems in chronic illness. In S.R. Leiblum & R.C. Rosey (Eds.), *Principles and Practice of Sex Therapy* (pp. 319–351). New York: Guilford.

Schover, L.R., & Jensen, S.B. (1988): *Sexuality and Chronic Illness: A Comprehensive Approach.* New York: Guilford.

Schubert, D.S.P., & Foliart, R.H. (1993): Increased depression in multiple sclerosis patients: A meta-analysis. *Psychosomatics,* 34:124–130.

Segraves, R.T. (1993): Treatment-emergent sexual dysfunction in affective disorder: A review and management strategies. *Journal of Clinical Psychiatry Monograph,* 11(1):57–60.

Sewell, D.D., Jeste, D.V., Atkinson, J.H., *et al.* (1994): HIV-associated psychosis: A study of 20 cases. *American Journal of Psychiatry,* 151:237–242.

Sharma, V., Persad, E., Mazmanian, D., *et al.* (1993): Treatment of rapid cycling bipolar disorder with combination therapy of valproate and lithium. *Canadian Journal of Psychiatry,* 38:137–139.

Sharpe, M., Peveler, R., & Mayou, R. (1992): The psychological treatment of patients with functional somatic symptoms. *Journal of Psychosomatic Research,* 36:515–519.

Sheard, M.H., Marini, J.L., Bridges, C.K., *et al.* (1976): The effect of lithium on impulsive aggressive behavior in man. *American Journal of Psychiatry,* 133:1409–1413.

Siever, J.J., Trestman, R.L., Coccaro, E.F., *et al.* (1993): Serotonin and impulsivity. In *1993 CME Syllabus and Proceedings Summary,* Annual Meeting, American Psychiatric Association, San Francisco, pp. 130–131.

Sloane, R.B., Stapes, F.R., & Schneider, L.S. (1985): Interpersonal therapy versus nortriptyline for depression in the elderly. In G.D. Burrows *et al.* (Eds.), *Clinical and Pharmacological Studies in Psychiatric Disorders.* (pp. 344–346). London: John Libbey.

Sluping, J.R., Rollinson, R.D., & Toole, J.F. (1980): Transient global amnesia. *Annals of Neurology,* 7:281–285.

Small, G.W., LaRue, A., Kaplan, A., *et al.* (1995): Decline predictors for age-related memory loss. *Proceedings,* Annual Meeting, American Psychiatric Association, Miami, pp. 19–20.

Smith, D.E., & Seymour, R.B. (1994): LSD: History and toxicity. *Psychiatric Annals,* 24:145–147.

Spiegel, D., Bloom, J.R., Kraemer, H.C., *et al.* (1989): Effect of psychosocial treatment on survival of patients with metastatic breast cancer. *Lancet,* 2:888–891.

Spitzer, R.L., First, M.B., Williams, J.B.W., *et al.* (1992): Now is the time to retire the term "organic mental disorders." *American Journal of Psychiatry,* 149:240–244.

Starkstein, S.E., Cohen, B.S., Fedoroff, P., *et al.* (1990): Relationship between anxiety disorder and depressive disorders in patients with cerebrovascular injury. *Archives of General Psychiatry,* 47:246–251.

Starkstein, S.E., Fedoroff, P., Berthier, M.I., & Robinson, R.G. (1991): Manic depressive and pure manic states after brain lesions. *Biological Psychiatry,* 29:149–158.

Steele, C., Lucas, M.J., & Tune, L. (1986): Haloperidol versus thioridazine in the treatment of behavioral symptoms in senile dementia of the Alzheimer type: Preliminary findings. *Journal of Clinical Psychiatry,* 47:310–312.

Stein, M.B., Heuser, I.J., Junkos, J.L., *et al.* (1990): Anxiety disorders in patients with Parkinson's disease. *American Journal of Psychiatry,* 147:217–220.

Stevens, J.R., & Herman, B.P. (1981): Temporal lobe epilepsy, psychopathology and violence: The state of the evidence. *Neurology,* 31:1127.

Stoddard, F.J. (1995): Psychiatric aspects of burns in children and adults. *Proceedings,* Annual Meeting, American Psychiatric Association, Miami.

Stoll, A.L., Mayer, P.V., Tohen, M., *et al.* (1993): Antidepressant-associated mania. In *1993 New Research Program and Abstracts,* 146th Meeting, American Psychiatric Association, San Francisco, p. 91.

Summers, W.K., Majovski, L.V., Marsh, G.M., *et al.* (1986): Oral tetrahydroaminoacridine in long-term treatment of senile dementia, Alzheimer type. *New England Journal of Medicine,* 315:1241–1245.

Sunderland T., Cohen, R.M., Molchan, S., *et al.* (1994): High dose selegiline in treatment-resistant older depressive patients, *Archives of General Psychiatry,* 51:607–615.

Swedo, S.E., Apoport, J.L., Cheslow, D.L., *et al.* (1989): High prevalence of obsessive compulsive symptoms in patients with Sydenham's chorea. *American Journal of Psychiatry,* 146:246–249.

Taclob, L., & Needle, M. (1976): Drug-induced encephalopathy in patients on maintenance hemodialysis. *Lancet,* 1:704–705.

Tariot, P.N., Schneider, L.S., Patel, S.V., & Golstein B. (1992): Alzheimer's disease and (-) Deprenyl: Rationale and findings. In I. Szelenyi (Ed.), : *Inhibitors of Monoamine Oxidase B: Pharmacology and Clinical Use in Neurodegenerative Disorders,* pp. 301–317. Basel: Birkhauser Verlag.

Taylor, M. (1990): Catatonia: A review of a behavioral neurologic syndrome. *Neuropsychiatry, Neuropsychology and Behavioral Neurology,* 3(1):48–72.

Thal, L.J., Rosen, W., Sharpless, N.S., *et al.* (1981): Choline chloride fails to improve cognition in Alzheimer's disease. *Neurobiology of Aging,* 2:205–208.

Thienhaus, O.J., & Khosla, N. (1984): Meningeal cryptococcosis misdiagnosed as a manic episode. *American Journal of Psychiatry,* 141:1459–1460.

Thomas, S.C., & Neale, T.J. (1991): Organic manic syndrome associated with advanced anaemia due to polycystic kidney disease. *British Journal of Psychiatry,* 158:119–121.

Tiefer, L., & Melman, A. (1990): Comprehensive evaluation of erectile dysfunction and medical treatments. In S.A. Lieblum & R.C. Rosen (Eds.), *Principles and Practice of Sex Therapy,* (pp. 207–236). New York: Guilford.

Tohen, M., Shulman, K.I., & Satlin, A. (1994): First-episode mania in late life. *American Journal of Psychiatry,* 151:130–132.

Tollefson, G.D. (1992): Short-term effects of the calcium channel blocker nimodipine. *Biological Psychiatry,* 27:1133–1142.

Tucker, D.M. (1981): Lateral brain function, emotion and conceptualization. *Psychological Bulletin,* 89:19.

Tupin, J.P., Smith, D.B., Cannon, T.L., *et al.* (1972): The long-term use of lithium in aggressive prisoners. *Comprehensive Psychiatry,* 14:311–317.

Umbricht, D., Degreef, G., Barr, W.B., *et al.* (1995): Postictal and chronic psychosis in patients with temporal lobe epilepsy. *American Journal of Psychiatry,* 152:224–231.

Varney, N.R., Alexander, B., & MacIndoe, J.H. (1984): Reversible steroid dementia in patients without steroid psychosis. *American Journal of Psychiatry,* 141:369–377.

Vartanian, G., Klementiev, B.I., Belokoskova, S.G., & Dorofeeva, S.A. (1993): Influence of vasopressin on patients with speech disturbance after cerebrovascular lesion. *Proceedings, Neuropsychopharmacology, Supplement/Abstracts* (p. 27). First International Congress of Hormones, Brain and Neuropsychopharmacology, Rhodes, Greece. New York: Elsevier.

Von Loveren-Huyben, C.M.S., Engelaar, H.F.W.J., Hermans, N.B.M., *et al.* (1984): Double-blind clinical and psychologic study of ergoloid mesylates (Hydergine) in subjects with senile mental deterioration. *Journal of the American Geriatric Society,* 32:584–588.

Walsh, J.K., & Engelhardt, C.L. (1992): Trends in the pharmacologic treatment of insomnia. *Journal of Clinical Psychiatry,* 53(12, suppl):10–17.

Watkins, P.B., Zimmerman, H.J., Knapp, M.J., *et al.* (1994): Hepatotoxic effects of tacrine administration in patients with Alzheimer's disease. *Journal of the American Medical Association,* 271:992–998.

Wehr, T.A., Sack, D.A., & Rosenthal, N.E. (1987): Sleep reduction as a first common pathway in the genesis of mania. *American Journal of Psychiatry,* 144:201–204.

Weilburg, J.B., Schacter, S., Pollack, M.H., *et al.* (1993): Focal paroxysmal EEG changes during atypical panic attacks. In *1993 New Research Program and Abstracts,* 146th Meeting, American Psychiatric Association, San Francisco, p. 115.

Weissman, M.M., & Markowitz, J.C. (1994): Interpersonal psychotherapy, current status. *Archives of General Psychiatry,* 51:599–606.

Whitlock, F.A., & Siskind, M.M. (1980): Depression as a major symptom of multiple sclerosis. *Journal of Neurology, Neurosurgery, Psychiatry,* 43:861–865.

Wilson, L.G. (1976): Viral encephalopathy mimicking functional psychosis. *American Journal of Psychiatry,* 133:165–170.

Wise, M.G., & Taylor, S.E. (1990): Anxiety and mood disorders in medically ill patients. *Journal of Clinical Psychiatry,* 51(1, suppl):27–32.

Witherington, R. (1988): Suction device therapy in the management of erectile impotence. *Neurologic Clinics of North America,* 15:123–128.

Wyszynski, A.M., & Wyszynski, B. (1993): Treatment of depression with fluoxetine in corticosteroid-dependent central nervous system Sjorgen's syndrome. *Psychosomatics,* 34:173–177.

Yager, J. (1977): Psychiatric eclecticism: A cognitive view. *American Journal of Psychiatry,* 134:736–741.

Yargic, I.L., Zubieta, J.K., Engleberg, C.N., & Demitrack, M.A. (1993): Psychiatric comorbidity and chronic fatigue. In *New Research Program and Abstracts,* Annual Meeting, American Psychiatric Association, San Francisco, pp. 89–90.

Yudofsky, S.C., Silver, J.M., & Hales, R.E. (1990): Pharmacologic management of aggression in the elderly. *Journal of Clinical Psychiatry,* 51(10 suppl):22–28.

Yudofsky, S.C., Williams, D., & Gounan, J. (1981): Propranolol in the treatment of rage and violent behavior in patients with chronic brain syndromes. *American Journal of Psychiatry,* 138:218–220.

Zielinski, R.J., Roose, S.P., Devanand, D.P., *et al.* (1993): Cardiovascular complications of ECT in depressed patients with cardiac disease. *American Journal of Psychiatry,* 150:904–909.

Part II

SUBSTANCE-RELATED DISORDERS

George Ulysses Balis, M.D.

All other specific substance-related disorders (delirium, dementia, amnestic disorder, psychotic disorder, mood disorder, anxiety disorder, personality change, sleep disorder, and sexual dysfunction) are discussed in **Part I.**

CHAPTER 13

INTOXICATION

Most intoxications are related to substance-use disorders and are particularly common among the young. Intoxication may also be the result of the use or misuse of prescribed medications, drug-drug interactions (especially among the elderly), or suicidal or accidental drug overdose. The severity of the syndrome is generally dose-related, although, in some instances, its severity or specific symptoms may be idiosyncratic, associated with the individual's ability to metabolize a certain drug (Balis, 1982).

GENERAL TREATMENT PRINCIPLES

The following general principles, formulated by Czechowicz (1978), are still applicable to acute, severe intoxications seen in hospital emergency rooms. Treatment should be supervised by a physician qualified in treating poisoning cases and in emergency procedures.

1. Adequacy of cardiopulmonary function and level of consciousness are the first concern.
2. The nature and seriousness of the intoxication should be determined through history, physical examination, urine and blood drug screening, and other laboratory tests.
3. The treatment plan must first address the need to eliminate the toxic substance from the body. In cases of ingested substances in which the overdose occurred within the preceding six hours, immediate measures may include induced emesis, gastric lavage, activated charcoal, and

cathartics. Induced vomiting is contraindicated in the presence of impaired consciousness or convulsions.

In the presence of central nervous system (CNS) depression, gastric lavage requires prior endotracheal intubation. Gastric lavage is contraindicated if the patient is convulsing. After lavage is completed, activated charcoal may be introduced into the stomach to absorb any remaining drug.

If toxic drug levels persist, other measures for elimination may be used, such as increasing urinary excretion or aqueous or lipid dialysis (peritoneal lavage or hemodialysis). Urinary excretion may be hastened by forcing fluids, by forced diuresis with intravenous (IV) 20% mannitol at the rate of 50 cc/hour or by the alkalinization of the urine with sodium bicarbonate (e.g., in phenobarbital poisoning).

4. Prompt, competent treatment of impaired respiration or circulation must be instituted. Upon stabilization of vital functions, an electrocardiogram (ECG) should be obtained to detect cardiac arrhythmias.

   In every stupor or coma for which the cause is questionable, the glucose-naloxone test should be administered (IV 500 cc of 50% glucose and 0.4 mg naloxone). Both agents are safe and readily reverse hypoglycemic or opioid-induced coma respectively. Physostigmine (1 to 2 mg IV) may serve as an antidote to anticholinergic coma; if successful, it will require frequent repeating. Symptomatic treatment may also include control of seizures, hyperthermia, cardiac arrhythmias, and so forth.

5. Adequacy of treatment should be regularly assessed by monitoring vital signs, arterial blood gases, drug blood levels, and level of consciousness. Continuous ECG monitoring may be necessary in intoxication with cardiotoxic drugs (e.g., tricyclics).

6. In less serious intoxications, the concomitant behavioral disturbances may become the major focus of management (see below), and may necessitate the cautious use of such medications as benzodiazepines (e.g., lorazepam) or neuroleptics (e.g., haloperidol), administered by mouth (P.O.), intramuscularly (IM), or IV.

PSYCHOSOCIAL MANAGEMENT

For patients seen in the emergency room, one must first place the patient in a quiet room and secure his or her safety (as well as that of the attending staff) by providing constant supervision and, if necessary, physical restraint. After any violent behavior is brought under control, special care may be needed to avoid provoking further violence and to maximize patient cooperation (Reid & Balis,

1987). Individuals with a substance-use disorder should be referred for specialized services.

SPECIFIC INTOXICATIONS

303.00 ALCOHOL INTOXICATION

Most cases of alcohol intoxication do not need special treatment. The most common problem requiring management is combative or assaultive behavior and, occasionally, suicidal behavior. The patient should be placed in a quiet room, under close supervision, and be handled with a nonprovocative, reassuring approach. Physical restraint may become necessary in combative individuals. Sedative drugs should be avoided because of the risk of potentiating the CNS depressant effects of alcohol. In more severe intoxications, CNS depressant effects may impair respiratory function (see "General Treatment Principles"). If there is evidence of recent drug use, gastric lavage and other symptomatic treatment may become necessary. In the case of an alcohol-disulfiram interaction, treatment consists of the IV administration of an antihistamine and symptomatic control of hypotension.

ALCOHOL IDIOSYNCRATIC INTOXICATION

An alcohol use disorder NOS, 291.9, also known as pathological intoxication, it consists of marked behavioral change (usually agitation, emotional lability, and aggressiveness) appearing within minutes of ingesting a subintoxicating amount of alcohol. Brain damage and temporal lobe epilepsy are thought to be predisposing factors. Treatment is primarily directed toward aggressive or agitated behavior, and may require the use of lorazepam or haloperidol.

305.40 SEDATIVE, HYPNOTIC, OR ANXIOLYTIC INTOXICATION

This is clinically similar to alcohol intoxication. Alcohol is cross-tolerant with sedative, hypnotic, and anxiolytic drugs.

In mild to moderate acute intoxication, if the patient is conscious and ambulatory, management is primarily directed toward monitoring vital signs and controlling agitation or aggressiveness. The patient should be placed in a quiet room under close supervision; physical restraints may become necessary. In more serious intoxications, treatment consists largely of supportive care and maintenance of vital functions (see "General Treatment Principles").

In an overdose of short-acting barbiturates, forced diuresis is of no value, although it can be very effective in meprobamate overdosage (e.g., IV 20% mannitol at 50 cc per hour). Urine alkalinization with sodium bicarbonate can be helpful in phenobarbital overdosage, by increasing the urinary excretion of the drug. In an overdose of nonbarbiturate sedative-hypnotics, forced diuresis and dialysis may be useful when response to other measures is unsatisfactory (Czechowicz, 1978). Aqueous dialysis is of little value in glutethimide poisoning, because of the drug's protein binding and storage in body fat. Glutethimide overdose may cause a coma-wakefulness cycle in which wakefulness is misinterpreted as improvement. Gastric lavage, if performed, should be done with a 1:1 mixture of castor oil and water. In methaqualone overdose, the presence of an intact gag reflex may cause difficulties during endotracheal intubation; dialysis may be helpful.

305.50 OPIOID INTOXICATION

Intoxication with an opioid presents with initial euphoria followed by apathy, dysphoria, agitation or retardation, impaired judgment, or impaired social functioning. It is accompanied by pupillary constriction (usually), slurred speech, impairment in attention or memory, and drowsiness or coma. It may also present with illusions or hallucinations with intact reality testing.

In mild to moderate intoxication, the management is primarily supervision, monitoring vital signs, and controlling agitation or aggressiveness. In more serious poisoning, medical complications include depressed respiration, depressed consciousness, hypotension, and pulmonary edema. Pupils may be dilated instead of constricted in cases with severe hypoxia or in mixed addictions. Meperidine may cause dilated pupils and is more frequently associated with convulsions. Heroin may remain active for six hours, methadone for 36 to 48 hours, and 1-α-acetylmethadol (LAAM) for 48 to 72 hours (Berger & Tinklenberg, 1979; Czechowicz, 1978).

The management of acute, severe opioid intoxication involves the prompt treatment of respiratory impairment and maintenance of vital functions (see "General Treatment Principles"). Naloxone (Narcan), 0.4 mg IV is effective in reversing both respiratory depression and coma. If the initial dose is ineffective, an additional dose may be given in about five minutes and again in 10 minutes. Failure to respond should raise consideration of other causes for the intoxication or coma. Narcotic antagonists are effective for about two to three hours; therefore, repeated doses may be necessary at regular intervals to continue to reverse respiratory depression. If withdrawal symptoms are precipitated, they should not be treated with methadone. The patient should remain hospitalized under continuous supervision for 24 to 48 hours (Czechowicz, 1978).

305.60 COCAINE INTOXICATION
305.70 AMPHETAMINE (OR RELATED SUBSTANCE) INTOXICATION

These produce very similar intoxication syndromes, often presenting with euphoria, hyperalertness, interpersonal sensitivity, anxiety, aggression, and/or impaired judgment developing during or shortly after use, and accompanied by various physical signs (e.g., tachycardia or bradycardia, pupillary dilation, elevated or lowered blood pressure, nausea or vomiting, confusion). An initial characteristic "rush" of well-being is followed in an hour or so by "crashing." Suicidal depression may complicate withdrawal. Medical complications in acute overdose consist of severe hypertension, hyperpyrexia, seizures, syncope, cardiac arrhythmias, or respiratory paralysis. The synthetic amphetamine DMDA, better known as "ecstasy," has been linked to the recent rise of the so-called "rave" phenomenon of all-night revelry under the influence of hallucinogens (Miller & Gold, 1991).

The management of a mild to moderate psychostimulant intoxication requires a quiet room where safety measures may be applied for the protection of the patient and staff. If reassurance is not sufficient to calm the patient, sedation with benzodiazepines (e.g., diazepam, 10 to 30 mg P.O. or lorazepam, 1 to 3 mg IM or IV) may control agitation. Physical restraints may become necessary. Vital signs should be monitored closely for rising blood pressure, pulse, and temperature. Treatment with neuroleptics is recommended when the blood pressure, pulse rate, or temperature is rising, or if acute paranoid behavior develops, provided no anticholinergic drugs were involved in the intoxication. It should be noted that chlorpromazine, although an effective antidote, has strong anticholinergic effects. The drug of choice is haloperidol in an initial dose of 3 to 5 mg P.O. or IM, with subsequent doses adjusted according to need. Increased fluids and acidification of urine with ammonium chloride can significantly enhance excretion of the drug (Berger & Tinklenberg, 1979). If psychosis is present or elevated vital signs persist in spite of adequate treatment, the patient requires hospitalization. The possibility of suicidal depression during withdrawal must be considered.

305.20 CANNABIS INTOXICATION

In moderate doses, cannabis acts as a sedative, while at high doses, it acts as an hallucinogen. Hashish, "hash oil," and tetrahydrocannabinol (THC) are much more potent than cannabis and are more likely to induce visual, auditory, or tactile illusions or hallucinations with intact reality testing (Balis, 1974).

Mild cannabis intoxication is relatively short-lived and does not generally require intervention. "Bad trips" resulting from cannabis-induced acute panic, hallucinations, and delusions are generally managed by "talk-down" or with a benzodiazepine (see "Hallucinogen Psychotic Disorder," Chapter 5).

305.90 PHENCYCLIDINE (PCP) (OR RELATED SUBSTANCE) INTOXICATION

This intoxication presents with belligerent, assaultive, impulsive, and unpredictable behavior; agitation; impaired judgment, and/or impaired social functioning during or shortly after use. It may be accompanied by nystagmus, hypertension, tachycardia, ataxia, dysarthria, hyperacusis, diminished responsiveness to pain, muscle rigidity, seizures, or coma. Illusions, altered perceptions, or hallucinations with intact reality testing may exist as well.

Severe PCP intoxication is characterized by motor inhibition and catatonic-like states, stupor, coma with eyes remaining open, seizures, opisthotonos, hyperreflexia, severe hypertension, and/or respiratory depression. Bloody vomiting suggests contamination by a synthetic intermediate that decomposes to hydrogen cyanide. The absence of mydriasis and the presence of ataxia, hypertension, and nystagmus differentiate PCP intoxication from hallucinogen intoxication. Delirium, mood disorder, and psychotic disorder may develop.

In low-dose intoxication, the key to management is sensory reduction and protection from self-harm. The patient should be kept in a quiet room, closely supervised from a distance. Physical restraint may be necessary. For sedation, diazepam or haloperidol is the drug of choice. In moderate to severe intoxication, close observation, with monitoring of blood pressure, respiration, and level of consciousness, is required. If status epilepticus develops, diazepam in 2- to 3-mg increments by slow IV is indicated. Acidification of the urine with ammonium chloride or vitamin C markedly enhances PCP excretion. Continuous or intermittent gastric suction has been recommended as a means of enhancing PCP excretion. Prolonged psychotic reactions following PCP intoxication are discussed under "Phencyclidine Psychotic Disorder" (Chapter 5).

305.90 CAFFEINE INTOXICATION

Presenting with restlessness, anxiety, excitement, insomnia, diuresis, agitation, tachycardia or cardiac arrhythmias, muscle twitching, and rambling speech, the toxic symptoms subside rapidly after reduction of intake or abstinence. Transient withdrawal symptoms may occur in chronic heavy users. No pharmacological treatment is necessary. A massive overdose may result in seizures that can be controlled with IV diazepam.

305.90 INHALANT INTOXICATION

This includes intoxication by inhaling the aliphatic and aromatic hydrocarbons found in gasoline, glue, paint, paint thinners, and spray paints, and, to a lesser extent, halogenated hydrocarbons found in cleaners, spray can propellants, and other volatile substances. The essential features are similar to those of alcohol and sedative-hypnotic-anxiolytic intoxication and include maladaptive behavior changes and physical signs of incoordination, nystagmus, slurred speech, unsteady gait, tremor, blurred vision or diplopia, generalized muscle weakness, depressed reflexes, and stupor or coma. The onset of intoxication is quick, and the course is short (one to one and a half hours). Medical complications of long-term solvent abuse include renal dysfunction, cardiac irregularity, and neurological complications that consist of cerebellar and cortical impairment and a potentially irreversible encephalopathy (Byrne *et al.*, 1991). Anecdotal case reports of serious psychiatric disorders, including psychosis, suggest the need for more studies.

During intoxication, treatment is primarily directed toward management of aggressive or assaultive behavior through behavioral interventions, or physical restraints, if necessary. In more serious intoxications involving CNS depression, cardiac arrhythmias, or seizures, treatment is largely supportive (see "General Treatment Principles").

Patients should be assessed for damage to the CNS, peripheral nervous system, kidneys, liver, lungs, heart, and bone marrow. Tests for heavy metal (e.g., lead) should be ordered, and chelating agents used as indicated. Although not well documented, withdrawal seizures and withdrawal delirium may occur in chronic heavy users (Barnes, 1979; Westermeyer, 1987). Long-term psychosocial treatment and rehabilitation are discussed in Chapter 15.

305.90 OTHER SUBSTANCE INTOXICATION

This classification includes intoxication with anesthetic gases (e.g., nitrous oxide, ether), short-acting vasodilator drugs (such as amyl or butyl nitrite), and anabolic steroids, as well as other intoxications that are relevant to psychiatric practice.

Anticholinergic drug intoxication is of particular interest because of the many prescription and over-the-counter drugs that have anticholinergic activity. Severe intoxication is characterized by (1) dilated and unreactive pupils, flushed face, warm and dry skin, dry mouth, paralytic ileus, urinary retention, tachycardia, hypertension or hypotension, increased respiratory rate, seizures, and/or hyperpyrexia; and (2) delirium, hallucinations, delusions, severe agitation and assaultiveness, stupor, and/or coma. Excessive use of anticholinergics, especially in association with other drugs, insufficient perspiration, the presence of heat-generating tremor; and/or elevated ambient temperature, can produce a hypermetabolic state or malignant hyperthermia similar to the neuroleptic malignant syndrome.

Patient management includes the usual measures for overdosage (emesis, gastric lavage, maintenance of cardiopulmonary functions, monitoring of vital signs), continuous ECG monitoring, and symptomatic treatment of anticholinergic effects. Physostigmine salicylate, 2 mg IV, reverses the coma and controls delirium, hyperthermia, and supraventricular tachycardia secondary to anticholinergic toxicity. A second dose of 1 to 2 mg of physostigmine may be given 15 minutes later. Physostigmine has a very short half-life; patients should be continuously monitored and additional doses provided as needed.

In milder cases, agitation may be controlled with diazepam, provided vital functions are stable and the patient is fully conscious. Seizures can be controlled with IV diazepam. In tricyclic intoxication, cardiac arrhythmias, other than supraventricular tachycardia, are treated with IV fluids and alkalinization with sodium bicarbonate or sodium lactate. If there is no improvement, propranolol and lidocaine may be useful. Prolonged ECG monitoring is extremely important for diagnosing cardiac arrhythmias and as a means of assessing the severity of tricyclic intoxication. The latter correlates with the degree of widening of the QRS complex and prolongation of the QT interval.

Anabolic-androgenic steroids are primarily used by athletes and young persons for body building (Yesalis *et al.*, 1993). Repeated use produces a sense of enhanced well-being and euphoria, increased energy, and altered libido, often followed by (or alternating with) dysphoria, irritability, suicidal thoughts, and/or aggressive behavior. Their long-term effects are largely unknown (Uzych, 1992 but may include hostility (Strauss, *et al.*, 1985; Yesalis *et al.*, 1993), aggressive behavior, and loss of control with minimal provocation ("roid rage") (Perry, *et al.*, 1990; Pope & Katz, 1990). Chronic use may also lead to depression, mania, psychosis, and liver disease (Pope & Katz, 1988). Psychosocial treatment and rehabilitation are discussed in Chapter 15.

Nitrous oxide (laughing gas) is used for its euphoriant effect; chronic use may cause paranoid states. Nitrite inhalants (poppers) are mild euphoriant drugs often used for their alleged aphrodisiac effect. Plant intoxicants include peyote, catnip, betel nut, kava, and absinthe. General treatment and rehabilitation principles are found in Chapter 15.

CHAPTER 14

WITHDRAWAL/DETOXIFICATION

Withdrawal includes all manifestations of the "abstinence sickness" except delirium. Common symptoms include anxiety, restlessness, irritability, insomnia, and impaired attention. The nature of the substance determines additional symptoms. The course is generally self-limited, unless it becomes complicated with delirium or seizures (e.g., in severe alcohol or sedative, hypnotic, anxiolytic withdrawal).

GENERAL TREATMENT PRINCIPLES

The treatment goal is to eliminate physiological dependence without allowing the development of the withdrawal syndrome. This procedure is based on decreasing doses, either of the abused drug or one that is cross-tolerant to it. Loss of physiological dependence does not necessarily cure underlying psychological dependence.

The site of detoxification (inpatient, outpatient, residential) is based on a number of considerations, including the type of substance, available resources, and the individual's lifestyle. In general, opiate detoxification can be done in an outpatient setting. Alcohol, in a severely addicted patient, should generally be withdrawn in a hospital setting; however, patients with mild to moderate withdrawal reactions can be managed at home or in a specialized residential setting. Serious barbiturate-type and/or polydrug dependence usually requires a hospital setting to prevent life-threatening complications. Amphetamine and cocaine withdrawal may require hospitalization in the presence of significant suicidal risk.

A detoxification treatment plan should follow certain general guidelines (Czechowicz, 1978). Whenever possible, a long-acting drug should be substituted for a cross-tolerant short-acting drug. The initial amount of the drug required to suppress withdrawal symptoms is determined empirically, by assessing symptom response to repeated drug dosages (e.g., in alcohol withdrawal) or through a challenge test (e.g., as in barbiturate withdrawal). The detoxification procedure should be safe and geared to provide a comfortable withdrawal. The patient should be closely monitored for signs and symptoms of withdrawal or intoxication in order to titrate dosage and the pacing of withdrawal. Provision should be made for an aftercare plan with appropriate further treatment and rehabilitation.

SPECIFIC WITHDRAWAL DISORDERS—DETOXIFICATION

291.80 ALCOHOL WITHDRAWAL

This disorder presents with autonomic hyperactivity (e.g., sweating, tachycardia), hand tremor, insomnia, nausea or vomiting, transient illusions or hallucinations, anxiety, and possible grand mal seizures. Illusions and hallucinations, if present, occur with intact reality testing and in a clear sensorium. The severity of the syndrome depends on the amount, frequency, and duration of prior alcohol consumption. Seizures occur in about 12% of inadequately treated patients. They are more likely to take place during delirium, and in those with a prior history of withdrawal seizures (Josephson & Sabatier, 1978). When they arise, they must be thoroughly evaluated to rule out other causes (e.g., head injury).

There are several pharmacological and nonpharmacological treatment regimens for alcohol withdrawal. Advocates of nonpharmacological management have claimed high success rates by capitalizing on the fact that most symptoms of alcohol withdrawal are evanescent, and can be managed with supportive care. The prudent clinician recognizes that supportive therapy is not effective against hallucinations, seizures, or cardiac arrhythmias, and that moderate to severe withdrawal should be managed pharmacologically.

Alcohol-dependent patients usually should be withdrawn in a hospital setting, such as a specialized detoxification unit, with cross-tolerant drugs. Any of several benzodiazepines are drugs of choice. In the loading dose technique, dosages are titrated to levels just suppressing withdrawal symptoms (e.g., lorazepam, 1 to 2 mg P.O. or IV; diazepam, 10 to 20 mg P.O.; or oxazepam, 30 to 60 mg P.O., administered every one or two hours until symptoms improve). Following stabilization, the benzediazepine is tapered and discontinued over several days. Some alcohol detoxification protocols are based on the as-needed use of benzodiazepines, administered when autonomic symptoms are present (tachycardia, high blood pressure). This technique may be more appropriate for milder withdrawal syndromes.

Additional treatment measures include metabolic interventions (for correcting hypoglycemia, hypophosphatemia, electrolyte and water imbalances) and nutrition supplementation (calories, thiamine and B complex vitamins, vitamin K for prothrombin deficiency). Seizures complicating alcohol withdrawal are treated with a loading dose of phenytoin, for example, 10 mg/kg infused IV at a rate of 50 mg/min, followed by 300 to 400 mg daily for one week. Prophylactic phenytoin probably has no routine value if seizures are absent, unless the patient has a history of epilepsy or prior episodes of withdrawal seizures. In such cases, the patient should receive 100 mg phenytoin, three times a day for five days, in combination with a benzodiazepine (Sellers *et al.*, 1983).

Many other drugs have been recommended by various practitioners. The evidence for their efficacy awaits more critical assessment. Neuroleptics have been used extensively to control symptoms other than seizures and delirium. They are especially indicated for hallucinations (Sellers & Kalant, 1982). Carbamazepine and valproic acid have been reported as effective and safe as oxazepam for alcohol withdrawal (Malcolm *et al.*, 1989); carbamazepine must not be prescribed for patients taking clozapine.

The capacity of α-adrenergic receptor agonists to reduce catecholamine levels has been used in alcohol withdrawal, as it has in opioid withdrawal. Thus, both clonidine (Baumgartner & Rowen, 1987) and lofexidine have been found effective in placebo-controlled studies of detoxification. The beta-blockers (e.g., propranolol) can also alleviate minor alcohol withdrawal symptoms (Sellers *et al.*, 1977), especially tremor, but their usefulness with regard to suppressing withdrawal seizures and delirium has been questioned (Luiskow & Reed, 1986). The same appears to be true of the α-adrenergic receptor agonists. On the other hand, a combination of the beta-blocker atenolol with oxazepam, in a random double-blind study, proved to be effective and safe (Kraus *et al.*, 1985).

Outmoded treatments for alcohol detoxification, such as paraldehyde and IV (pure) or oral (beverage) ethanol, continue to be seen, particularly in non-psychiatric departments (Howell & Kane, 1993).

291.1X, 292.89 COMPLICATED ALCOHOL WITHDRAWAL

Alcohol withdrawal delirium (delirium tremens, or DTs) is a serious complication that occurs in about 5% of cases and may occasionally lead to death from other intercurrent complications. Treatment is discussed under withdrawal-related delirium in Chapter 3. Psychotic, mood, anxiety, and sleep disorders with onset during alcohol withdrawal are also discussed in their respective chapters in **Part I.**

292.00 SEDATIVE, HYPNOTIC, OR ANXIOLYTIC WITHDRAWAL

Barbiturates, similarly acting sedative-hypnotic drugs (e.g., ethchlorvynol, glutethimide, methyprylon, chloral hydrate, paraldehyde, methaqualone), and anxiolytic drugs (meprobamate and benzodiazepines) produce a withdrawal syndrome almost identical to that of alcohol. As with alcohol, it may lead to grand mal seizures and may progress to a delirium.

Withdrawal from short-acting barbiturate dependence (e.g., pentobarbital, amobarbital) begins 12 to 24 hours after the last dose. Seizures most often take place between the third and seventh day; status epilepticus may occur if seizures are not prevented. Withdrawal delirium most often happens between the fourth and sixth day. Convulsions associated with withdrawal from long-acting benzodiazepines (especially diazepam) can occur several weeks after discontinuing the drug. In severely addicted patients, detoxification should generally be carried out in a hospital setting. Tapered withdrawal may be accomplished by phenobarbital substitution, pentobarbital substitution, or slow withdrawal of the addicting agent (Czechowicz, 1978).

Phenobarbital Substitution

The stabilization dose of phenobarbital is tentatively calculated on the basis of the patient's history and by monitoring response to the drug. The initial daily requirement is calculated by substituting one sedative dose (30 mg) of phenobarbital for each hypnotic dose of any reported sedative-hypnotic. Thirty milligrams of phenobarbital is equivalent to about 100 mg of most short-acting barbiturates (e.g., amobarbital, pentobarbital, secobarbital), 500 mg chloral hydrate, 350 mg of ethchlorvynol, 250 mg of glutethimide, 400 to 600 mg of meprobamate, 250 to 300 mg of methaqualone, or 300 mg of methyprylon.

The initial total daily dose of phenobarbital should never exceed 600 mg, regardless of the dosage claimed by the patient. The established daily requirement is given in divided doses, three or four times daily. If toxic symptoms occur (sedation, slurred speech, nystagmus, ataxia), the daily dose should be reduced. The patient should be maintained on the stabilization dosage for two days before graded withdrawal is initiated. Once this is achieved, the total daily dose of phenobarbital is reduced by 30 mg/day. During this period, the patient should be closely monitored for signs of acute withdrawal or phenobarbital toxicity, so that the dosage can be titrated accordingly.

Pentobarbital Substitution

In cases involving dependence on a short-acting barbiturate, the pentobarbital challenge test helps to establish the degree of barbiturate tolerance (and thus dependence) and to determine the initial pentobarbital requirement. A standard dose of 200 mg is given orally at two-hour intervals until signs of barbiturate toxicity are elicited. No further treatment is necessary if 400 mg or less results in intoxication. If no signs of intoxication are present, one continues the challenge until signs of mild intoxication are produced. The total amount of pentobarbital given becomes the stabilization dose. After a two-day period of stabilization, the pentobarbital is gradually withdrawn by 10% of the total drug dosage per day, not to exceed 100 mg/day. The rate and amount of reduction may need to be adjusted if withdrawal or toxic signs occur. Once the stabilization dose is established with pentobarbital, an equivalent dose of phenobarbital may be used instead of pentobarbital, because of its longer half-life. In the case of barbiturate withdrawal delirium, the patient should be sedated to the point of mild intoxication and stabilized (suppression of all withdrawal symptoms) for two days before detoxification is started. In extreme agitation, the initial dose of sedative is given IV (e.g., 5 mg lorazepam, 10 mg diazepam, or 500 mg amobarbital).

Slow withdrawal without substitution may be used in patients dependent on benzodiazepines, long-acting sedative-hypnotics, or mixed sedative-hypnotics. Detoxification of reliable patients may be accomplished in an outpatient setting if appropriate monitoring is available. The patient is initially given the addicting drug at his or her current daily intake level, and then is gradually withdrawn at a rate of about 20% of the total dosage per day. Benzodiazepines require special consideration. Withdrawal from benzodiazepines must be differentiated from rebound, the latter being defined as recurrence of the original symptoms of illness at a level greater than baseline. As with all cross-tolerant members of this class of drugs, the high-dose withdrawal syndrome is more likely to be associated with delirium and seizures. Short-acting benzodiazepines produce more severe withdrawal symptoms than do long-acting ones (Busto, *et al.*, 1986). Short-acting benzodiazepines are also more frequently implicated in seizures during withdrawal (Perry & Alexander, 1986).

Seizures tend to occur early in the withdrawal of short-acting benzodiazepines (e.g., after one to four days with lorazepam) and later with the longer-acting (up to 27 days with diazepam) (Busto *et al.*, 1986). Alexander and Perry (1991) estimate that when seizures are destined to occur, a short-acting benzodiazepines with a half-life that is 25% that of a long-acting benzodiazepine results in the occurrence of seizures in half the time of a long-acting drug. Patients often describe particular difficulty in withdrawing from alprazolam; delirium and seizures are relatively common in those who are not slowly tapered from previously high doses.

When withdrawing from therapeutic doses of benzodiazepines, the drug should be gradually tapered over a one- to two-week period, on an outpatient basis. If the patient has been taking a short-acting benzodiazepine (e.g., alprazolam), he or she should usually be placed on an equivalent dose of a long-acting benzodiazepine (e.g., diazepam), and then tapered at about 20% per week (Alexander & Perry, 1991). Reports on the use of propranolol, clonidine, carbamazepine, and antidepressants in withdrawing patients from benzodiazepines are interesting, but require further research.

Several DSM-IV psychotic, mood, and anxiety syndromes present additional withdrawal phenomena associated with this class of drugs, and are listed under different codes (e.g., with or without hallucinations or delusions). They must be differentiated from similar syndromes that occur during intoxication, and are discussed in their respective chapters in **Part I.**

292.0 OPIOID WITHDRAWAL

Such withdrawal presents with dysphoric mood, nausea or vomiting, diarrhea, lacrimation or rhinorrhea, pupillary dilation, piloerection or sweating, yawning, insomnia, muscle aches, and/or fever. Opioid drugs include morphine and codeine; the semisynthetics heroin, oxymorphone, and hydromorphone; and the purely synthetic meperidine, methadone, levomethadyl acetate, and fentanyl. They also include some designer drugs (analogues of meperidine and fentanyl acetate).

The time of onset and duration of the syndrome vary with the drug (e.g., shortest course with hydromorphone, longest with levomethadyl). Heroin and morphine withdrawal syndromes begin 8 to 12 hours following the last dose and gradually subside over 7 to 10 days. Dependence may be demonstrated by the naloxone test (0.4 mg IM naloxone, which will precipitate withdrawal symptoms in opioid-dependent individuals), although most clinicians no longer rely on naloxone challenge to diagnose opioid dependence.

Detoxification can be carried out in an inpatient, residential, or outpatient setting, using opioid agonists (e.g., methadone, LAAM) or certain nonopioids (e.g., clonidine).

Opioid Agonists

The methadone method uses methadone substitution. When carried out in a hospital setting, the standard approach is to give an initial dose of 10 to 20 mg of oral methadone. If withdrawal symptoms are not suppressed, an additional 5 to 10 mg may be given. Most patients require no more than 20 to 40 mg per day (Jaffe, 1995); the total daily dose should not exceed 40 mg. Once the stabilizing dose of methadone is estimated, the patient is maintained on that level, with divided doses twice a day, for two or three days. Detoxification then begins, with a reduction each day by 15 to 20% of the total daily dose. Withdrawal is completed in 5 to 10 days.

Detoxification from methadone itself is commonly done on an outpatient basis in methadone treatment clinics. Patients with concurrent drug dependencies or medical or psychiatric problems may require inpatient care. Inpatient detoxification requires prior confirmation of maintenance dosage and enrollment in a methadone maintenance program. In these patients, the detoxification period should last longer, extending over several weeks at a reduction rate of 3 to 5 mg/day. Some clinicians recommend outpatient withdrawal from methadone maintenance by a process of gradual detoxification over four to six months, with a dose decrement of approximately 3% per week. A recent study by Kanof, and associates (1993) found that the development of an organic mood syndrome is common in patients undergoing slow detoxification, and is associated with a poor outcome. The prophylactic use of antidepressants in these patients has not been well studied.

Levomethadyl (LAAM) has been successfully used in outpatient withdrawal from heroin. It may be given infrequently (e.g., only three times per week); however, LAAM takes longer to achieve initial stabilization than does methadone (Jaffe, 1995). Buprenorphine, in injectable form, has also been successfully used for the detoxification of hospitalized opioid-dependent patients (Parran *et al.*, 1994).

Nonopioids

Clonidine Method. Numerous reports have documented the effectiveness of the α-adrenergic receptor agonist clonidine for suppressing the symptoms of opioid withdrawal (Cami *et al.*, 1985). Compared with methadone, clonidine appears to be more effective in suppressing autonomic signs of abstinence, but less effective in reducing subject-reported symptoms and discomfort (Jasinski, *et al.*, 1985). Major side effects include hypotension and sedation. One recommended regimen is to begin with clonidine, 0.2 mg every six hours P.O. the first day, adjust the dose to 0.8 to 1.2 mg/day in divided doses for the next 7 to 10 days, and then taper downward over two to three days. A transdermal clonidine patch has been used at doses ranging from 0.4 to 0.6 mg per day. Clonidine is withheld if the blood pressure drops to 90/60 mmHg or below. The usual dosage for outpatient use is 0.1 to 0.3 mg three times a day, with an upper limit of 1.2 mg per day.

It appears that clonidine is a reasonably safe and effective drug for detoxifying selected opiate addicts, especially those being directly detoxified from illicit opioids or patients who have been stabilized on relatively low doses of methadone. It may be best suited for detoxifying patients selected pending naltrexone therapy. Clonidine has no effect on relapse rates following detoxification (Jaffe, 1995). Hartman *et al.* (1991) found that acetorphan, an enkephalinase inhibitor, may be safe and effective in opioid withdrawal.

Accelerated Withdrawal/Rapid Detoxification

Opioid antagonists (e.g., naltrexone) have been used to precipitate opioid withdrawal as a means of shortening the time it takes for the acute withdrawal symptoms to resolve (thus shortening hospitalization). The method can be used in either an inpatient or a day hospital setting. Clonidine (0.1 mg three times daily), augmented by a benzodiazepine for nighttime sedation, is used to control the withdrawal syndrome precipitated by naltrexone (Jaffe, 1995).

The DSM-IV provides a separate code for opioid sleep disorder with onset during withdrawal (292.89). See Chapter 12.

292.0 AMPHETAMINE (OR RELATED SUBSTANCE) WITHDRAWAL

It consists of a dysphoric mood accompanied by fatigue; vivid, unpleasant dreams; insomnia or hypersomnia; increased appetite; agitation; and/or psychomotor retardation. It may progress during the first two weeks to a major depression with significant suicidal risk, which may persist for weeks or longer. In the presence of suicidal risk, detoxification should be carried out in a controlled environment and under close observation, preferably in a psychiatric hospital. The addicting drug should be promptly discontinued and the patient placed on suicide precautions if necessary.

Severe agitation or delirium upon admission may be treated initially with moderate doses of a neuroleptic, which should be tapered and discontinued shortly after control of the target symptoms. The presence of concurrent and persisting delusions (amphetamine psychotic disorder) calls for a neuroleptic. If a persistent depressive episode develops, antidepressants may be necessary, following guidelines applicable to depressive disorders. Psychotherapeutic management and psychosocial counseling should also be provided (Berger & Tinklenberg, 1979), as well as referral to a drug or mood disorders treatment program prior to discharge. Treatment of amphetamine intoxication and dependence is discussed in Chapters 13 and 15.

292.0 COCAINE WITHDRAWAL

Contrary to earlier reports, the prolonged use of cocaine causes physiological dependence and a characteristic withdrawal syndrome upon abrupt discontinuation, which has been described as triphasic withdrawal (Kleber & Gawin, 1987). More recent investigators (Satel, et al., 1991) have argued that only the early "crash" represents a short-term abstinence. In our view, cocaine and amphetamine withdrawal can best be understood as depletion syndromes (most likely involving dopamine), rather than as syndromes involving the classic mechanism of abstinence. In this regard, they are analogous to the model of reserpine-induced depression. Past suggestions for using dopamine agonists (e.g., bromocriptine, amantadine) in cocaine detoxification (Giannini, et al., 1989) as a means of correcting an alleged central dopamine dysfunction have not received support from more recent studies (Satel et al., 1991).

The clinical syndrome, as well as the treatment and management of cocaine withdrawal, similar to that of amphetamine withdrawal (see above). Cocaine intoxication and dependence are discussed in Chapters 13 and 15.

292.0 NICOTINE WITHDRAWAL

This withdrawal presents with dysphoric mood, insomnia, irritability or anger, anxiety, restlessness, difficulty concentrating, decreased heart rate, and increased appetite or weight gain. Treatment is discussed in Chapter 15.

MIXED-DRUG WITHDRAWAL

In mixed-substance dependencies, detoxification should proceed with the gradual withdrawal of one drug at a time, while stabilizing the patient on the other drug(s) on which he or she is dependent. In combined heroin and barbiturate dependence, it is preferable to withdraw the barbiturate first, while stabilizing the patient on methadone. In combined alcohol and barbiturate dependence, the detoxification procedure is similar to that for other sedative-hypnotic-anxiolytic dependence, since the substances are cross-tolerant and have an additive effect. One must calculate the phenobarbital equivalent of alcohol (about 15 mg of phenobarbital per ounce of 80 to 100 proof alcohol) and add it to the phenobarbital equivalent of the sedative-hypnotic. In combined opiate and alcohol dependence, one should begin with alcohol detoxification while stabilizing the patient on methadone, and then proceed with methadone withdrawal (Czechowicz, 1978).

CHAPTER 15

SUBSTANCE DEPENDENCE/ABUSE

This diagnostic class defines disorders with maladaptive behavioral changes associated with the pathologic use of psychoactive substances. They are divided into substance dependence and substance abuse. Other Axis I and Axis II mental disorders are often comorbid (dual diagnosis).

Substance dependence has been redefined by new criteria in the DSM-IV. The essential feature is a cluster of cognitive, behavioral, and physiological symptoms that constitute a dependence syndrome. Substance abuse is a residual category in which maladaptive patterns of psychoactive substance use have never met the criteria for dependence.

In addition to syndromes of intoxication, withdrawal, and dependence/abuse, substance use may also become complicated by a number of substance-specific mental disorders, including delirium, dementia, amnestic disorder, mood disorder, psychotic disorder, anxiety disorder, personality change, sleep disorder, and sexual dysfunction. These are discussed in **Part I.**

GENERAL THERAPEUTIC PRINCIPLES

The field is replete with treatment approaches based on diverse theories and ideologies, with claims of therapeutic successes that, for the most part, lack objective substantiation. Most are founded on the disease concept of alcoholism and drug addiction.

Currently available treatment modalities include:

- Pharmacological methods, such as disulfiram for alcoholism, narcotic maintenance and narcotic antagonists for opioid dependence, and various psychotropic drugs for the short-term management of targeted symptoms following detoxification.

- Psychosocial methods, such as individual, group, family, and conjoint psychotherapy; contingency contracting; behavior modification; aversive conditioning; community reinforcement; and relaxation techniques.
- Sociotherapies, such as specialized therapeutic communities (e.g., Synanon) and other residential programs.
- Self-support groups, such as Alcoholics Anonymous (AA), Narcotics Anonymous (NA), Dual Recovery Anonymous, and such groups as Al-Anon and Alateen for family members.
- Various therapeutic, educational, occupational, inspirational, or humane programs supported or sponsored by government agencies, private industry, religious groups, or volunteer organizations.
- Systems for the regular monitoring of urine for drugs, through employee assistance programs and other organizations.

Seven general guidelines should be considered in treatment planning.

1. No single treatment modality can claim high effectiveness for chemical dependence; a combination is usually required to achieve a measure of therapeutic success.
2. The choice of treatment modalities must be tailored to the individual, taking into consideration his or her specific problems, response to previous treatment attempts, and available resources.
3. Different treatment approaches are administered by a great variety of professionals, nonprofessional practitioners, and lay groups. The physician should play a central role in the initial evaluation and diagnosis, management of physical-psychiatric complications, detoxification, and appropriate referral. In follow-up care, the physician may apply some of the specific methods available, or may collaborate with other practitioners and agencies involved in treatment and rehabilitation.
4. Detoxification is a prerequisite for any treatment plan (see "Withdrawal," Chapter 14).
5. Chemical dependency treatment programs based on 12-step principles are widespread, reporting a 50% response rate 12 months after discharge. There is good evidence to suggest that some chemically dependent individuals can recover without adherence to the 12 steps, if alternative methods are strictly applied.
6. The presence of associated psychopathology (dual diagnosis) requires specialized psychiatric treatment, especially in mood disorders and some personality disorders (e.g., antisocial or borderline personality).

7. The socially dislocated individual (e.g., unemployed, homeless, legally entangled, or culturally alienated) requires social and vocational rehabilitation aimed toward reintegration into family, community, and/or work.

Most treatment models rely on 12-step programs as the cornerstone of recovery support, and incorporate elements of intervention, education, empathic confrontation of denial, training in relapse prevention skills, and developing an intensive, ongoing program of recovery based on use of both self-help and professionally led groups (Minkoff, 1994). Pharmacotherapy for addiction continues to be an adjunctive rather than primary tool in rehabilitation.

Factors suggesting good treatment outcome include:

- Patience and perseverance in the face of very difficult and frustrating patients and chronic and relapsing disorders. These should be tempered by a realistic appraisal of the patient's potential and limitations, and by an awareness of transference-countertransference problems.
- Maintenance of abstinence during treatment. Abstinence, not controlled substance use, is the ultimate treatment goal.
- A degree of program coerciveness, which may range, as clinically appropriate, from subtle measures of substance control to involuntary commitment to a treatment facility. Coerciveness may take the form of "contracts" that the patient is persuaded or forced to make with the therapist, spouse, or employer. Structured environments and disulfiram administered under supervision are other examples.
- Regular and/or random urine testing. This is a key aspect of successful management.
- Breaking through massive denial. Strong efforts must be made during the initial phase of treatment to help the patient recognize and accept the full scope of the problem.
- Maintaining wavering motivation. The patient must stay in treatment and remain abstinent. Some therapists have adopted cognitive-behavioral models (e.g., network therapy), in which "social cohesiveness" is used as a vehicle for engaging patients in office treatment, avoiding dropping out, and increasing compliance. Family members and peers may join the therapy process to increase the therapeutic network.
- Developing alternative coping styles to handle intense dysphoric affects, especially rage, guilt, anxiety, and depression. Self-esteem must be bolstered and maintained. Whenever feasible, environmental contingencies and social factors that may precipitate relapse should be controlled, either by the patient (e.g., by avoiding them) or by the treatment program.

TREATING THE DUALLY DIAGNOSED PATIENT

Minkoff (1994) suggests a unified framework for dually diagnosed patients that subdivides the recovery process into four specific phases: acute stabilization, engagement, prolonged rehabilitation, and rehabilitation/recovery. This model proposes that the treatment of addiction in psychiatric populations is basically the same as in nonpsychiatric populations, with such modifications as special preparation and training for 12-step programs, a modified 12-step program called Dual Recovery Anonymous (DRA), and a comprehensive range of services for each disease (e.g., crisis stabilization/detoxification, recovery/rehabilitation support, case management, family support and education, positive social networks, and residential/day programs) (Ridgely, 1991; Minkoff, 1994). For some dually diagnosed patients, especially those with a comorbid major psychiatric disorder, pharmacotherapy is important, and requires special considerations of medication choice and treatment compliance.

SPECIFIC SUBSTANCE USE DISORDERS

303.90 ALCOHOL DEPENDENCE
305.00 ALCOHOL ABUSE

Detoxification must take place before treatment (see "Withdrawal," Chapter 14).

Basic Principles

A professionally led comprehensive treatment program is the best approach. Such a program may include inpatient and free-standing rehabilitation programs, day hospitals, outpatient programs, office practice, and self-help programs. Residential treatment for two to four weeks is often the first step following detoxification. In addition to a 12-step model, the treatment plan may also include individual, group, family, and/or conjoint therapy; disulfiram; and short-term tranquilizers or antidepressants for targeted psychopathology. The patient should be urged to join AA and to attend meetings regularly. Al-Anon provides assistance to spouses of alcoholics, while Alateen serves the needs of children of alcoholic parents. A good prognosis is correlated with higher socioeconomic status and social class, the absence of medical and psychiatric problems, a positive work history, previous AA contact, and the absence of a family history of alcoholism.

The primary physician plays a crucial role in diagnosis and treatment. Dealing with the patient's denial is an early and decisive task. One strategy is to give the patient the Michigan Alcoholism Screening Test (MAST), a reliable and valid test for diagnosing alcoholism. An authoritative demonstration of the problem may serve as the first step in weakening the patient's defensive armor. With acceptance of the problem and the establishment of a therapeutic alliance, the physician can proceed to negotiate a therapeutic contract. In the absence of a therapeutic alliance, coercion by the patient's employer, family, probation officer, or teacher, coupled with breathalyzer monitoring is a prerequisite in the early stages of care.

Long-term abstinence should be the goal. If this is not possible, a trial period of abstinence is an acceptable compromise. The contract should include a means to deter drinking and ways to monitor compliance. Disulfiram may prove helpful as a temporary deterrent in selected cases; a challenge dose of alcohol after disulfiram is not necessary. The patient must be fully instructed about the consequences of drinking within four days of ingestion of the drug.

Disulfiram is given at bedtime in a loading dose of 500 mg daily for five to seven days, then continued on a daily maintenance dose of 250 mg. A spouse or some other person should be involved in administering the disulfiram at least every three or four days to ensure compliance. Another method is to have the patient visit the therapist every three or four days during the first month to monitor ingestion of the drug. During these brief visits, the emphasis is on talking about problems most alcoholics face when they stop drinking. After a month or so, a new contract is negotiated, with the patient assuming responsibility for controlling the drinking.

Psychotherapies

The usual psychotherapeutic approach is primarily supportive. The therapist plays an active and nurturing role while maintaining clear boundaries of separateness and setting firm limits that discourage acting out. So-called recovery-oriented psychotherapy (Zweben, 1986) operationalizes the changing ways in which the therapist can assist the patient in the phase-specific tasks of recovery. Intensive insight-oriented psychotherapy has not been effective in maintaining abstinence.

Family therapy is a valuable and often necessary adjunct to treatment of the substance-dependent individual, particularly when integrated into a comprehensive program. It can be crucial in the treatment of dysfunctional family systems associated with alcohol abuse.

Pharmacotherapy

When clinical conditions allow, a drug-free treatment regimen is recommended, especially during the first two to three weeks following detoxification (Pattison, 1986). Recent studies have shown the opiate antagonist naltrexone to be an effective adjunct in the treatment of alcohol dependence, significantly reducing relapse rates, drinking days, and craving (O'Malley *et al.*, 1992; Volpicelli, *et al.*, 1992). Lower alcohol consumption may be the result of naltrexone's blockage of the "high" produced by alcohol, or its influence on the "priming effect" of an initial drink or craving (O'Malley *et al.*, 1995).

Social Support

Halfway houses are often important for patients with placement problems following detoxification and hospital discharge. Referral to vocational rehabilitation and social support agencies may be required in selected cases. In most communities, a multimodal treatment approach is available.

Dual Diagnosis

A primary psychiatric disorder may play a causative role in the development of alcoholism or, conversely, alcoholism may be a destabilizing factor in a primary psychiatric disorder. Schizophrenia, mood disorders, severe anxiety, borderline personality, antisocial personality, and bulimia nervosa are common. Treatment should be provided concurrently with that for the substance-related disorder. Outcome studies of tricyclic antidepressants and lithium for depression in alcoholics show equivocal success, except for patients in whom a primary mood disorder can be diagnosed (Weiss & Mirin, 1989). A placebo-controlled trial showed that although fluoxetine (60 mg/day) does not prevent alcohol abuse relapse in nondepressed alcoholics, it does improve depressive symptoms in those with comorbid major depression. A 12-week trial of buspirone in anxious alcoholics resulted in reduced anxiety, a slower return to heavy drinking, and fewer drinking days during a follow-up period (Kranzler *et al.*, 1994).

304.00 OPIOID DEPENDENCE
305.50 OPIOID ABUSE

Treatment programs for the opioid (mainly heroin) addict include maintenance with opioid agonists, maintenance with opioid antagonists, therapeutic communities, and abstinence-oriented recovery programs. Most of these provide a combination of adjunctive approaches, such as group therapy, improvement of social skills, vocational training, job placement, and family counseling.

Treatment

Methadone. Methadone maintenance is the most common and most successful treatment for opioid dependence. It is offered in federally regulated clinics under close supervision and monitoring. Unlike heroin, methadone is long-acting (24 hours) and is orally effective. In the usual doses (40 to 50 mg), it blocks opioid craving, whereas in much higher doses (100 to 120 mg), it blocks their euphoriant effect. The former is more significant for maintenance. In spite of some criticism, methadone maintenance is an effective and safe treatment that allows the addict to change his or her lifestyle, stabilize functioning, reduce exposure to the human immunodeficiency virus (HIV), and reintegrate himself or herself into the community. Treatment goals are the reduction of illicit drug use, reduction of criminal activity, increased employability, increased self-esteem, and improvement in family and community functioning (Berger & Tinklenberg, 1979). According to Food and Drug Administration (FDA) regulations, those eligible for methadone maintenance are individuals whose dependence on heroin has lasted longer than two years. It is indicated for addicts who have an extensive history of drug use and antisocial behavior and who have repeatedly failed to maintain abstinence.

A typical methadone maintenance clinic provides the daily administration of oral methadone, monitored with urinalysis, plus drug counseling and ancillary services, such as individual and group psychotherapy. The preferred dosage is 60 to 100 mg/day (Jaffe, 1995). In spite of the acknowledged success of these programs, several authors suggest that this approach tends to reinforce the addict's identity as a member of the drug subculture and to perpetuate detrimental attitudes toward the drug. Many methadone-maintenance patients, especially those treated with lower doses of methadone alone, continue to abuse other licit and illicit drugs, most commonly alcohol.

Levo-α-acetylemthadol. Levomethadyl (LAAM) is a long-acting and clinically safe congener of methadone that can be administered three times per week, thus affording greater treatment flexibility (Ling & Blaine, 1979; Judson *et al.*, 1983). Unfortunately, LAAM remains an "orphan" drug despite efforts by the National Institute on Drug Abuse (NIDA) to make it available for general clinical use.

Opioid Antagonists. Maintenance with opioid antagonists is a novel approach that attempts to decondition behaviors related to opioid use and relapse. By blocking both heroin-induced euphoria and heroin-induced relief of conditioned abstinence in the former opioid abuser, narcotic antagonists, such as cyclazocine, naloxone, naltrexone, and buprenorphine, may help extinguish the behaviors of opioid injection. Buprenorphine, a mixed agonist-antagonist, appears to be effective for opioid detoxification as well as maintenance, and may prove acceptable to abusers who refuse methadone maintenance. At higher doses (8 to 30 mg), buprenorphine appears to reduce the frequency of clinic visits, and may be an alternative to dispensing take-home doses (Resnick *et al.*, 1993). A flexible dosing procedure using buprenorphine has been shown to be as effective as methadone in opioid dependence. Neither buprenorphine nor methadone appears to influence cocaine use.

Naltrexone, a nearly pure long-acting opioid antagonist, seems to be the most promising opioid antagonist. Naltrexone induction therapy consists of the following steps.

- Detoxification from heroin or methadone and the establishment of a drug-free period for at least seven days postheroin or ten days post-methadone.
- Administration of a naloxone challenge dose to the abstinent patient (e.g., 0.8 mg subcutaneously or IV of naloxone should elicit no withdrawal).
- Administrating of an initial dose of 25 or 50 mg of naltrexone.
- Maintenance naltrexone of 350 mg/week, given in a daily (50 mg/day), twice-weekly (150 mg on Mondays and 200 mg on Thursdays), or thrice-weekly (100 mg on Mondays and Wednesdays and 150 mg on Fridays) regimen.
- Weekly urine screening for drugs of abuse during the initial several months of treatment, with periodic physical examinations.

This treatment model is based on the hypothesis that drug-seeking behavior is perpetuated by the reinforcing effects of acute opioid effects, and that failure to experience these effects will result in extinction of the conditioned craving and related behaviors. Once a naltrexone regimen is initiated, patients cease craving opiates. Noncompliance is a major problem; most patients quit treatment within a few weeks (Jaffe, 1995). Patients most likely to benefit typically are socially stable (employed, married), self-motivated, and stabilized on low-dose methadone before detoxification from methadone and induction of naltrexone.

Abstinence-Oriented Recovery Models.   Such models in various addiction treatment centers are based on the alcoholic recovery model (AA) and derivative self-help groups. Confrontation is essential to break the addict's denial of the seriousness of the illness. Later, adding an educational approach helps the person learn about his or her illness. Residential programs, in which group therapy is the primary treatment modality and family participation is actively sought, are routine. Discharge planning should provide for continued support and structure, required NA attendance, urine screening, aftercare groups, and, as appropriate, postprogram individual or family therapy. This approach is most successful for patients who are in the early stages of addiction and are motivated to change.

Therapeutic Communities.   Communities such as Synanon, Odyssey House, Daytop, and Phoenix House are drug-free, full-time residential programs that attempt to rehabilitate and resocialize the drug addict through a rigidly defined lifestyle that emphasizes group interaction, peer pressure, and self-government. Treatment in the typical therapeutic community lasts one to two years, and generally uses a forceful confrontational approach. Some have criticized the model as excessively authoritarian. Others note that there is little methodologically vigorous evidence to substantiate its effectiveness. This model is thought to be most effective for the highly motivated individual who can complete the required program (Sells, 1979). It is impractical for many addicts; however, it may be a good choice for the those with legal entanglements and court referral. Daytime (nonresidential) therapeutic communities also exist, but have not been carefully studied (Sells, 1979).

Psychotherapy. In spite of the widespread opinion that individual psychotherapy is ineffective with opiate addicts, several recent studies indicate that professional psychotherapy can add benefit to standard drug counseling in a methadone-maintenance program. Short-term interpersonal psychotherapy has both proponents and detractors. Supportive-expressive and cognitive-behavioral psychotherapies can be useful in the context of a methadone program. Several studies suggest that psychodynamic, cognitive-behavioral, and implosive group therapy may be helpful (Abrahms, 1979). Psychotherapy is particularly indicated in patients with amenable psychiatric symptoms.

Psychopharmacotherapy may be indicated in dually diagnosed addicts presenting serious psychiatric symptoms, especially depression. Doxepin may reduce depressive symptoms in opiate addicts in a methadone program. Experience with imipramine is inconsistent, although one recent uncontrolled study suggests that depressed methadone-maintenance patients improved in both mood and abuse behavior after imipramine (Nunes *et al.*, 1991). The newer antidepressants (e.g., SSRIs) have not been well studied in this population.

404.10 SEDATIVE, HYPNOTIC, OR ANXIOLYTIC DEPENDENCE
305.40 ABUSE

These disorders are often initiated or maintained through indiscriminate or poorly supervised prescribing practices, especially in the elderly. Younger people abuse these drugs for their intoxicating effect, to enhance opioid euphoria, or to counteract the stimulant effects of cocaine and amphetamine. The concurrent abuse of alcohol is very common.

There is a paucity of studies on treatment and rehabilitation. Detoxification is a prerequisite of any treatment approach (see "Withdrawal"). Following detoxification, the patient should be evaluated to rule out primary psychopathology (e.g., depression), which should be treated if present. When the presenting symptom is chronic insomnia, the patient should be directed toward nonpharmacological therapies, such as progressive relaxation or biofeedback. Trazedone, 50 mg at bedtime p.r.n., is a safe and effective alternative.

There are no controlled studies on the efficacy of psychotherapy for this form of abuse. A few older studies indicate poor outcome, except in patients with comorbid psychiatric illness.

Benzodiazepines are the most commonly abused drugs in this group. Rickels and associates (1991), summarizing a three-year follow-up of 123 long-term prescription benzodiazepine users, found that 73% were benzodiazepine-free at follow-up, after successfully completing a discontinuation program. The only predictors of benzodiazepine-free outcome were participation in the taper program, shorter duration of use, and younger age. Variables found to have no predictive value included half-life of the drug, mode of withdrawal (abrupt versus gradual), and daily dose.

304.50 HALLUCINOGEN DEPENDENCE
305.30 HALLUCINOGEN ABUSE
304.30 CANNABIS DEPENDENCE
304.20 CANNABIS ABUSE
304.90 PHENCYCLIDINE (OR RELATED SUBSTANCE) DEPENDENCE
305.90 PHENCYCLIDINE ABUSE

These classes of substances share common aspects of epidemiology and pattern of use. They are often used in the context of a characteristic drug subculture.

The severity of the disorder varies according to the type of substance, degree of dependence, and concomitant psychopathology. Polydrug abuse often includes alcohol and cocaine. Underlying psychopathology is a common problem, and usually involves depression and/or personality disorders. Treatment of the underlying psychiatric disorder is a necessary condition of long-term rehabilitation.

Following thorough psychiatric evaluation, patients with psychiatric pathology should be referred for additional treatment. Both individual and group psychotherapy are often recommended, although their efficacy has not been completely established. Referral to drug-free outpatient treatment programs and utilization of community service support agencies are important. Unfortunately, most patients are not sufficiently motivated to pursue treatment; the majority drop out after the initial evaluation. Treatment in residential programs, and especially in a therapeutic community with a rigorously structured resocialization program, provides the greatest chance for success, especially for the highly motivated individual. Generally, the longer a person stays in treatment, the more favorable is the outcome.

304.20 COCAINE DEPENDENCE
305.60 COCAINE ABUSE

There is no consensus regarding the optimal treatment for cocaine use (Kleber & Gawin, 1987). In general, programs use the 12-step recovery method of AA, contingency contracting, and urine screening. Contingency contracting is based on the patient's agreement to participate in a urine monitoring program and to accept an aversive contingency in the event of either a cocaine-positive urine or failure to produce a urine sample (Higgins *et al.*, 1993). Hospitalization is necessary for those with chronic free-base or IV use, significant medical or psychiatric complications, and/or concurrent dependence on other drugs.

Nonbiological treatments have emphasized psychological strategies (individual, group, and/or family therapy) aimed at modifying addictive behaviors, with reported initial success rates in the range of 40 to 45%. A behavioral treatment program consisting of contingency procedures and community reinforcement may offer promise for initial cocaine abstinence (Higgins *et al.*, 1991). In one study, a multicomponent behavioral treatment program based on a community reinforcement approach, coupled with incentives contingent on cocaine-free urine specimens, was effective in retaining outpatients in treatment and establishing cocaine abstinence (Higgins *et al.*, 1993, 1994). In another, Covi, *et al.* (1993) reported that weekly interpersonal/cognitive/behavioral psychotherapy led to 50% "improvement." A one-year naturalistic follow-up study using psychotherapy and desipramine for cocaine dependence showed a delayed improvement response for patients who received cognitive-behavioral relapse prevention, as compared with supportive clinical management (Carroll *et al.*, 1994).

Pharmacological approaches have been reported as useful for initial cocaine abstinence (Rao *et al.*, 1995). Several older studies found desipramine effective as an adjunct to psychotherapy in decreasing craving and facilitating initial abstinence (Gawin & Kleber, 1984; Gawin *et al.*, 1989; Kleber & Gawin, 1987). Fluoxetine was recently found to improve concurrent depression in cocaine addicts (Batki *et al.*, 1993). Available evidence does not appear to support the claim that antidepressants are effective in maintaining cocaine abstinence.

Nunes and colleagues (1990) found lithium ineffective in cocaine abusers with bipolar spectrum disorders. Early reports suggesting that carbamazepine may be useful in treating cocaine abusers have not been supported by more recent studies (Crosby *et al.*, 1993). The serotonin agonist m-CPP has been shown to decrease cocaine craving, suggesting a possible 5-HT dysfunction in cocaine addicts (Branchey *et al.*, 1993). Clinically distinct subgroups of cocaine abusers may respond differentially to pharmacotherapy and psychotherapy (Carroll *et al.*, 1994). So far, studies have failed to provide evidence that drugs are useful in the treatment of cocaine dependence.

Abuse of cocaine, especially crack cocaine, is most common among (although not limited to) characteristic subcultures. An understanding of sociocultural issues is important to the success of follow-up care.

304.40 AMPHETAMINE OR SIMILARLY ACTING SYMPATHOMIMETIC DRUG DEPENDENCE
305.70 AMPHETAMINE ABUSE

There are no established treatment guidelines for this class of psychoactive drugs. Treatment approaches are similar to the psychosocial methods described in cocaine abuse.

304.60 INHALANT DEPENDENCE
305.90 INHALANT ABUSE

Inhalant intoxication is discussed in Chapter 13.

Family assessment is critical for obtaining collateral information and for ruling out child abuse or neglect in the younger abuser (Westermeyer, 1987).

Once abstinence is achieved, psychosocial interventions are necessary to prevent recurrence. Concomitant psychopathology must be recognized and treated. Various psychotherapies, sociodrama, and vocational rehabilitation have been used to treat adolescent abusers. Family intervention and mobilization of community resources are particularly important (Westermeyer, 1987).

305.10 NICOTINE DEPENDENCE

In contrast to other substance-use disorders, nicotine dependence is not associated with impairment in social or occupational functioning. There are many treatment methods, reporting varying rates of success.

Behavioral and Psychotherapeutic Techniques

These include hypnosis, aversive conditioning, desensitization, symptom substitution, covert desensitization, group therapy, relaxation training, supportive therapy, and education. Assessment of motivation and readiness to quit are important first steps. Among nonbiological techniques, none has proved superior to others, and none has consistently shown long-term success rates in excess of 20% (Mann *et al.*, 1986).

Pharmacotherapies

Nicotine replacement, using either a nicotine-containing gum or a transdermal patch, is currently the most important medication approach. There is some evidence that subjects with high nicotine tolerance are more apt to benefit (Hall *et al.*, 1985). The transdermal nicotine patch has some advantages over the gum (Hartman *et al.*, 1991). Nicotine replacement should be combined with physician intervention, counseling, follow-up, and relapse prevention (Hurt *et al.*, 1994).

Other pharmacological approaches to smoking cessation have been reviewed by Jarvick and Henningfield (1988).

Before nicotine replacement was available in the United States, Farebrother and colleges (1980) found propranolol effective, but lobeline sulfate (a nicotine agonist), sedatives, and psychostimulants have not proved helpful. Glassman and associates (1984) found that clonidine, which may block nicotine withdrawal symptoms, reduced the craving for cigarette smoking. Silver acetate chewing gums and lozenges, used as an aversive deterrent, may have some effectiveness (Fey *et al.*, 1991; Hymonowitz, *et al.*, 1993).

Educational Programs

Widely available for smokers interested in giving up the habit, the best results are seen in programs that combine education with group therapy and support, and those that incorporate behavioral techniques and nicotine chewing gum. In spite of reported high rates of success for some programs, the majority of smokers eventually relapse.

When motivation is high, abrupt abstinence ("cold turkey") may be the best method. Clinicians should emphasize the importance of total abstinence after an attempt to quit smoking, and follow up with patients within the first two weeks (Kenford *et al.*, 1994).

304.80 POLYSUBSTANCE DEPENDENCE

Many polysubstance abusers use multiple drugs indiscriminantly; others follow a characteristic pattern of alternating psychostimulant drugs with sedative-hypnotic-anxiolytic drugs or alcohol.

It appears that polysubstance abusers are more likely to show significant psychopathology than are single-substance abusers. Treatment of the concomitant psychiatric disorder is very important. Detoxification of patients with mixed-drug dependence is discussed in the section on "Withdrawal." There are no established specific guidelines for the long-term treatment and rehabilitation of the polysubstance abuser. In general, treatment is similar to that described in single-substance dependence, with an emphasis on treating the underlying psychopathology, when present.

304.90 OTHER SUBSTANCE DEPENDENCE
305.90 OTHER SUBSTANCE ABUSE

This classification includes inhalant anesthetic gases (e.g., nitrous oxide, ether), short-acting vasodilators (e.g., amyl, butyl, or isobutyl nitrite), anabolic-androgenic steroids, cortisol, various over-the-counter drugs (e.g., antihistamines, anticholinergics, anorectics, and cough syrups, some containing pseudoephedrine), and plant intoxicants (e.g., catnip, betel nut, kava). There are no established specific guidelines for the treatment and rehabilitation of patients abusing these substances. Treatment should be individualized, taking into consideration the various psychosocial and motivational determinants of substance-abusing behavior, the general principles outlined at the beginning of this chapter, and, when present, comorbid psychopathology.

References for Part II

Abrahms, J. L. (1979): A cognitive behavioral versus nondirective group treatment program for opioid addicted persons: An adjunct to methadone maintenance. *International Journal of Addictions,* 14:503–511.

Alexander, B., & Perry, P. J. (1991): Detoxification from benzodiazepines. *Journal of Substance Abuse and Treatment,* 8:9–17.

Balis, G. U. (1974): The use of psychotomimetic and related consciousness-altering drugs. In S. Arieti (Ed.), *American Handbook of Psychiatry,* vol 3. New York: Basic Books.

Balis, G. U. (1982): Criterion value of atypical drug responses in the diagnosis of atypical psychiatric disorders. *Journal of Nervous and Mental Diseases,* 170(12):737–743.

Barnes, G. E. (1979): Solvent abuse: A review. *International Journal of the Addictions,* 14:1–26.

Batki, S. L., Wasburn, A. M., Manfredi, L. B., *et al.* (1993): Fluoxetine for cocaine abuse: Depression and antisocial personality. *Proceedings,* Annual Meeting, American Psychiatric Association, San Francisco.

Baumgartner, G. R., & Rowen, R. C. (1987): Clonidine versus chlordiazepoxide in the management of acute alcohol withdrawal syndrome. *Archives of Internal Medicine,* 147:1223–1226.

Berger, P. A., & Tinklenberg, J. R. (1979): Medical management of the drug abuser. In A. M. Freeman, R. L. Sack, & P. L. Berger (Eds.), *Psychiatry for the Primary Care Physician.* Baltimore: Williams & Wilkins.

Branchey, M. H., Buydens-Branchey, L. B., & Fergeson, P. (1993): Serotonin agonist M-CPP decreases cocaine craving. *Proceedings,* Annual Meeting, American Psychiatric Association, San Francisco.

Busto, U., Sellers, E. M., Naranjo, C. A., *et al.* (1986): Withdrawal reaction after long-term use of benzodiazepines. *New England Journal of Medicine,* 315:854–859.

Byrne, A., Kirby B., Zubin, & Ensminger, S. (1991): Psychiatric and neurological effects of chronic solvent. *Canadian Journal of Psychiatry,* 36:735–738.

Cami, J., Torres, S., San, L., *et al.* (1985): Efficacy of clonidine and methadone in the rapid detoxification of patients dependent on heroin. *Clinical Pharmacology and Therapeutics,* 38:336–341.

Carroll, K. M., Rounsaville, B. J., Gordon, L. T., *et al.* (1994): Psychotherapy and pharmacotherapy for ambulatory cocaine abusers. *Archives of General Psychiatry,* 51:177–187.

Covi, L., Hess, J., & Kreiter, N. (1993): Psychotherapy dosage affects cocaine dependence. *Proceedings,* Annual Meeting, American Psychiatric Association, San Francisco, p. 192.

Crosby, R.D., Halikas, J.A., Graves, N.M., *et al.* (1993): Carbamazepine in the treatment of cocaine abuse. *Proceedings,* Annual Meeting, American Psychiatric Association, San Francisco.

Czechowicz, D. (1978): *Detoxification treatment manual.* Rockville, MD: National Institute of Drug Abuse, U.S. Department of Health, Education, and Welfare.

Farebrother, M., Pearce, S., Turner, P., *et al.* (1980): Propranolol and giving up smoking. *British Journal of Diseases of the Chest,* 74:95–96.

Fey, M., Hollander, M., & Hymonowitz, N. (1991): Silver-acetate deterrent therapy: A minimal-intervention self-help aid. In J.A. Cocores (Ed.), *The Clinical Management of Nicotine Dependence.* New York: Springer-Verlag.

Gawin, F. H., & Kleber, H. D. (1984): Cocaine abuse treatment. *Archives of General Psychiatry,* 41:903–909.

Gawin, F. N., Kleber, N. D., Byck, R., *et al.* (1989): Desipramine facilitation of initial cocaine abstinence. *Archives of General Psychiatry,* 46:117–121.

Giannini, A. J., Folts, D. J., Feather, J. N., & Sullivan, B. S. (1989): Bromocriptine and amantadine in cocaine detoxification. *Psychiatric Research,* 29:11–16.

Glassman, A. H., Jackson, W. K., Walsh, B. T., *et al.* (1984): Cigarette craving, smoking withdrawal, and clonidine. *Science,* 226:864–866.

Hall, S.M., Tunstall, C., Rugg, D, *et al.* (1985): Nicotine gum and behavioral treatment in smoking cessation. *Journal of Consulting and Clinical Psychology,* 53:256–258.

Hartman, N., Leong, G.B., Glynn, S.M., *et al.* (1991): Transdermal nicotine and smoking behavior in psychiatric patients. *American Journal of Psychiatry,* 148:374–375.

Higgins, S. T., Budney, A. J., Bickel, W. K., *et al.* (1994): Incentives improve outcome in outpatient behavioral treatment of cocaine dependence. *Archives of General Psychiatry,* 51:568–576.

Higgins, S. T., Budney, A. J., Bickel, W. K., *et al.* (1993): Achieving cocaine abstinence with a behavioral approach. *American Journal of Psychiatry,* 150:763–769.

Higgins, S. T., Delaney, D. D., Budney, A. J., *et al.* (1991): A behavioral approach to achieving initial cocaine abstinence. *American Journal of Psychiatry,* 149:1218–1224.

Hirt, M., & Greenfield, H. (1979): Implosive therapy treatment of heroin addicts during methadone detoxification. *Journal of Consulting and Clinical Psychology,* 47:982–983.

Howell, E. F., & Kane, F. J. (1993): Outmoded treatments for alcohol detoxification. *Proceedings,* Annual Meeting, American Psychiatric Association, San Francisco.

Hurt, R. D., Dale, L. C., Fredrickson, P. A., *et al.* (1994): Nicotine patch therapy for smoking cessation combined with physician advice and nurse follow-up. *Journal of the American Medical Association,* 371:595–600.

Hymonowitz, N., Feuerman, M., Hollander, M., & Frances, R. J. (1993): Smoking deterrence using silver acetate. *Hospital and Community Psychiatry,* 44:113–114.

Jaffe, J. H. (1995): Pharmacologic treatment of opioid dependence: Current techniques and new findings. *Psychiatric Annals,* 25:369–375.

Jarvik, M. E., Cullen, J. W., Gritz, E. R., *et al.* (1977): *Research on smoking behavior.* National Institute on Drug Abuse, Research Monograph Series 17, DHEW. Washington, D.C.: U.S. Government Printing Office.

Jarvik, M. E., & Henningfield, J. E. (1988): Pharmacological treatment of tobacco dependence. *Pharmacology, Biochemistry and Behavior,* 30:279–294.

Jasinski, D. R., Johnson, R. E., & Kocher, T. R. *et al.* (1985): Clonidine in morphine withdrawal. *Archives of General Psychiatry,* 42:1063–1066.

Josephson, G. W., & Sabatier, H. S. (1978): Rational management of alcohol withdrawal seizures. *Southern Medical Journal,* 71:1095–1097.

Judson, B. A., Goldstein, A., & Inturrisi, C. E. (1993): Methadyl acetate (LAAM) in the treatment of heroin addicts. *Archives of General Psychiatry,* 408:834–840.

Kanof, P. D., Aronson, M. J., Ness, R. (1993): Organic mood syndrome associated with detoxification from methadone maintenance. *American Journal of Psychiatry,* 150:423–428.

Katz, N. W. (1980): Hypnosis and the addictions: A critical review. *Addictive Behaviors,* 5:41–47.

Kenford, S. L., Fiore, M. C., Jorenby, D. E., *et al.* (1994): Predicting smoking cessation. *Journal of the American Medical Association,* 271:589–594.

Kleber, N. D., & Gawin, F. N. (1987): Pharmacological treatments of cocaine abuse. In A. M. Washton & M. S. Gold (Eds.), *Cocaine: A Clinician's Handbook.* New York: Guilford.

Kranzler, H. R., Burleson, J. A., Del Boca, F. K., *et al.* (1994): Buspirone treatment of anxious alcoholics: A placebo-controlled trial. *Archives of General Psychiatry,* 51(9):720–731.

Kraus, M. L., Gottlieb, L. D., Horwitz, R. I., *et al.* (1985): Randomized clinical trial of atenolol in alcohol withdrawal. *New England Journal of Medicine,* 313:905–909.

Ling, W., & Blaine, J. D. (1979): The use of LAAM in treatment. In R. I. DuPont, A. Goldstein, & J. O'Donnell (Eds.), *Handbook on Drug Abuse* (pp. 87–96). Washington, D.C.: U.S. Government Printing Office, National Institute on Drug Abuse.

Luiskow, B. I., & Reed, J. (1986): Atenolol for alcohol withdrawal. *New England Journal of Medicine,* 314:783–785.

Malcolm, R., Ballanger, J. C., Sturgis, E. T., *et al.* (1989): Double-blind controlled trial comparing carbamazepine to oxazepam treatment of alcohol withdrawal. *American Journal of Psychiatry,* 146:617–621.

Mann, L. S., Johnson, R. W., & Levine, D. J. (1986): Tobacco dependence: Psychology, biology, and treatment strategies. *Psychosomatics,* 27:713–718.

Miller, N. S., & Gold, M. S. (1991): *Drugs of abuse: A comprehensive series for clinicians,* Vol. 2. New York: Plenum.

Minkoff, K. (1994): Models for addiction treatment in psychiatric populations. *Psychiatric Annals,* 24:412–417.

Nunes, E. V., McGrath, P. J., Wager, S., & Quitkin, F. D. (1990): Lithium treatment for cocaine abusers with bipolar spectrum disorders. *American Journal of Psychiatry,* 147:655–657.

Nunes, E. V., Quitkin, F. M., Brady, R., & Stewart, J. W. (1991): Imipramine treatment of methadone maintenance patients with affective disorder and illicit drug use. *American Journal of Psychiatry,* 148:667–669.

O'Malley, S. S., Jaffe, A. J., Chang, G., *et al.* (1992): Naltrexone and coping skills therapy for alcohol dependence: A controlled study. *Archives of General Psychiatry,* 49:881–887.

O'Malley, S. S., Jaffe, A. J., & Rounsaville, B. J. (1995): Naltrexone: Matching patients and treatments. *Proceedings,* Annual Meeting, American Psychiatric Association, Washington, D.C.

Parran, T. V., Adelman, C. L., Jasinski, D. R. (1994): A buprenorphine stabilization and rapid-taper protocol for the detoxification of opioid-dependent patients. *American Journal of Addictions,* 3:306–313.

Pattison, E. M. (1986): Clinical approaches to the alcoholic patient. *Psychosomatics,* 27:262–270.

Perry, P. J., & Alexander, B. (1986): Sedative/hypnotic dependence: Patient stabilization, tolerance testing and withdrawal. *Drug Intelligence and Clinical Pharmacy,* 20:532–537.

Perry, P. J., Anderson, K., & Yates, W. (1990): Illicit anabolic steroid use in athletes. *American Journal of Sports Medicine,* 18:422–428.

Pope, H. G., & Katz, D. L. (1988): Affective and psychotic symptoms associated with anabolic steroid use. *American Journal of Psychiatry,* 145:487–490.

Pope, H. G., & Katz, D. L. (1990): Homicide and near-homicide by anabolic steroid users. *Journal of Clinical Psychiatry,* 51:28–31.

Rao, S., Ziedonis, D., & Kosten, T. (1995): The pharmacotherapy of cocaine dependence. *Psychiatric Annals,* 25:363–369.

Reid, W. H., & Balis, G. U. (1987): Evaluation of the violent patient. In R. E. Hales & A. J. Frances (Eds.), *Annual Review of Psychiatry,* Vol. 6 (pp. 491–509). Washington, D.C.: American Psychiatric Association Press.

Resnick, R. B., Pycha, C., & Ganter, M. (1993): Buprenorphine: Reducing dosing frequency. *New Research Program and Abstracts,* Annual Meeting, American Psychiatric Association, San Francisco, p. 163.

Rickels, K., Case, W. G., Schwizer, E., *et al.* (1981): Long-term benzodiazepine users 3 years after participation in a discontinuation program. *American Journal of Psychiatry,* 148:757–761.

Ridgely, M. S. (1991): Creating integrated programs for severely mentally ill persons with substance disorders. In K. Mincoff & R. E. Drake (Eds.), *An Overview in Dual Diagnosis of Major Mental Illness and Substance Disorder.* San Francisco: Jossey-Bass.

Satel, S. L., Price, L. H., Palumbo, J. M., *et al.* (1991): Clinical phenomenology and neurobiology of cocaine abstinence: A perspective inpatient study. *American Journal of Psychiatry,* 148:1712–1716.

Sellers, E. M., & Kalant, H. (1982): Alcohol withdrawal and delirium tremens. In E. M. Pattison & E. Kaufman (Eds.), *Encyclopedic Handbook of Alcoholism* (pp. 147–166). New York: Gardner.

Sellers, E. M., Naranjo, C. A., Harrison, M., *et al.* (1983): Oral diazepam loading: Simplified treatment of alcohol withdrawal. *Clinical Pharmacology Therapy,* 34(6):822–826.

Sellers, E. M., Zilm, D. H., & Degani, N. C. (1977): Comparative effects of propranolol and chlordiazepoxide in alcohol withdrawal. *Journal of Studies in Alcohol,* 38:2096–2108.

Sells, S. B. (1979): Treatment effectiveness. In R. I. DuPont, A. Goldstein, & J. O'Donnell (Eds.), *Handbook on Drug Abuse* (pp. 105–181). Washington, D.C.: U.S. Government Printing Office, National Institute on Drug Abuse.

Strauss, R. H., Ligget, M., & Lanese, R. (1985): Anabolic steroid use and perceived effects in ten weight-trained women athletes. *Journal of the American Medical Association,* 253:2871–2873.

Uzych, L. (1992): Anabolic-androgenic steroids and psychiatric-related effects: A review. *Canadian Journal of Psychiatry,* 37:23–28.

Volpicelli, J. R., Alterman, A. I., Hayashida, M., & O'Brian, C. P. (1992): Naltrexane in the treatment of alcohol dependence. *Archives of General Psychiatry,* 49:876–880.

Weiss, R. D., & Mirin, S. M. (1989): Tricyclic antidepressants in the treatment of alcoholism and drug abuse. *Journal of Clinical Psychiatry,* 50(7, suppl):4–9.

Westermeyer, J. (1987): The psychiatrist and solvent-inhalant abuse: Recognition, assessment, and treatment. *American Journal of Psychiatry,* 144:903–907.

Yesalis, C. E., Kennedy, N. J., Kopstein, A. N., & Bahrke, M. S. (1993): Anabolic-androgenic steroid use in the United States. *Journal of the American Medical Association,* 270:1217–1221.

Zweben, J.E. (1986): Recovery oriented psychotherapy. *Journal of Substance Abuse Treatment,* 3:255–262.

Part III

OTHER DISORDERS PRIMARILY SEEN IN ADULTS

William H. Reid, M.D., M.P.H.

CHAPTER 16

SCHIZOPHRENIA AND OTHER
PSYCHOTIC DISORDERS

Psychotic disorders share one of the most distressing characteristics of psychiatric syndromes: loss of contact with, or inappropriate response to, the real world. Psychosis may occur with disorders not found in this chapter (e.g., in mood disorders); however, here we are referring to conditions in which it is a core symptom of the disturbance.

"Psychosis" is a generic term, a symptom, and not a disorder in itself. It often responds to generic antipsychotic treatment (e.g., neuroleptic medication or electroconvulsive therapy [ECT]). The underlying causes of schizophreniform and similar psychoses, and their treatments, are complex, however, and almost always warrant more than a symptomatic approach.

295.XX SCHIZOPHRENIA

General Principles

Schizophrenia is a very serious illness. Its victims require the best available treatment in order to forestall or prevent devastating exacerbations and chronic disability. Adequate drug therapy is almost always the backbone of such efforts. Early and vigorous treatment is important to long-term outcome.

Just a few years ago, adequate drug treatment usually meant good compliance with a traditional neuroleptic regimen, and acceptance of significant social and mental disability in 75 to 90% of patients. Today, however, partial success with phenothiazine, thioxanthene, or butyrophenone drugs should not satisfy the psychiatrist. Early trials of newer antipsychotic medications are critical to finding large numbers of patients with the potential for further—sometimes dramatic—improvement.

The treatment of schizophrenia illustrates the importance of psychosocial approaches as well. Although their effects on long-term outcome and the illness itself have not yet been established, active community programs, creative crisis intervention, and a variety of supported housing and employment options increase the quality of life and, in some (but not all) studies, decrease the need for hospitalization.

EARLY AND ACUTE TREATMENT

Provided other causes of psychosis are ruled out, the treatment of an acute exacerbation of schizophrenia is similar to that for acute schizophreniform psychosis and brief psychotic disorder. Alleviation of the acute psychosis is the primary goal in any case.

If the patient is known to have schizophrenia, acute treatment is carried out in a context of preparation for maintenance and long-term care. The history generally suggests which approaches (e.g., which medications) have been successful in the past and what follow-up drugs and other treatments are likely to be needed in the future. In brief psychotic and schizophreniforn disorders, one does not know whether or not the psychosis will continue and meet the duration criteria for more chronic illness, so the general rule of vigorous and complete somatic treatment applies. As mentioned above, there is ample evidence that rapid and complete early treatment is associated with better social and clinical prognosis in those patients destined for a schizophrenic diagnosis.

Pharmacologic and milieu treatment should begin as soon as an appropriate history, examination, observation, and protection from self-harm or aggressive behaviors have been completed. Since psychotic patients are difficult to assess comprehensively, it is not unusual for the patient's discomfort and psychosis to require some form of management before the evaluation can be completed. Conservative approaches, such as physical containment or restraint, may be the safest early measures, although antipsychotic medications can usually be prescribed if carefully monitored.

Treatment Setting

The acute exacerbation of schizophrenic or schizophreniform psychosis should be treated in a medical environment unless there is a compelling reason to do otherwise. Patients who are well known to the treating physician, or for other reasons do not immediately require inpatient treatment, protection, or stabilization, can sometimes be treated outside the hospital, but the risks are significant. Some emergency rooms and psychiatric emergency services are equipped to manage and observe such patients for several hours. A few facilities have beds and specialized nursing care available without complete admission to the hospital. Either may be used in situations in which the patient responds quickly and has a safe and sophisticated environment to which he or she can return.

Nevertheless, the overall treatment of acute schizophrenia usually requires a multifaceted approach and medical monitoring during and shortly after intensive initial treatment. Inpatient care, preferably with an experienced nursing staff, is recommended. Less experienced staff members, such as are those on a general medical ward or in a nursing home, often are not qualified to provide intensive psychiatric care. They may misinterpret (or not recognize) important symptoms or effects of treatment (e.g., mistake sedation for antipsychotic response).

Medications in Acute Treatment

For almost all patients, antipsychotic medication is the clinician's most effective means to alleviate or attenuate symptoms and shorten the hospital stay. Adequate drug treatment during hospitalization promotes social adjustment after discharge and increases the patient's potential for continued remission during outpatient care.

The "traditional" medications (phenothiazines [e.g., fluphenazine and others], thioxanthenes [e.g., thiothixene], haloperidol, loxapine) still have a place in the treatment of schizophreniform psychosis, although the proportion of patients with truly good response—one that pleases the patient, doctor, and family—is probably less than one-third. Most have more troublesome side-effects profiles than clozapine, olanzapine, or risperidone, and the probability of serious adverse effects, given proper monitoring of whichever medication is chosen, is likely to be greater with the traditional drugs. The route of administration is one advantage of the older medications; rapidly absorbed injections, easy-to-swallow liquids, and compliance-improving depot forms are all available. Rapidity of action is another advantage; parenteral and some oral forms act much more quickly than does risperidone or, especially, clozapine.

The author believes that the newer, so-called atypical antipsychotic medications should be considered early in treatment. In spite of their cost, there is ample evidence that clozapine, olanzapine, and perhaps risperidone, should be the drugs of choice for many, perhaps most, schizophrenic patients early in the course of their disease. Although not as rapidly effective, they may be started as soon as the need for crisis symptom control has passed. Traditional and atypical neuroleptics should overlap during the process.

If a traditional drug is chosen, the particular choice is generally less important than are proper, consistent administration and appropriate monitoring for drug response and side effects. Most drug classes have some level of documented effectiveness. The dihydroindolone molindone has not gained much popularity in the United States, and has not shown any therapeutic advantage over the more established medications.

Among traditional neuroleptics, most clinicians usually prefer "high-potency" drugs. The sedative and other side effects of such medications as chlorpromazine make them second choices during the acute treatment phase. When very rapid response is needed, parental haloperidol is among the fastest-acting drugs, with significant blood levels and therapeutic response sometimes coming within 30 minutes. Rapid neuroleptization techniques, in which repeated doses of high-potency medication are given every 30 to 60 minutes, are no longer considered more effective than lower-dose procedures, and are associated with increased side effects and adverse effects. Short-acting, high-potency benzodiazepines (e.g., lorazepam) can augment the antipsychotic effect of traditional neuroleptics during the initial phase of treatment. They usually are not helpful later.

Many recent studies show no consistent advantage to very high medication doses, at least in some groups of patients (Rifkin *et al.*, 1991). Nevertheless, it is important to "give enough, long enough." In the acute phase, at least "standard" doses are usually necessary; low doses of antipsychotic drug (e.g., less than about 10 mg/day of haloperidol or the equivalent) are insufficient for most patients (Levinson *et al.*, 1990; Rifkin *et al.*, 1991; Van Putten *et al.*, 1990).

Fear of extrapyramidal or other side effects should not lead one to an inappropriately low dose, since the therapeutic level of traditional neuroleptics (but not clozapine or other "atypical" ones) is often one at which extrapyramidal effects are to be expected. The prophylactic use of antiparkinsonian medication is often indicated, particularly in younger patients, in order to smooth the patient's experience with the neuroleptic, increase the probability of future compliance, and prevent uncomfortable reactions, such as significant akathisia or dystonia.

Nonresponders. About half of new schizophrenic or schizophreniform patients will have some acceptable response within three to four weeks of beginning standard-dose traditional neuroleptic treatment. This does not imply *optimal* response, but positive symptoms will have remitted and the patient will be amenable to the next steps in treatment. For those who do not respond adequately, one may wait a bit longer; increase the dose beyond standard ranges; prescribe an augmenting drug, such as lorazepam or lithium; change to a different class of neuroleptic; or prescribe ECT. Many refractory patients will respond to one or more of these; the psychiatrist should not hesitate to use them when necessary.

In one of the best fairly recent reviews on this topic, Christison *et al.* (1991) examined several alternative and adjunctive biological therapies. Switching to clozapine offered the best opportunity for marked benefit; additional prescribing experience since the Christison *et al.* review confirms that clozapine should be considered early in patients who respond poorly. Olanzapine is another choice. There is probably a subgroup of patients for whom risperidone is an excellent drug, but its onset of action and monitoring convenience appear to be its only advantages over clozapine at present. Several other new neuroleptics are being studied (e.g., quetiapine [Seroquel], sertindole [Serlect, Serdolect], ziprasidone, amisulpride), many of which are currently available in Europe. Some are likely to appear on the U.S. market within the next several months or years.

The Christison *et al.* review found augmentation of traditional neuroleptics to be useful as well, with lithium a first choice (regardless of the presence or absence of affective symptoms), followed in preference by a high-potency benzodiazepine. The need for sedation, the possibility of a paradoxical reaction, and the propensity for drug abuse should be considered. The augmenting drug can usually be discontinued in the eventual maintenance regimen. Carbamazepine may be tried as well, although it must not be combined with clozapine.

Electroconvulsive Therapy. Acute psychosis, particularly with catatonia, severe withdrawal, or affective disturbance, often responds to ECT. The technique should also be considered in patients for whom neuroleptics may be contraindicated, such as pregnant, nursing, elderly, or debilitated patients; those with significant liver problems; or patients who have previously experienced neuroleptic malignant syndrome. Although acutely effective for many patients, ECT probably does not change the course of the illness (Koehler & Sauer, 1983; Sarker *et al.,* 1994).

Patience. Although some patients respond soon after reaching therapeutic levels of medication, a positive outcome often takes considerable time. Once one has reached a dose that is likely to be effective, it may be necessary to continue the drug for several weeks, in an appropriate therapeutic environment, to assess complete response. In some patients, clozapine may require over six months to show its therapeutic effects (Lieberman *et al.,* 1994), but almost all who will respond show potential for improvement within a few weeks after reaching a therapeutic dose (Carpenter *et al.,* 1995). Many patients, particularly those treated early in their disorders rather than after months or years on other drugs, respond much sooner.

Although a patient at times may need additional, or different treatment, and although the patient, his or her family, and/or the ward staff may press for a change in treatment, clinical experience and the available literature both suggest that early medication changes and the premature stopping of a potentially successful medication usually confuse treatment rather than help it (Nurnberg & Levine, 1986).

Other Target Symptoms

Acute agitation, aggressive behavior, acute depression, or sleeplessness may be treated separately from the target psychosis. If sedation is needed, for example, sedative drugs may be added to the antipsychotic regimen in such a way that physiologic REM cycles are conserved. The wrenching anxiety often seen in acutely ill patients can be treated with any of several short-acting benzodiaz-epines. Although these may alter the bioavailability of the neuroleptic or even cause a rare paradoxical response, the advantage of symptom specificity—and the possibility of neuroleptic augmentation separate from anxiolytic effects—often mitigates toward their use.

Acute Hospital Treatment

The inpatient milieu for early or brief hospital treatment of the schizophrenias should include a therapeutic combination of architecture, staffing, programs, social structure, respite, patient participation, and transition to the next level of care. Each has a place in a dynamic inpatient experience that will lead to a suc-cessful transition to either outpatient care or extended residential treatment.

Architectural requirements vary with clinical philosophy and the needs of the patient population. Persons treated under court order or involuntary commit-ment may require a closed unit, although the rationale for locked doors is some-times more legal, administrative, or political than therapeutic. Modern treatment environments combine patient and staff safety with pleasing design, using durable materials to provide warmth, color, texture, adequate illumination, and commu-nication in the unit. Properly chosen materials can also decrease unit noise and confusion. There should be space for gathering together as well as for patient privacy.

The need to observe patients for evaluation and protection should be tem-pered to avoid their feeling of being in a fishbowl. Nursing stations should be highly accessible, not hidden away where they are likely to be used as retreats by some staff members. The glassed-in type of nursing station is a counterthera-peutic anachronism that should be avoided on all but the intensive-care ward. It combines the worst aspects of the fishbowl, "us versus them," and a tempting staff retreat.

Access to other aspects of the treatment program, such as dining facilities, group rooms, occupational therapy, or recreation, should be as open as is fea-sible. Meals, for example, should be served in a cafeteria or dining room setting, and bedroom or day room meal service avoided whenever possible.

Staffing should reflect the number and variety of mental health profession-als needed for medical, social, and educational treatment; rehabilitation and administration; and ward maintenance and the like. Architecture should not be a substitute for adequate staff. Staffing ratios vary with patient care needs; how-ever, a quality inpatient environment will not substitute locked doors, extra seclu-sion rooms, highly regimented activities, or other barriers for individual observation and care.

Each staff member should be competent in his or her particular field and be sensitive to the needs of patients with acutely disturbed thought processes. Sometimes these needs are for intervention or redirection; sometimes they are for intrusive presence. Staff sex, age, or cultural background may be relevant to some treatment issues. The administrative hierarchy and attending professionals should express their support for the ward staff through mutual respect, professional use of their expertise, opportunities for additional education and training, and fair compensation. The hospital should be alert to the toll taken on the staff by continuous work with difficult, sometimes frustrating patients.

Administrative policies that interfere with clinical care should be kept to a minimum. In this era of regulations, cost containment, bureaucracy, and lack of trust, particularly in the public sector, employee dissatisfaction (and sometimes a literal fear of managers and overseers) is a significant source of job dissatisfaction. Nevertheless, incompetent or abusive care should not be tolerated. One must strive to recognize and deal with any staff member who is exploitative, hostile, or otherwise unprofessional.

Therapeutic programs—required, encouraged, and elective—are a part of every active inpatient milieu during most of the patient's day. Several hours of structured activity should be available, including therapeutically oriented ward meetings or groups. In other activities, organization is evident, but the structure is less pronounced, such as in occupational therapy (OT), in recreational therapy (RT), or at meals. Even free periods may have some organization by virtue of the fact that they are scheduled or contain optional alternatives.

Structure. Therapeutic programs must fit the needs and abilities of the patient. They should allow for individual needs and preferences, rather than assuming a sameness among all patients. They should be neither intrusive nor overstimulating, but rather should provide an atmosphere of security and consistency, in which the patient's world is one of predictability, caring, and growth.

The primary effort during hospitalization for acute psychosis should be toward alleviation of psychosis and the restoration of rational thinking, and not toward restructuring the patient's behavior patterns, understanding the illness, or complete resocialization. Many "psychoeducation" programs, for example, are not very useful early in treatment, when the patient's thought process cannot yet take advantage of the lessons. Similarly, discussions of medication compliance are unlikely to affect health behaviors months hence, when the patient is beset by complex and forceful pressures and impulses to stop his or her medication. Psychotherapy should focus on supporting the current acute treatment process (and later on return to the community), not on complex issues or psychodynamics.

The brief treatment unit must provide a therapeutic and structuring environment that is dynamic, not static. Although medication and shelter from the outside world will often lead to improvement, the patient should not be expected merely to remain on a ward while the medication does its work. In the best of circumstances, the patient is engaged in a multimodal environment from which he or she emerges as either an outpatient or an extended-stay patient with the best possible opportunity for continued improvement. This implies that transition or discharge planning should begin early, often within the first few days of hospitalization.

The *respite* function of brief hospitalization is often overlooked in descriptions of the clinical milieu. When patients respond to the shelter or protective setting in which psychic reorganization and healing can occur, we sometimes accuse them of being "dependent." However, a significant part of the patient's psychotic deterioration may be related to special stresses, sometimes from the environment, but more often from a combination of idiosyncratic internal and external conflict. It is thus reasonable for the patient to accept, and make use of, the soothing, protective aspects of the hospital. Careful attention to the discharge or transition process becomes all the more important in this regard.

Somewhere between discussions of "structure" and "respite," one must address the issue of the chaos that sometimes marks acute care wards. The hospital setting, which is intended to decrease psychotic symptoms, reassure patients, and promote structure, should not be one that is full of noise, confusion, or fear. When teaching psychiatry trainees, the author often recommends that they spend a couple of days and nights on their own wards, a suggestion that may be met with uncomfortable giggles but should not engender great anxiety. If the acute unit is an uncomfortable or fearful place for the doctor, is it suitable for patient care?

Patient Participation. The patient is usually expected to become an active participant in hospital treatment. The dynamic inpatient milieu has certain expectations of even the most disorganized person. At the least, he or she is expected to behave within broad human guidelines, dressing rather than remaining naked, refraining from striking others, and the like. These are not always within the control of the most acutely disturbed patients, but denying basic responsibilities over long periods because of "illness" can usurp many of the patient's human rights, and communicate the expectation that he or she will remain sick. One must not endanger others while expecting an agitated patient to contain himself; however, there must be a basic implication that the patient is a legitimate part of the ward environment, with its reassuring consistency and rules. Although the patient, other patients, and staff members will be protected as necessary, the patient's responsibilities, as far as possible, are those of an adult. He or she is not patronized or treated as a child, and is expected to participate in his own care to the extent practicable.

Transition and Discharge. External forces, such as insurance limitations or managed care guidelines, often press the psychiatrist to discharge the patient before he or she is clinically ready. The length of stay for acute schizophrenic or schizophreniform psychosis is often less than 30 days (sometimes under two weeks); however, the patient should not be pushed into the outside world prematurely. Financial or administrative considerations must not displace clinical judgment.

Whenever feasible, the physician and ward staff should have some knowledge of the post-hospital environment to which the patient will be returning, in order to prepare him or her to leave eventually, and to prepare the family and community to receive and work with the patient. Family visits and meetings, practical counseling, and realistic transition plans are important parts of the treatment program. Extensive or uncovering psychotherapy, individually or in groups, should not be started in the hospital unless either the inpatient stay can be extended to accommodate it or the therapy can continue after the patient leaves. Relationships formed with staff members and other patients are important, but should be pursued as temporary alliances that may soon be broken. Reintegration into the family and/or community should begin soon after the psychosis abates, with appropriate attention to how forbidding the outside world may seem.

Transition to the next level of care should be done with attention to detail, particularly if the patient will leave the hospital, and especially if he or she will be living far away. The patient and others should understand all aspects of any follow-up that is offered. A transitional aftercare group or program in which the patient may work with the staff and/or patients from the inpatient milieu may be helpful, although most patients should direct their energies away from attachments with the hospital. Whenever feasible, the future physician, psychotherapist, or clinic should contact the patient before actual discharge.

Structured follow-up is not always possible. Some patients refuse it; others drift away in a few weeks or months. Still others leave to go to a setting where it is simply not practical to make definitive contacts or to follow the patient into the outpatient world. Occasionally, recommendations and good wishes are all that one can offer.

Conservative Treatment of Acute Schizophreniform Psychosis

Inpatient. The mere presence of a stable, consistent, protective inpatient milieu that is structurally different from the patient's community living situation may help some patients with schizophreniform psychosis. Although many patients who respond dramatically to environmental change will later be found to have some diagnosis other than schizophrenia, the idea that the patient deserves an opportunity to improve before receiving biological treatment is often worth exploring. The psychiatric inpatient ward should be a place that can tolerate moderate agitation and inappropriate behavior, thus lessening the level of crisis felt by family and nonpsychiatric professionals. For many psychotic patients, particularly those for whom a complete history is not available, a day or two of observation without drugs is the initial treatment of choice.

Outpatient. Crisis intervention outside the hospital, with supportive "holding" of the acutely decompensating patient in a safe (perhaps familiar) setting by trained intervenors, has had its proponents off and on for many years. While it is clear that schizophreniform psychosis is a biological phenomenon, requiring neurochemical repair and stabilization, nonbiological approaches have occasionally been suggested. When the thought disorder has clearly been exacerbated by external forces (e.g., intractable external stresses), this may constitute reasonable treatment; however, we recommend that any psychotic episode be evaluated, and treatment be directed, by a competent psychiatrist.

SUBACUTE/INTERMEDIATE CARE

Medications

Once crisis or emergency treatment has taken place, the drug initially used to control the acute psychosis usually can be continued for intermediate treatment. Initial dosage levels of traditional medications (but probably not clozapine) can often be reduced up to 50% once the patient has been stabilized; however, one should observe the patient on the lower dose for several days before assuming it is sufficient. Augmenting drugs, such as benzodiazepines or lithium, should be discontinued cautiously. Significant changes in medication or dose should be avoided just before transfer or discharge.

Several studies and considerable clinical experience with traditional neuroleptics indicate that after the acute psychosis has abated, much lower doses can and should be tried. While most reports describe maintenance populations and prevention of relapse (see below), the equivalent of 5 to 10 mg/day of haloperidol is effective for many subacute patients. Treatment decisions are highly individual, however; higher doses are necessary for many, perhaps most, patients.

It should be noted that clozapine has *not* proved effective in low doses for most patients. In the author's experience, decreasing the dose to levels very much below the initial response dose, often to save money, is a significant cause of relapse. There is little clinical experience with decreasing risperidone doses early in treatment, although most patients who respond will do so at 6 mg/day or less.

The oral administration of antipsychotic medication is preferable for most patients at this stage of care. Although more rapidly acting and predictable for crisis use, injection carries a number of countertherapeutic connotations, including penetration, assault, and infantilization. Oral medication should be substituted whenever possible. Depot preparations, such as fluphenazine or haloperidol decanoate, should be used with caution at this stage of treatment, since any adverse reactions and side effects may not be reversed as easily as those of other dosage forms. Nonetheless, as the patient prepares to leave the hospital, there may be reason to prescribe a depot neuroleptic.

Surreptitious administration of medication, in fruit juice, for example, usually leads to more problems than solutions. "Odorless, tasteless" preparations advertised for acute patients belie a basic atmosphere of manipulation and distrust. It is usually better to deal directly with an issue of medication refusal, and address the reasons for it, than to circumvent the problem. When given openly, however, a liquid form may be preferred for a variety of reasons.

Drug Choice. Prior drug effectiveness is often the best predictor of current response. "Challenge doses" and other methods of predicting dosage or therapeutic response have not been shown to be accurate or effective enough for general use with neuroleptics. With a few exceptions, plasma levels of antipsychotic drugs have not proved to be reliable predictors of bioavailability or therapeutic response. It should be noted, however, that clozapine plasma levels above 350 to 400 ng/ml are far more likely to be associated with positive response than lower levels (Kronig *et al.*, 1995). Nonresponding patients, and those suspected of not taking their medication, may benefit from testing of blood levels, if only to establish gross bioavailability and compliance.

Depot injections of fluphenazine or haloperidol are helpful for many patients, particularly those for whom medication compliance problems are anticipated (Glazer & Kane, 1992). Several authors suggest that the depot medication be instituted *before* compliance problems arise, and that oral test doses and injections be started before the patient leaves the hospital. Patient response should be observed and side effects alleviated before discharging the patient.

Psychotherapy

All major types of psychotherapy have found some use in the treatment of schizophrenia. McGlashan (1994) reminds us that psychotherapy has evolved along with our understanding of schizophrenia, and that the patient can be considered and reconsidered for various kinds of intervention as the illness waxes and wanes. In spite of the biological themes of many psychiatry training programs and research efforts, any sophisticated treatment program should recognize psychotherapeutic approaches beyond simple support and education (Gabbard, 1994).

Therapy is often used to support the biological and social parts of the treatment plan, such as medication compliance and discharge transition. Problem-solving approaches, perhaps aimed at rehabilitation, are sometimes useful for patients who are stable at this point in treatment. Exploration of conflictual material is rarely possible, although it may be appropriate for some people in highly specialized programs.

Group therapy in some form is commonly recommended, and may focus on education, support, reality testing, skill development, communication, or problem solving. Group goals and process should be titrated to patients' abilities and prognoses, although involving patients at slightly different levels of stability and improvement is often useful. Many techniques and leadership styles have been described (Fenton & Cole, 1995); structure and directiveness are important in most settings.

Patients are often receptive to information about their illness, treatment, or adaptive needs. Individually chosen and structured, this can be very helpful and support the overall treatment effort. Unfortunately, some inpatient settings have a rigid schedule of individual or group psychoeducation and required "programming" that is unrelated to the patient's ability to use or retain the information.

Family intervention and therapy can begin very early in treatment. At first, families need to understand what is happening to their loved one, receive optimistic but realistic information, and learn how best to participate in his or her care.

Family "intervention" is different from family "therapy," generally connoting more directive intercession. Tarrier *et al.* (1994) described significantly fewer relapses five and eight years after admission and family intervention in a cohort of particularly stable patients. Families with high "expressed emotion" (EE), an overly stimulating environment associated with relapse in some studies, showed more positive response to the intervention. McFarlane (1994) reviewed a number of studies and concluded that psychoeducation in multiple family groups is a cost-effective rehabilitation vehicle.

Psychosocial Techniques

At this point in care, such things as community support and case management exist more as plans than as realities for the patient. The clinician's experience with them should suggest which ones are appropriate for a given patient and thus should be included in discharge planning. While it is tempting to offer an entire menu of supports and interventions to every patient, it is better (and more cost-effective) to tailor them to individual needs, with the knowledge that plans can be changed after the patient has had a chance to experience community care for a while.

When combined with a comprehensive program of medication and other service delivery, social skills training improves some coping skills and symptoms, and perhaps outcome as well (Liberman, 1994). Nevertheless, Dobson (1995) found that specific social skills training, sometimes associated with decreases in negative symptoms, did not improve relapse rates over social milieu treatment. A more detailed discussion of psychosocial treatments is presented in the following section.

COMMUNITY AND MAINTENANCE CARE, RELAPSE PREVENTION

Almost all schizophrenic patients are outpatients most of the time. Although crisis and hospital treatments are important, most patients spend their lives outside hospitals. Appropriate outpatient and community treatment increases—sometimes dramatically—the probability that those lives will be satisfying and productive.

Medication and Other Biological Treatments

Maintenance medication is the cornerstone of relapse prevention and improved quality of life. The patient should have had a successful introduction to his or her drug regimen, with attention to a smooth transition to the maintenance prescription, control of side effects, and understanding the importance of treatment compliance.

Until a few years ago, the choice of a maintenance neuroleptic was not considered as important as consistent administration and follow-up. Clozapine, other new and atypical antipsychotic drugs, and a new appreciation of depot preparations have changed this view. At this writing, the superiority of clozapine over traditional medications for most patients—not only refractory ones—is all but established. How clozapine will compare with other new drugs, such as risperidone, olanzapine, and those likely to follow on the U.S. market, is less clear. Efficacy and side-effect profiles suggest that none will immediately replace it in the clinical armamentarium. The author's experience, largely anecdotal, indicates that clozapine is probably superior to risperidone for most patients. In Europe, it is often the neuroleptic of first choice and is not reserved for treatment-refractory patients (Neuhalfen & Kaplan, 1994).

One does not lightly displace the traditional medications that have been so important in the fight against chronic mental disability. Nonetheless, among those patients (up to 80%) who tolerate maintenance clozapine, one-third to one-half improve dramatically and, in some studies, another 50% fare better than they did on older neuroleptics (Carpenter *et al.*, 1995; Lieberman *et al.*, 1994; Reid *et al.*, 1994; Reid & Mason, 1995; Meltzer & Okayli, 1995; Chow *et al.*, 1995). Some of these studies highlight improvements in relapse and rehospitalization rates; all associate the improvements with actual, lasting symptom decreases. Some reports describe lower patient tolerance but positive group response in clinical efficacy for those patients who continue to take the medication (Chow *et al.*, 1995).

Several studies imply that clozapine is useful for negative and, especially, cognitive symptoms (Meltzer & Okayli, 1995). A critical review by Carpenter *et al.* (1995) found clearly superior response in about 50% of refractory patients, but associated that superiority with overall efficacy rather than with targeted response to negative or cognitive symptoms.

A number of atypical neuroleptics other than clozapine, olanzapine, and risperidone have completed phase III U.S. trials and/or are available in Europe. Quetiapine, sertindole, olanzapine, ziprasidone, and amisulpride all show signs of effectiveness against negative symptoms compared with traditional drugs (usually haloperidol), less potential for extrapyramidal symptoms, implied protection from tardive dyskinesia, and little anticholinergic activity.

All of the clozapine studies and reports cited describe *group* results. In each, there were a number of patients who did not respond to, or perhaps could not tolerate, clozapine. The choice of medication must be an individual process, founded in effectiveness but with a careful consideration of side effects, likely adverse effects, future compliance, route of administration, and individual response characteristics. For example, the psychiatrist may strongly recommend the compliance security of depot haloperidol or fluphenazine. Some patients find that low doses of risperidone are effective and have few or no side effects. Others refuse the weekly blood count required with clozapine or are concerned about the possibility, however small, of lethal agranulocytosis. Still others experience intractable side effects or adverse effects that necessitate a change.

Electroconvulsive Therapy. The psychiatrist must be prepared to offer, or at least to consider and refer the patient for, the entire range of biological treatments. Although medications are the treatment of choice for most patients and ECT is usually not a useful augmentation for neuroleptics (Sarkar *et al.*, 1994), it still has a role in the therapy of refractory or drug-intolerant patients. Stiebel (1995) recently described a small series in which ECT was a safe, effective, and well-tolerated maintenance treatment for chronic patients.

Psychosocial Interventions

Psychosocial techniques have virtually revolutionized community care and the rehabilitation of chronic psychotic illness. Relatively passive approaches, such as regular clinic follow-up, support groups, case management, and clinic-sponsored social clubs, available for many years, assist in community adaptation and decrease rehospitalization to some extent. Several more active strategies have emerged during the past decade that can have a measurable positive impact on the patient.

Non-hospital Settings

Therapeutic Environments. Day clubs and "inns" provide healthy alternatives to less savory environments or the streets. They can offer skills training, group therapy, and respite, as well as social support, and can be operated by a few staff members and stable, trained patients (perhaps as supported work; see below). More intensive group homes, such as Soteria House (Mosher, 1991), offer non-hospital growth for young patients in order to encourage a better prognosis (e.g., after a first psychotic break). These strategies should not be confused with day hospitals, which are usually active, medical/therapeutic "stepdown" programs for patients in transition from inpatient care, or are attempts to prevent hospitalization. Similarly, psychiatric crisis intervention should be differentiated from what some authors call crisis respite. Lay staff or volunteer intervention not supervised by a psychiatrist should be reserved for minor or social crises (e.g., family discord, housing problems). If acute psychosis, threat of suicide or violence, adverse medication reaction, or comparable problems are present, psychiatric assessment should be sought.

Education and Personal Skills Training. There is little doubt that stable patients can, to some extent, learn to monitor their symptoms and reacquire skills related to social interaction, getting along in public, taking their own medication, and the like. Patient training in illness understanding and symptom recognition may be effective for relapse recognition and prevention in some fairly stable patients. Family involvement is often helpful (Eckman *et al.*, 1992). Special teaching techniques are necessary, especially when cognitive deficits are prominent. Cognitive deficits must be recognized in order to individualize other psychosocial programs as well, and create the greatest potential for success.

There is considerable question about patients' ability to generalize their skills outside the clinical or rehabilitation setting, particularly when the consequences of failure (e.g., failure to take medication properly) are significant. Generalization is often unsuccessful, especially in skills training programs that do not continue training into the patient's real living environment (Benton & Schroeder, 1990). When the patient's natural environment can be changed to meet rehabilitation needs, or when special training can be provided there instead of in an artificial setting, success is more likely. Unfortunately, most studies still find that community skills are not apt to reach the level temporarily demonstrated in the "classroom" (Liberman, 1992; Wong, 1993).

Assertive Community Treatment (ACT). Also described as active community treatment or assertive continuous treatment, ACT uses principles of aggressive outreach by a small team of clinical and support staff members, often including a psychiatrist and specially trained and stable patients. The ACT team becomes a consistent part of the patient's environment, continually available and sometimes inserting itself into the patient's life in order to encourage him or her to take advantage of clinical, support, and rehabilitative opportunities. The U.S. Veterans Administration recently published results of a two-year, multicenter study of successful intensive psychiatric community care (IPCC) in which programs diligently applied four principles—intensity, flexibility and community orientation, focus on rehabilitation, and continuity of care (Rosenheck *et al.*, 1995).

Supported Housing. Housing for the chronically mentally ill need not always consist solely of what patients can find on their own. Cheap, unmonitored rooming houses and residential hotels are giving way to the mental health community's recognition that one's living environment is an important part of one's ability to remain out of the hospital, one's quality of life, and often one's safety. Supported housing blends well with continuity of care, and can thus benefit patients even though there is little evidence that the programs change the symptoms or course of severe mental illness.

There are many kinds of supported housing. Sometimes, it takes the form of simple rent and utility payments, with minimal case management or supervision. In other forms, it may include group living, assisted living, or settings that also offer the psychiatric and psychosocial services that the patient needs. Housing and related costs themselves are often paid from the patient's disability income or other social entitlements. There is some controversy about whether or not scarce dollars earmarked for treatment—as contrasted with social welfare dollars—should be spent for supported housing or for supported-work salaries (see below).

Supported Employment. Supported employment implies more than a sheltered workshop. Patients are trained in the skills they need to find and keep real, paying jobs, and then provided with intensive supervision and support to encourage both generic work behaviors (e.g., regular attendance, acceptable appearance and affect) and specific job performance (e.g., through on-the-job coaching). Most programs include the development of relationships between the clinic or mental health center and various potential employers, illustrating the benefits to companies' participating in the program. Social supports, such as targeted group therapy (including family groups), may be offered.

Outcome. Combined with appropriate medication and clinical follow-up, ACT, supported housing, and supported work all improve the quality of life. Many studies suggest that intensive community care and attention decrease hospital readmissions as well (Rosenheck *et al.,* 1995; Liberman, 1994; Quinliven *et al.,* 1995). In the Rosenheck study, 9 of 10 VA treatment sites decreased their need for inpatient services, lessening them overall by 33%. Some reports, however, describe few significant differences between intensive case management (not identical to classical ACT) and routine case management (Sands & Canaan, 1994). Tyrer *et al.* (1995) found that British community patients under "close observation" for 18 months were hospitalized more often than were those with routine follow-up, suggesting that such individual scrutiny was superior in recognizing important psychotic symptoms and thus the need for admission. Although ACT is moderately expensive, it is probably cost-effective.

In spite of the several other reasons to consider ACT, supported environments, and similar approaches, there is little indication thus far that even aggressive psychosocial treatments affect the long-term course of schizophrenia. Improvement in psychotic symptoms is modest, if present at all. Dencker and Dencker (1994) remind us that in this era of hospital downsizing throughout the Western world, "schizophrenia in all phases must be treated as the disease it is, not as a social problem."

Advocacy for Patients and Families

Patient and family organizations, such as the National Alliance for the Mentally Ill (NAMI), and other advocates, such as the National Mental Health Association (MHA), gather both dollar and human resources to battle severe mental illness. Schizophrenia is a prominent target for such groups, although not the only one. These are not merely support groups. NAMI, for example, provides information for patients and families, informs and encourages professionals, stimulates research on severe and chronic mental illness, and has become a prominent participant in local and national mental health policy. The NAMI psychoeducation curriculum *A Journey of Hope* is a useful part of many treatment programs. There are also primary support groups that limit themselves to current and former patients, such as the various state Mental Health Consumers. Unfortunately, a few such groups actually discourage their members and others from taking advantage of modern psychiatric treatment.

SIDE EFFECTS AND ADVERSE EFFECTS OF NEUROLEPTIC DRUGS[1]

The side effects and adverse effects of antipsychotic medications must be understood by the clinician before the drugs are prescribed. The ward staff should be trained in the recognition of these, and of signs of toxicity. The patient and his or her family should receive complete information, unless such a discussion cannot be understood because of psychosis or would not be in the best interest of recovery, including which side effects or adverse effects are common and which occur only rarely. It is often useful to provide simple, clear, written materials and to encourage discussion with caregivers.

Fortunately, most side effects of antipsychotic medications are benign and little more than an inconvenience for the patient. Some, however, such as acute dystonia, can be quite painful, and many others may be frightening or misunderstood by the patient and family. Without appropriate attention, any side effect can become a patient's rationalization for stopping the medication, a motive for treatment noncompliance or severing the doctor-patient relationship.

Most common side effects can be controlled by either titrating the dosage downward or prescribing an additional medication. It is often unwise to decrease the neuroleptic dose below standard levels early in the acute treatment of the psychosis, since such doses are associated with significantly lower antipsychotic effect (Rifkin *et al.*, 1991). The prophylactic addition of such drugs as benztropine, trihexyphenidyl, or amantadine is often recommended. One must understand, however, that they add clinical considerations, including new side effects (e.g., anticholinergic effects), drug-drug interactions, other alterations of clinical response to the neuroleptic, and the patient's psychological reaction to the change in treatment.

---

[1]In this text, the term "side effects" refers to benign conditions that may, nevertheless, be inconvenient, frightening, or painful (e.g., mild tremor or sedation). Adverse effects are associated with significant potential for harm (e.g., tardive dyskinesia or agranulocytosis). The distinction is not always completely clear.

Traditional ("Conventional") Neuroleptics

Neurologic and nonneurologic side effects and adverse effects are discussed briefly below. Neuroleptic malignant syndrome, clozapine-related agranulocytosis and cardiovascular/respiratory effects, and tardive dyskinesia are discussed in greater detail at the end of this section.

Sedation. A common side effect, even with the so-called nonsedating neuroleptics, sedation dissipates after a few days or weeks, as tolerance develops. This side effect is often used as a substitute for a hypnotic agent, although it does not provide physiologic sleep cycles.

Autonomic Effects. Such effects, not mentioned elsewhere in this section, are most commonly represented by postural hypotension. Most are dose related. Both orthostatic hypotension and persistent hypotension are more common with the low-potency neuroleptics, although geriatric patients in particular may have difficulties with haloperidol and other high-potency drugs as well.

Anticholinergic Effects. Since the antipsychotic, antidepressant, and antiparkinsonian drugs all have anticholinergic effects, and since two or more may be prescribed together, considerations of dose and additive effects are important. For most patients, these represent only an inconvenience, such as dry mouth or mild constipation. For some, such as middle-aged or older men, they may be significant (e.g., prostate enlargement). Blurred vision related to problems with accommodation is common, and should not be confused with exacerbation of glaucoma (see below). Serious symptoms, including anticholinergic delirium, which may be confused with functional psychosis, are often related more to antiparkinsonian drugs than to the neuroleptics themselves.

Severe syndromes, such as those related to drug overdose or (rarely) abuse of antiparkinsonian agents, can be treated with physostigmine 0.5 to 2.0 mg every 15 to 30 minutes, intramuscularly (IM) or by slow intravenous (IV) drip, until central nervous system (CNS) or cardiac symptoms abate. Because physostigmine is rapidly metabolized, the patient should be closely observed and the dose repeated as needed to maintain improvement until the anticholinergic medications have been metabolized. If a trial of physostigmine at the above doses does not have a positive effect, other sources for the patient's symptoms, including stroke or neuroleptic malignant syndrome, should be strongly considered.

Neuroleptic-Induced Pseudoparkinsonism. Similar to Parkinson's disease, it generally begins within a few weeks of the onset of treatment. Akinetic symptoms may be mistaken for schizophrenic symptoms or depression, and include shuffling gait, flattening of expression, and general psychomotor retardation. Severe rigidity may be confused with catatonia, and may eventually lead to muscle damage, difficulty in breathing, or difficulty with eating. Pill rolling and intention tremors are common.

Oral antiparkinsonian (benztropine, trihexyphenidyl, etc.) or anticholinergic (diphenhydramine, etc.) drugs are the primary treatment; amantadine works as well. Intramuscular anticholinergic agents are generally quite effective for acute discomfort, but if they are not, dopamine agonists, such as bromocriptine, may be used (Levinson & Simpson, 1987). Thioridazine has few extrapyramidal side effects.

The "rabbit syndrome," with rapid lip tremors, is an unusual form of extrapyramidal effects, and should not be confused with tardive dyskinesia. It will usually respond to antiparkinsonian drugs.

Akathisia. This can easily be mistaken for anxiety or worsened psychosis. Restlessness is generally felt, primarily in the legs, or as difficulty in sitting still. It is a major source of discomfort, and should be treated. When found in the absence of pseudoparkinsonism, it may respond poorly to the usual antiparkinsonian, anticholinergic, or antihistaminic preparations, but often yields to benzodiazepines.

Acute Dystonia. Most of acute dystonic reactions occur within 24 hours of treatment, 90% by the third day (Sranek *et al.*, 1986). They are painful and frightening, often include torsion of the trunk and oculogyric crisis, and are more common in young males. Dystonic reactions (and other side effects, as well) are often confused by the patient with "allergy." Patients who say they are allergic or hypersensitive to neuroleptics should be carefully questioned, since these effects are easily preventable in most cases and there are few alternatives to antipsychotic treatment.

Symptoms should be treated immediately with IM or IV medication. Benztropine, 1 to 2 mg IM, is usually sufficient, and acts about as rapidly as an IV injection. Diphenhydramine or biperiden is effective as well. Oral antiparkinsonian drugs are preventive, and should be considered prophylactically for young male patients, both to prevent the dystonia and to enhance medication compliance.

Endocrine Abnormalities. Many patients taking antipsychotics for long periods gain modest amounts of weight, and sometimes develop a fuller facies. Some of these effects, particularly in men, are related to increased prolactin levels, which in turn may lead to gynecomastia and/or lactation. Treatment with amantadine or bromocriptine is usually helpful. Thioridazine is the neuroleptic most commonly associated with sexual dysfunction, including occasional impotence or retrograde ejaculation.

Increased Seizure Potential. An increased potential for seizures is frequently a concern in patients taking neuroleptic drugs, particularly the low-potency drugs and promazine (rarely psychiatrically prescribed). In traditional neuroleptics, seizures are rare with proper medication dosage; however, patients with seizure disorders should be monitored until their stability is established. Patients who have taken overdoses or very large amounts of neuroleptics should be considered at risk.

Dose-related seizures occur in about 1 to 5% of new clozapine patients, primarily in those whose dose has been rapidly increased. Very slow upward titration can eliminate most seizure risk. It is prudent to obtain a baseline electroencephalogram (EEG) in patients whose dose exceeds 600 mg/day. The majority of patients who have had a clozapine-related seizure can continue the drug, with or without prophylactic anticonvulsants. Valproic acid or phenobarbital is recommended for some, but not carbamazepine (which is associated with an increased risk of agranulocytosis). The clozapine dose should be decreased by one-half for a week, and then slowly increased to therapeutic levels.

Electrocardiographic Changes. Thioridazine is the conventional antipsychotic drug most likely to alter the electrocardiogram (ECG). Serious arrhythmias are quite unusual, although a pretreatment ECG may be advisable when high doses are anticipated, or in patients at cardiac risk.

Ophthalmic Effects. As already mentioned, anticholinergic effects frequently cause mild accommodation problems, particularly in the elderly. Thioridazine is associated with a well-known, serious retinopathy, almost always in doses above 800 mg/day. Small deposits of melanin in the lens or cornea, usually of no clinical significance, may appear with any of the phenothiazines, but are uncommon in other neuroleptics. Glaucoma is listed as a possible side effect for most of these drugs, primarily because of the anticholinergic effects and the theoretical vulnerability to narrow-angle disease. This potential has probably been considerably overstated in the literature (Reid *et al.*, 1976).

Photosensitivity and Other Skin Reactions. Patients taking neuroleptics, particularly chlorpromazine, are often vulnerable to sunburn (which may exacerbate other temperature-regulation problems). Sunscreens are recommended. Inconvenient rashes, usually maculopapular, are common. Although these may represent real allergies or hypersensitivities, their importance should not be overplayed to the patient. An antihistamine (e.g., diphenhydramine) is usually effective, as is switching to another medication. If the rash continues, a clinical decision can be made as to whether treatment of the psychosis is more important than the dermatitis.

Liver Toxicity. Because all of the neuroleptics are metabolized through the liver, most with some difficulty, it is important to establish baseline liver function and to be alert for clinical signs of hepatotoxicity. Mild elevations of liver enzymes are generally not contraindications to neuroleptic use. The phenothiazines are the most likely offenders, and probably should not be used for patients with significant cholestasis.

Agranulocytosis. With conventional neuroleptics (not clozapine), onset is usually within three months of the beginning of drug therapy, and most often involves high doses. Death is unusual, with recovery following standard supportive and antibiotic treatment for one to three weeks. Suddenness of onset precludes the effectiveness of serial monitoring of the white blood count; however, a baseline complete blood count is prudent. Patients frequently relapse if the phenothiazine is reinstituted; switching to a nonphenothiazine antipsychotic is recommended. Clozapine-related agranulocytosis is discussed below.

Tardive Dystonia. This involves the rare, rapid onset of abnormal movements that are similar to those seen in tardive dyskinesia, but are more rapidly disabling, after even a brief prescription of antipsychotic medication. Treatment is unclear. Very high doses of antiparkinsonian medications (e.g., 60 mg/day of trihexyphenidyl) may be helpful for some patients. Stereotaxic surgery may be necessary in extreme cases (Goldman *et al.*, 1985).

Neuroleptic-Induced Catatonia. This is an unusual syndrome that is difficult to differentiate from schizophrenic symptoms. A change of neuroleptic or prescription of amantadine is the accepted treatment. This syndrome is not the same as malignant or lethal catatonia, although it appears similar and the physiologic reactions may simply have different (i.e., medication versus internal) causes. They are often discussed together.

Neuroleptics in Pregnancy or During Lactation. There appears to be little risk in becoming pregnant while taking therapeutic doses of neuroleptics, although a few cases of congenital malformation possibly related to antipsychotic drugs have been reported. It is probably prudent to postpone drug treatment until the second trimester when clinically feasible; however, no definitive studies regarding the pros and cons of this practice have been done. Postnatal syndromes may be prevented by discontinuing medication at least 10 days before delivery. Since antipsychotic drugs enter breast milk, breast feeding should be discouraged.

Drug-Drug Interactions. As implied above, neuroleptics add to the sedative, CNS depressant, and anticholinergic effects of other drugs. They may decrease blood levels of tricyclic antidepressants, and may decrease either the blood level or the anticonvulsant effect of phenytoin. The interactions of neuroleptics with cardiac preparations or pressor drugs must be considered for the individual agents involved. They increase the analgesic effects of pain relievers, including narcotics, either through drug interaction or through their own pain-dulling effects.

Neuroleptic Malignant Syndrome

Neuroleptic malignant syndrome (NMS) is the most serious acute adverse effect of traditional antipsychotic medications. Although rare, it is regularly reported in the literature, and has been seen at least a few times by most experienced clinicians. It affects all age groups, and, depending on early recognition and treatment, has a mortality of up to 20%. Age under 40, male sex, nonschizophrenic mental illness, physical or neurological debilitation, and significant doses of high-potency conventional neuroleptics may increase the risk of NMS, but, except for physical debilitation, not to a striking extent. In some cases, severe extrapyramidal symptoms interact with a medical condition to increase vulnerability. Many similar syndromes with a nonneuroleptic etiology may be misdiagnosed as NMS, perhaps up to 25% of the time, including fulminating forms of catatonia variously called malignant or lethal (Sewell & Jeste, 1992; Philbrick & Rummans, 1994).

Symptoms may appear early in antipsychotic treatment, but are sometimes delayed for many months. They include a rapid rise in body temperature (up to 105 to 107°F), severe extrapyramidal symptoms, severe muscle rigidity, sweating, hypertension, alterations of mental status, elevated creatinine phosphokinase (CPK), and elevated white count.

Significant mortality or morbidity is almost always associated with medical complications. Patients treated rapidly for their extrapyramidal symptoms, and promptly supported medically, are very likely to survive.

Treatment is fairly straightforward, and often successful. Neuroleptics should be discontinued and the patient immediately treated with bromocriptine, amantadine, or dantrolene. Intensive medical support, hydration, and body cooling must be instituted as well. The decision about future antipsychotic treatment may include carefully monitored rechallenge with a dopamine-blocking neuroleptic after at least two weeks, but atypical neuroleptics, such as clozapine or risperidone, are safer and likely to be more effective.

Electroconvulsive therapy is effective in many cases of NMS. It has the additional advantage of being effective for malignant (lethal) catatonia and being relatively safe for patients with other NMS-mimicking syndromes.

Clozapine-Related Agranulocytosis and Cardiovascular/Respiratory Syndromes

Idiosyncratic agranulocytosis is seen in just under 1% of patients taking clozapine. It is not dose related. The manufacturer currently does not allow prescribing in the United States without a weekly white blood count (WBC) and monitors the results for leukopenia through a national registry. This process has kept the number of severe cases of agranulocytosis to a minimum, with only 12 deaths among over 77,000 patients through September 1994 (Honigfeld, 1994).

Clozapine-related agranulocytosis is seen most often during the first 4 to 18 weeks of treatment. Leukopenia under 3,500 WBC/mm^3 has occurred in 2.5 to 3% of patients, about 20 to 25% of whom have developed granulocyte counts under 500/mm^3. Almost all cases remit quickly after discontinuing the drug (Sandoz, 1993). The syndrome is almost never seen after the first year of clozapine treatment, although monitoring is required.

Patients who have died generally have been those whose blood counts dropped extremely rapidly, a condition sometimes related to combinations of clozapine and other medications associated with blood dyscrasia (e.g., carbamazepine), and with middle or advanced age. The patient should not be rechallenged, as there is increased probability of a second episode, which may occur more precipitously than the first. Carbamazepine is currently considered an absolute contraindication to clozapine.

Severe hypotension occurs in a very small portion of the roughly 9% of patients who develop some hypotension, usually early in treatment. About 0.03% of patients experience severe respiratory collapse, sometimes with cardiac arrest. Some association with benzodiazepine-clozapine combinations has been suggested, but the relationship is far from proven. Nonetheless, some caution with this combination is advised. As with other drugs that may cause hypotension, elderly patients may require additional monitoring.

There are indications that adverse cardiovascular events are much more common in normal, nonpsychotic individuals than in those with psychotic disorders. One should thus be cautious when using normal control subjects in clozapine research.

Tardive Dyskinesia

Although generally associated with total cumulative dose of conventional neuroleptic drugs, tardive dyskinesia can appear in any patient, even early in treatment. Most cases appear slowly, offering time to consider therapeutic alternatives. There is no broadly effective treatment. Prevention, through using the lowest effective neuroleptic doses, frequent monitoring with an abnormal involuntary movements scale (AIMS) or similar instrument, and/or use of atypical neuroleptics, is recommended.

The first step in treatment is to decrease or discontinue the neuroleptic, if clinically feasible. Clozapine or low doses of risperidone may be substituted for many patients. One should expect the dyskinesia to worsen temporarily. If the benefits of the conventional antipsychotic drug outweigh the risks of worsening tardive dyskinesia, the medication may be continued after careful discussion with the patient and/or guardian. Some patients have what Gardos *et al.* (1994) describe as a benign long-term course of tardive dyskinesia, and deteriorate very slowly if medication is carefully managed.

About one-third of patients with tardive dyskinesia improve spontaneously (up to 50% better ratings on AIMS scales) within several months of discontinuing neuroleptic medication (Glazer *et al.,* 1990). In the Glazer study, spontaneous improvement was much more likely in nonschizophrenic patients, however, and some dyskinesias worsen of their own accord.

Pharmacotherapy is at least partially effective for about half of patients. Initial conservative treatment may be with a relatively benign medication, such as high doses of vitamin E (which is not as likely to be helpful as some other choices, but has few side effects). After a reasonable period without effect, consider levodopa (L-Dopa) with carbidopa, which has shown markedly different results in studies but may be effective for many patients within three months (Simpson *et al.,* 1988; Ludatscher, 1989), or clonazepam. Other benzodiazepines are sometimes effective; the mechanism of action is unclear, and their sedative effect may account for some of the improvement. Patients taking dopamine agonists, such as L-Dopa, should be monitored for worsening of their psychosis.

Several other medications have limited success in tardive dyskinesia. Clozapine is probably not directly effective; initial reports of improvements may have been due to spontaneous remissions. Remoxipride, not available in the United States, may have some positive effects. There are several descriptions of improvement with clonidine and propranolol, both adrenergic drugs, but no recent studies. Cholinergic supplements, such as lecithin and choline, have shown inconsistent results.

ECT may be considered in severe cases of tardive dyskinesia, either as an adjunctive effort to decrease the neuroleptic dose or as a primary treatment of the dyskinesia. Results are variable.

Increasing the dose of conventional neuroleptic in an effort to suppress symptoms of tardive dyskinesia is usually inappropriate, but may be necessary in carefully selected situations. Appropriate informed consent, with an understanding by the patient and/or guardian of the potential risks and benefits, should be obtained.

SPECIAL CONSIDERATIONS

Suicide

The risk of completed suicide in schizophrenia is probably surpassed only by that in hopeless medical illness and major mood disorders. The addition of an affective component to acute or subacute psychosis increases the likelihood of suicide attempts. Psychotic thinking makes attempts less predictable by clinicians or families, less organized, more impulsive, and more likely to be successful. Hopelessness about one's disease or social adaptation is a contributing factor. Most schizophrenics are aware of their illness, and of the fact that it usually responds incompletely to treatment. Withdrawal and ostracism by the community often lead to isolation.

Suicide should be considered a possibility for all patients, and a probability for those who are particularly withdrawn, are hopeless, or have a history of previous attempts. Gesture-like—or even bizarre—previous attempts should not decrease one's caution about the seriousness of the patient's impulses. Schizophrenics may confuse self-directed and other-directed aggressive impulses, with a concomitant danger to others, particularly during acute psychosis.

Acute Catatonia

Acute and severe catatonia can be a life-threatening syndrome. While catatonic schizophrenia is considered a subtype of the diagnosis, catatonia has neurological connotations that deserve special diagnostic and treatment attention. When not responsive to initial medications, such as potent neuroleptics, severe catatonia often remits quickly with ECT, which is especially indicated for the malignant or lethal type. Benzodiazepine muscle relaxants may be helpful symptomatically and may prevent rhabdomyolysis.

295.40 SCHIZOPHRENIFORM DISORDER

Schizophreniform disorder should be treated using the principles described for acute and subacute schizophrenic psychosis. Special attention should be focused on whether or not the patient eventually will meet the duration criteria for schizophrenia; follow-up is important.

Neuroleptic medication may be cautiously tapered if the psychosis remits completely for several weeks. It is tempting to be conservative in the hope that the symptoms will not recur; however, one must remember that if the patient does eventually merit a schizophrenic diagnosis, his or her prognosis is improved considerably by vigorous treatment during the first psychotic presentation and the prevention of another acute exacerbation, if possible.

295.70 SCHIZOAFFECTIVE DISORDER

General Principles

Primary treatment should be focused on the schizophreniform nature of the primary illness, using the treatment principles described for schizophrenia. Schizoaffective patients are often more difficult to keep in remission than are schizophrenics, and their mood symptoms do not respond as well as those in patients with pure mood disorders. The affective component sometimes appears after schizophrenia has been diagnosed for several years, and should be treated with biological techniques according to its presentation (i.e., manic or depressive type) after antipsychotic medication has been stabilized.

The *manic* type may be treated with a neuroleptic and a mood stabilizer, such as lithium, carbamazepine (provided clozapine is not being used), or valproic acid. Carbamazepine's enzyme induction decreases the bioavailability of antipsychotic drugs and carbamazepine itself, so that dose and balance must be carefully monitored at the beginning of therapy. Mood stabilizers alone are not recommended, even when current symptoms appear entirely affective. Except for clozapine, neuroleptics alone are usually insufficient.

Atypical neuroleptics, such as clozapine or risperidone, should be considered early in treatment, as well as for refractory patients. Clozapine alone is suitable for some patients, although the extent of its ability to treat both psychotic and affective symptoms in schizoaffective disorders is not yet clear. If augmentation is required, carbamazepine should not be used.

Patients with the *depressed* type require an antidepressant medication in addition to a neuroleptic, but antidepressants alone are not sufficient. Although all of the popular antidepressants have been found useful in group studies, monoamine oxidase inhibitors should probably be reserved for atypical presentations. Fixed-dose preparations should be avoided. Mood stabilizers may be used to prevent affective relapse, but do not address depression itself as well as do other drugs.

The relative unpredictability and impulsivity of chronically psychotic and depressed patients make suicide a significant danger for many of them. Overdose potential is a consideration with all drugs, especially those associated with higher lethality, either alone or in combination (e.g., tricyclics).

ECT may be helpful for either depressed or manic types of schizoaffective disorder, particularly patients with severe depression, intractable agitation, and/or failure to respond adequately to reasonable trials of medication. It is the safest effective alternative for some elderly or debilitated patients.

Finally, one should note that dysphoria is a common symptom in schizophrenia. Drug-induced or postpsychotic depressions are common. These and the akinetic effects of antipsychotic drugs may be mistaken for schizoaffective withdrawal and psychomotor retardation.

297.1 DELUSIONAL DISORDER

The treatment of delusional disorder has been best studied in patients with somatic delusions, since they tend to seek medical help far more than do other subtypes. The treatment of other subtypes is rarely reported in the literature. Erotomanic patients may come to psychiatric attention when their victims report them to the police. Those with jealous delusions may be referred by a spouse.

Some young delusional patients can accept supportive treatment and low or maintenance doses of neuroleptics. Many do not improve and some go on to meet the criteria for schizophrenia, but there have been several case reports of patients who were able to continue working or attending school. There is little doubt that many patients live relatively uneventful, if uncomfortable, lives away from psychiatric care.

Psychotherapy

Supportive therapy may be helpful, with therapists neither supporting nor strongly refuting the delusions. Confidentiality should be stressed, but with clearly stated disclaimers should significant danger to others arise. A slow questioning of the ways the delusions interfere with one's life can be introduced after the therapeutic alliance has been well established. Neither direct confrontation nor dynamic interpretation has been reported to be useful; either may damage the tenuous doctor-patient relationship.

Although hospitalization is not routinely suggested or required, preventing disturbing behaviors, particularly in erotomanic patients, may be necessary. If the safety of others, including the therapist, is threatened, other steps must be taken (see below).

Medications

Most reports address the somatic subtype of delusional disorder and do not clarify the diagnosis; patient groups may include those with a somatoform disorder or, occasionally, another psychosis. Except for those with somatoform delusions, most patients either do not accept or do not continue psychiatric treatment (Rockwell *et al.*, 1994; Opjordsmoen, 1988).

Neuroleptics are the most commonly reported medications. Pimozide has been successful in a number of cases involving erotomania, pathological jealousy, and somatoform delusions (especially delusions of infestation) (Lynch, 1993; Munro, 1988; Opler & Feinberg, 1991; Lindskov & Baadsgaard, 1985; Munro *et al.*, 1985; Byrne & Yatham, 1989); the diagnoses in some of these cases were not clear. Ungvari and Vladar (1986) performed the only known controlled study, which found positive results at 2 to 8 mg/day in 10 patients with delusions of infestation. Andrews *et al.* (1986) noted that pimozide is not popular in the United States, although it is available, and reported three cases of delusional infestation that were successfully treated with haloperidol. When neuroleptics are accepted and effective for nonsomatic delusions, depot forms may be considered to enhance compliance (especially in cases of socially inappropriate behavior, such as erotomanic stalking).

Mok and Yatham (1994) reported that two patients with long-standing persecutory delusions, who met the criteria for delusional disorder, responded to clozapine (one at 175 mg/day and one at 500 mg/day). Both had been unsuccessfully treated with a variety of other neuroleptics. Response was not complete, but modest improvement was corroborated by family and caregivers. Stein *et al.* (1994) prescribed fluoxetine for four patients with pathological jealousy (not necessarily within a true delusional disorder). Three responded well to 80 mg/day, and one to 20 to 30 mg/day. The same article reported a patient whose unreasonable jealousy remitted with pimozide at 1 mg/day and another who had only a partial response to sertraline, 200 mg/day. All responses were sustained for 12 weeks of treatment. Reports of treatment with tricyclic antidepressants or lithium treatment are few and pessimistic.

Most medications are more likely to be helpful for superimposed symptoms, such as anxiety or depression, or for acute psychotic crisis. Paranoid sensitivity to side effects and the possibility of disinhibition should be considered.

Follow-up and Prognosis

The resilience of delusional disorder and the potential for some patients to harm others suggest regular follow-up whenever feasible. A Danish prospective study of 88 delusional patients indicated little change in symptoms over six to eight years. Patients whose delusions were less severe and those with ideas of reference had the best outcomes. Those whose primary delusions were of persecution or influence had the worst. Delusional content changed little over the study period. Over 50% of the patients received a schizophrenic diagnosis at some point. The rate of suicide was much higher than that of the general population (Jorgensen, 1994).

SPECIAL CONSIDERATIONS FOR POTENTIALLY DANGEROUS PATIENTS

Patients who are a distinct danger to others (e.g., erotomanic stalkers with violent intent or persons with persecutory delusions who have clearly intimated significant threats to others), and who are in a position to carry out their threats, should, in the author's opinion, be reported to a law enforcement agency or the potential victim. Many clinicians believe that it is safer—for both the potential victim and the therapist—to continue treatment without reporting, in the hope that the risk will decrease. The author respectfully disagrees, and believes that when significant danger is reasonably predictable, the patient is not contained, and treatment is not rapidly decreasing the risk, the duty to both the patient and the public requires some form of protective effort. Disclosure is one alternative. Attempting to have the patient hospitalized (voluntarily or involuntarily) is another. The latter is more restrictive for the patient, but has the advantage of greater protection from civil liability when done in good faith. As mentioned above, hospital treatment may or may not alter the delusional condition.

Unless there is good reason to act without the patient's knowledge, he or she should be made aware that disclosure (or some other protective measure) is necessary, and, if possible, should participate in it. However, discussing disclosure or hospitalization with the patient can precipitate feelings of betrayal and anger, and so should be carried out in safe circumstances. The clinician may explain that it is unrealistic to attempt treatment when risk to others is such a weighty concern, and that if any violence were to take place, it would affect the patient as well.

298.8 BRIEF PSYCHOTIC DISORDER

Crisis management and the initial treatment of brief psychotic disorder are similar to those for schizophreniform or schizophrenic exacerbations, except that the clinician does not know at the time of the diagnosis whether or not the disorder is destined to evolve into a more chronic condition. It is prudent to avoid treatments that cannot easily be reversed (e.g., depot medications), and, when feasible, to choose those that will allow one to differentiate this disorder and its relatively benign course from those of more ominous prognosis. Cautious discontinuation of neuroleptics should be part of the treatment plan, with careful monitoring for symptom return and attention to the status of possible psychotogenic stressors (e.g., childbirth, aberrant grief).

Special Considerations

The postpartum subtype of brief psychotic disorder is a serious condition that at best renders mothering inadequate and can portend significant physical danger for both mother and child. Biological treatment is almost always required. Patients often respond well to neuroleptics, but the affective components of the disorder suggest antidepressant or mood-stabilizing measures as well. One must be aware that neuroleptics appear in mothers' milk in concentrations that may affect nursing children. Electroconvulsive therapy may be the treatment of choice in some depressive presentations, and should be considered for others as well, particularly when a rapid response is required.

Prevention is often possible. Parents should be counseled about the likelihood of postpartum psychosis or other severe disturbance if either the prospective mother or her family has a history of such symptoms. Prophylactic lithium has been effective, although it crosses the placental barrier and should be considered only if the physician believes the potential benefits outweigh the risk to the fetus. Lithium and carbamazepine are particularly contraindicated during the first trimester. A few reports suggest verapamil as an alternative for patients with histories of pregnancy and postpartum mania (Goodnick, 1993). (See Chapter 17 on Mood Disorders for a further discussion of postpartum affective syndromes.)

297.3 SHARED PSYCHOTIC DISORDER *(FOLIE À DEUX)*

The first treatment principle in shared psychotic disorder (induced paranoid disorder, *folie à deux*), whenever feasible, is separation of the persons involved. The primary patient should be treated using whatever antipsychotic measures are appropriate.

The secondary patient, whose psychosis began after that of the person with the primary disorder, may improve, or even clear completely, after separation, especially if the secondary patient is the child of the psychotic primary. Successful treatment of the primary can have the same effect. Measures to prevent reuniting of the two patients, or to provide appropriate monitoring of their relationship, should be instituted if possible.

Hospitalization of the secondary should be considered in order to provide a supportive environment in which the patient's loss can be resolved and more productive defenses strengthened. Medication may be necessary, either for psychosis or for the affective symptoms that may develop. Although the patient may not wish vigorous treatment, and may avoid it, the clinician should remember that sooner or later the patient will separate from the primary, for example, through the death of a psychotic parent. Preparation for this event, and support when it occurs, may prevent further decompensation.

293.XX PSYCHOTIC DISORDER DUE TO A GENERAL MEDICAL CONDITION

Treatment of these disorders is discussed in **Part I,** Chapter 6 under "Psychotic Disorders Due to a General Medical Condition."

SUBSTANCE-INDUCED PSYCHOTIC DISORDER

Treatment of these disorders is discussed in **Part I,** Chapter 6 under "Substance-Induced Psychotic Related Disorders".

298.9 PSYCHOTIC DISORDER NOS

The treatment of psychotic symptoms or disorders not specified above generally includes treating a known source of the symptoms (cf., reversal of heavy metal poisoning, alleviation of major depression with psychosis), using a biological antipsychotic treatment (e.g., a neuroleptic drug), or both. In some cases, supporting the patient while a self-limited psychotic episode runs its course is the best approach (cf., severe acute stress reactions, some intoxications). When the source of the symptoms is not known, one should be cautious about prescribing intrusive or potentially damaging forms of therapy, or treatments that may mask important symptoms or recovery.

CHAPTER 17

MOOD DISORDERS

The treatment of mood disorders often involves both the treatment of acute mood episodes and the management of chronic, waxing and waning illness. Although some patients present singular, nonrecurring depressive or other mood events, many have chronic neurochemical imbalances that appropriate treatment does not cure, but usually attenuates. Complete alleviation of acute symptoms is often an attainable goal, as is preventing or attenuating their recurrence.

DEPRESSIVE DISORDERS

Depressions may present at any age, in many forms, and with varying severity. Most are eminently treatable, with response rates of 70 to 90% for appropriate strategies. Only characterologic dysphorias, and perhaps dysthymia, are less amenable to today's therapies. Age, the type and severity of depression, past treatment response, general medical status, life circumstances, and several other factors may affect the choice of treatment.

Like some other psychiatric disorders, depression clouds the patient's ability to view his or her world realistically. This often means that, despite great discomfort, he or she does not see the problem as resulting from a treatable condition. Such hopelessness or misperception is sometimes described as "seeing the world through black-colored glasses."

SUICIDE

The unwarranted perception of hopelessness that depression often produces is a major cause of serious suicidal ideation. Although this text will not address suicidality in great detail, it is important to evaluate risk, discuss it with the patient (and often the family), and tell the patient that once the depressive symptoms are alleviated, self-destructive impulses are very likely to dissipate as well.

Suicide danger may come from several sources. One of the most potentially lethal is the deep feeling that life is so excruciating that only death can ease the pain. Such patients often experience a kind of "tunnel vision" in which death is the only visible alternative. Other scenarios include depressive psychoses in which one's self-sacrifice will somehow save others, and delusions of saving oneself or others (e.g., one's children in severe postpartum syndromes) by "taking them to heaven."

Statistically, older and medically ill depressed patients are at greater risk for suicide than most other groups. The extent to which this reflects a logical way of dealing with terminal illness or severe and permanent disability, as contrasted with treatable depression or a temporary impulse, is not always clear. In any event, one should strongly recommend that the patient retain some hope as the clinician searches for depression or some other treatable cause for the suicidal ideation.

Assessment of suicide danger is important; however, many commonly quoted indices for prediction are not very useful—and sometimes irrelevant— for individual patients. Statistics that discuss, for example, different rates of suicide by age, sex, marital status, employment status, or availability of a particular method of self-harm are almost always based on retrospective reviews of large groups. One should note that although the *correlates* of rare events, such as suicide, may be statistically significant in large groups, the actual numerical disparities are often small.

The psychiatrist and/or treatment team must make judgments about patient care that involve a *balance* of pursuit of therapeutic objectives, necessary patient protection, and other aspects of treatment. While the clinician should be aware of the more important risk factors, a statistical "correlate" of suicide is not necessarily a useful clinical "predictor." It is thus more reasonable to speak of relative risk than of suicide prediction. Individual patients, real-life situations, and the treatment considerations in which doctor and patient are engaged are much more complex than mere actuarial charts or tables.

Once a significant risk of suicide is suspected, the clinician should change his or her view of treatment necessity from voluntary and patient-controlled to (at least partially) involuntary and other-controlled. One should take steps to prevent the patient's unrealistic self-destructive impulses from endangering self or others.

The nature of those steps varies with the situation. Sometimes, a physician can and should directly restrict the patient's freedom and arrange for appropriate monitoring (e.g., when the patient is in a hospital). More often, less direct measures are all that are possible or appropriate, as when the clinician must petition for emergency admission to the hospital or communicate his concern to the patient's family. The important thing is that the clinician gather as much information as feasible in order to understand the patient and circumstances, be aware of reasonably foreseeable suicide danger, and consider all relevant approaches to the situation.

The phrase "suicide gesture" deserves comment. From time to time, health care or mental health professionals say such things as, "She cut her wrist but it wasn't serious"; "She couldn't have died from that small overdose of aspirin"; or "His behavior was just a suicide gesture." Unless one knows the patient very well, it is good practice never to try to differentiate a suicide gesture from an attempt. The chance of death from minor lacerations or a small overdose may be low, but the stakes are very high. Patients who seem to be looking for "attention" often increase the potential lethality of their behavior the next time. Patients whose actions are based in psychosis may do seemingly silly things in the name of suicide, but their next attempt may be fatal. Finally, unsophisticated patients with severe depression may not realize that a small overdose will not kill them.

A state hospital inpatient with schizophrenia was found lying in a service road on the facility campus. He said he was trying to commit suicide, but his behavior was discounted because the campus speed limit was only 5 mph. Less than 24 hours later, he was killed after lying down on a nearby highway.

An uneducated woman was brought to the emergency room after taking an overdose of her husband's vitamins. The staff noted that the vitamins were harmless *per se,* but referred her to a psychiatrist, who found that she was morbidly depressed. It later became clear that she thought the pills were "powerful medicine," since they had been prescribed by doctors at the local VA hospital.

The recognition and management of suicide potential in "VIP" patients is particularly important. Like cancer and heart disease, serious depression and suicide do not respect prominence, profession, education, or income. It is not uncommon to see a colleague, a well-known person, or member of such a person's family suffering from depression or other mental illness, with serious risk of suicide. In such instances, one must be very careful to treat this patient as any other, to judge the situation objectively, and not to accede to such exhortations as, "Going to the mental hospital would ruin my career" or "I'll *really* be suicidal if you try to commit me."

A physician took an overdose after being accused of supplying illegal drugs to undercover agents. During treatment on the medical unit of a local hospital, both he and his wife said that the overdose was "just a stupid impulse," and that he should be discharged at once. They were furious at the psychiatric consultant who recommended involuntary psychiatric hospitalization (since the patient would not admit himself). Nevertheless, a temporary observation order was obtained and he was transferred to a private facility about 100 miles away. At the end of the initial observation period, he petitioned for release. The private hospital psychiatrist, believing the patient, did not contact the original referring psychiatrist for additional information. The patient killed himself the day he was discharged.

Discharge planning for the potentially suicidal hospital patient is sometimes seen as a Catch-22. The patient may not be able to grow further in the hospital and should be treated in the least restrictive clinically appropriate setting, yet there is always some possibility of suicide. Graduated, hierarchical efforts at increased responsibility and freedom are the hallmarks of both good treatment and good risk management. Decisions of this kind often should include treatment team participation. This allows input from many different people, who see the patient in many different settings from day to day. Unaccompanied passes and discharge should be considered thoughtfully, not impulsively. It is usually prudent to go slowly after a significant recent change in patient behavior, staffing, or treatment. Similarly, one should not increase the freedom or decrease the monitoring of severely ill patients merely for special occasions, such as a holiday or a visit from a family member.

Finally, suicide and suicide risk are not concepts that lend themselves to medical cost containment. The role of the clinician is to advocate for the best patient care possible. It is sometimes necessary to decrease the quality of *elective* care for financial reasons (as when a patient's insurance policy does not cover certain procedures and the patient is unwilling or unable to be responsible for the cost); however, when life or limb is at risk, one must not allow financial or administrative decisions to outweigh medical ones. Our ethics and, more and more, malpractice case law demand that we call loudly for those things our patients truly need.

296.XX MAJOR DEPRESSIVE DISORDER

We will address major depression in two steps: treatment of the acute depressive episode and follow-up for additional symptom remission and/or prevention of subsequent episodes. The principles of treating acute depression are similar whether the episode is isolated, a recurrence of chronic depression, or part of a bipolar disorder. Some of the following sections will thus refer to this section, after specific diagnosis-related considerations, to discuss severe depressive symptoms.

Biological treatment—medication or electroconvulsive therapy (ECT)— provides the best chance for prompt and complete symptom alleviation. Psychotherapeutic techniques are useful in several ways, but should not be the primary treatment modality unless the patient cannot tolerate biological treatment or some other unusual circumstance exists. Nevertheless, the best overall response is often attained with a combination of biological and psychological or psychodynamic treatment.

ACUTE DEPRESSIVE EPISODES

One of the first steps in the treatment of severe depression is to let the patient and family know that although depression is very painful, the prognosis is usually quite good. About 80% of patients will feel much better within one or two months, and many will experience complete remission or recovery, provided they receive appropriate treatment and follow clinical recommendations. Nevertheless, the hopelessness and cognitive impairment that are part of major depression often keep patients from anticipating improvement.

Biological Therapies

Antidepressant Medications. Medication choice is affected by several things, including safety and effectiveness data, prior medication response in patient and family, and special patient sensitivity to or tolerance of particular medications. Good past patient response, without serious adverse effects, is one of the most important predictors of current response, and may overrule consideration of more modern drugs. In the absence of personal data, the knowledge that a particular medication has helped a close relative with similar symptoms is important in eventual drug choice. Some patients cannot tolerate medication that otherwise would be effective, either acutely or for the extended periods usually necessary to prevent relapse; ECT is a safe and usually effective alternative. In experienced hands, cognitive or cognitive-behavioral psychotherapy (CBT) may be an appropriate intervention for a few such patients (Beck *et al.*, 1979; Hollon *et al.*, 1992; McKnight *et al.*, 1992), although some controlled studies question this position (Elkin *et al.*, 1989).

Several types of antidepressants are safe and effective for many patients who experience an acute major depressive episode. All other things being equal, selective serotonin reuptake inhibitors (SSRIs) and other "third-generation" antidepressants are usually the drugs of first choice; studies have shown them to be at least as effective in most (but not all) patients as the older antidepressants, with better tolerance, fewer side effects, and less likelihood of overdose lethality (Dantzler & Salzman, 1995). Individual factors may make tricyclics (TCAs), trazodone, amoxapine, or, in unusual circumstances, maprotiline or irreversible monoamine oxidase inhibitors (MAOIs), a rational early choice as well.

Overdose potential must be considered with all antidepressants, especially the tricyclics and MAOIs. Large prescriptions should not be given to patients who are severely depressed, have recently recovered, or are recovering from depressive episodes, or are a known suicide risk. Several of the newer antidepressants are safer in overdose; however, the clinician must not become complacent about prescribing.

Specific Medication Strategies. Traditional clinical wisdom suggests that patients with agitated or retarded depressions may first receive sedating or activating medication, respectively. Among the TCAs and other older drugs, the more sedating include amitriptyline and trazodone. "Activating" is a relative term, which often simply implies lack of sedative effect; it should not be confused with the true stimulating effect of methylphenidate or amphetamine. Several third-generation drugs are sometimes associated with initially increased activity and decreased sleep, which may or may not be viewed as helpful in a particular patient. Moclobemide, a reversible MAO-A inhibitor (RIMA) not yet available in the United States, has been found as effective in agitated depression as traditional sedative antidepressants and imipramine in several European studies (Delini-Stula *et al.*, 1995). In any event, antidepressant properties, separate from more peripheral activating or sedating effects, should be the primary interest.

For patients with medical conditions that limit antidepressant drug tolerance, or who must take other medications that interact with antidepressants, an SSRI or venlafaxine is often the drug of first choice. Bupropion and maprotiline are generally well tolerated, but may not have sufficient antidepressant effect. The MAOIs, particularly the reversible moclobemide and brofaramine, show promise in some studies. For many (e.g., pregnant patients), ECT or nonbiological treatments should be considered (see below).

Depression with delusions or other psychosis (but not a comorbid psychotic disorder) often either relapses with, or does not respond to, antidepressant monotherapy. Most authors suggest ECT or a combination of antidepressant and antipsychotic drugs in relatively high doses (Dubovsky & Thomas, 1992). ECT is safer for, and better tolerated by, many (perhaps most) patients, especially the elderly or debilitated (Meyers, 1995). Amoxapine has antipsychotic properties in some patients.

In melancholia, TCAs are still the preferred medication, particularly as noted in some studies of elderly patients (Roose *et al.*, 1994). Some reports, however, suggest that SSRIs and MAOIs are just as effective on average, provided one uses an adequate dose (Rosenbaum *et al.*, 1993).

So-called double depression, a major depression overlying chronic dysthymia, may represent two separate disorders. The major depressive episode often responds fairly well to biological therapy, but the dysthymia usually remains. Psychotherapy, particularly CBT and interpersonal approaches, may significantly increase the overall response. See "Dysthymic Disorder," on page 224.

In the various forms of atypical depressions, in which patients have reactive moods, sensitivity to rejection, and increased sleep, appetite, and/or tiredness, MAOIs (Liebowitz *et al.*, 1988) and SSRIs (Pande *et al.*, 1992) are usually more effective than the TCAs. The MAOIs have been more thoroughly compared with TCAs. Other new antidepressants show some promise, but have not been sufficiently studied for this indication. Thase *et al.* (1992) found tranylcypromine especially effective in anergic depression. Atypical depressive features are common in seasonal major depression. Fluoxetine has been successful for such patients (Lam *et al.*, 1995), as has bright-light therapy (see discussion of "Seasonal Pattern Specifier" on page 235).

M. Fava *et al.* (1993) describe "angry depression," in which some depressed patients are outwardly quite hostile and present with angry or markedly cynical affect. Third-generation medications such as SSRIs or venlafaxine are generally the treatment of choice; their study reported success with moderate doses of fluoxetine. Psychotherapy is often disappointing, since the problem is not directly caused by internal conflict, misinterpretation, or the external environment.

"Give enough, long enough" should be a catch phrase for the pharmacologic therapy of depression. Many "treatment failures" occur because the physician—often, but not always, a nonpsychiatrist—does not raise the dose to appropriate levels and/or the physician or patient discontinues the drug before it has had an opportunity to work. Although eventual response can sometimes be predicted by early partial drug effect, the depression should not be considered nonresponsive to any of the common antidepressants until at least six weeks have passed. When a more rapid effect is needed, one should consider ECT or, in some cases, a central nervous system (CNS) stimulant.

Plasma levels of antidepressants are indicated to monitor a therapeutic window for a few TCAs (e.g., nortriptyline, desipramine); however, their main utility is in establishing general medication compliance, gross absorption and bioavailability, and toxicity. If the patient is not responding as expected at a usually effective dose, one may wish to verify a reasonable (but not necessarily clinically predictive) plasma level.

"Start low and go slow" is a traditional approach for some illnesses and patients (such as the elderly or debilitated); however, different classes of medication require different dosing schedules. The TCAs are often initially prescribed at about one-fourth of the usual maintenance dose, then increased every two or three days (Richelson, 1993). The dose and rate of increase vary for other drugs and different kinds of patients. For new patients especially, the physician should monitor the dose, tolerance, and side effects carefully during the first several weeks, since one of the most common reasons for lack of improvement is patient discontinuation of the medication.

Treatment-refractory patients—those who have not responded to an adequate dosage and duration of usually appropriate treatment—may be approached with one of several augmentation or combination protocols. Merely changing to another medication group and/or searching for predictors of success with other drugs (e.g., family history) may help. After that, ECT is often the most effective and safest alternative. Combining ECT and an antidepressant medication (or neuroleptic in psychotic syndromes) is sometimes necessary. Adding lithium, thyroid hormone, or small amounts of a CNS stimulant, such as methylphenidate or *d*-amphetamine, to an antidepressant drug is useful in some forms of anergic depression, melancholia, and late-life depression in which it is difficult to attain therapeutic levels of antidepressant. Careful combinations of a MAOI and a TCA (but not imipramine) may be considered if several other approaches have failed. Sleep deprivation protocols may potentiate medication effects as well (Leibenluft & Wehr, 1992; Hemmeter *et al.*, 1995).

Side Effects and/or Adverse Effects. Serious adverse effects of antidepressants are uncommon in physically healthy patients. Complete prescribing information is beyond the scope of this text; however, we will summarize some common or clinically significant information. One should note that elderly or debilitated patients, in whom severe depression is proportionately common, are at significantly higher risk of unwanted medication effects. Some can cause serious health problems, mimic general medical illness, or render the drug intolerable. Nevertheless, when choosing a medication, one should focus on probable effectiveness, and not merely on the side-effect profile.

The induction of manic or hypomanic episodes in patients not known to be bipolar, or acceleration of manic or hypomanic cycles, may occur with any antidepressive treatment. The psychiatrist should monitor the patient's recovery for manic or hypomanic symptoms (particularly decreased total sleep time) and adjust treatment accordingly. Some studies suggest that cycle acceleration may occur in almost one-third of bipolar patients who are being maintained on antidepressants alone (Altshuler *et al.*, 1995).

Mixtures of major antidepressant groups (e.g., TCAs, MAOIs, SSRIs) should always be approached with caution, and are sometimes broadly contraindicated. At least two weeks of "washout" should take place between MAOIs and SSRIs and *vice versa*, longer with drugs of extended half-lives, such as fluoxetine (allow about six weeks). Similar washout should be accomplished between MAOIs and TCAs (and *vice versa*), unless one is considering combination treatment of a severe and refractory depression. In such cases, one may cautiously add phenelzine or isocarboxazid to an existing TCA regimen (not the other way around) or, perhaps safer, discontinue all antidepressants and start the TCA and MAOI at the same time. The use of SSRIs may increase clozapine levels (Centorrino *et al.*, 1996).

Anticholinergic effects (most commonly, dry mouth, constipation, or blurred vision) are routinely seen with the tricyclics, and occasionally reach serious proportions (e.g., significant prostate enlargement, delirium), especially in elderly or debilitated patients. Glaucoma is often considered a relative contraindication to anticholinergic drugs; however, only the (rare) narrow-angle type presents a serious risk.

Cardiac complications of TCAs, some serious, are not uncommon in elderly or predisposed patients; MAOIs may be problematic as well. The TCAs, MAOIs, and trazodone are associated with orthostatic hypotension in some patients; the effect is not usually dose related.

Many TCAs and trazodone are quite sedative. SSRIs and MAOIs may produce insomnia. The SSRIs are associated with decreased appetite and weight loss early in therapy, but weight *gain* is possible with any antidepressant, especially later in treatment. Sexual dysfunction may occur with most drugs, but is seen more often with the SSRIs. Bupropion has few side or adverse effects.

The common irreversible MAOIs are associated with well-known restriction of foods that contain large amounts of tyramine, meperidine and related pain medications, imipramine, fluoxetine, and carbamazepine, any of which may pre-cipitate a hypertensive crisis. Practical clinical concern regarding dietary restric-tions has probably been overstated in the past, with patients given long lists of prohibited foods, only a few of which contain enough tyramine to cause the unwanted histamine response under ordinary circumstances. The most impor-tant offenders, which should be eliminated from the diet, are aged cheeses, most red wines, beer, many kinds of sausage, fava beans, liver, smoked or pickled fish, and brewer's yeast. Large amounts of other sources of alcohol; some overripe fruits, such as bananas or avocados; and some soured dairy products, such as yogurt or sour cream, should be avoided. The newer, reversible MAO-A inhibi-tors (moclobemide and brofaramine), when used in appropriate doses, do not precipitate the histamine response and thus avoid the problem of hypertensive crisis. MAOIs should be discontinued slowly to prevent a withdrawal syndrome, which can mimic relapse of depression.

One should consider possible nervousness, insomnia, headache, or sexual dysfunction when prescribing SSRIs. Amoxapine, closely related to the phenothi-azines, carries some risk of extrapyramidal symptoms, dose-related seizures, and, rarely, drug-related dyskinesias. Trazodone may cause painful priapism.

The use of cyclic and MAOI antidepressants is relatively contraindicated in pregnant patients, particularly in the first trimester, and in those who are nurs-ing. There is insufficient experience or research to suggest the safety of newer drugs, such as the SSRIs and venlafaxine, in such patients. On the other hand, severe depression itself is dangerous to the mother and fetus/infant; definitive treatment usually should not be postponed. The use of CBT or ECT may be a safer alternative for pregnant patients who require immediate treatment.

Electroconvulsive Therapy. A safe and effective treatment for major depressive episodes, ECT is usually considered after one or more unsuccessful trials of medication in patients who cannot tolerate—or do not wish—antidepressant drugs, or when acute depression must be alleviated quickly to pre-vent suicide or physical deterioration. Its use may also be indicated for patients who have a personal or family history of a good response. There are few abso-lute contraindications; particular attention must be paid to space-occupying intracranial lesions and conditions that preclude the use of brief, light anesthe-sia.

Like antidepressant medication, ECT should usually be considered a treat-ment for a depressive episode, and not as a cure for the affective disorder itself. Most patients require some form of maintenance medication or ECT to prevent relapse or recurrence. Maintenance ECT is recommended for, or preferred by, many patients for whom chronic antidepressant drugs are problematic. It is usu-ally provided on an outpatient basis, every two to four weeks, with minimal dis-ruption of the patient's work or other day-to-day activities. After the initial ECT series, some patients respond to antidepressant drugs that were not effective before ECT.

Detailed discussions of ECT and ECT procedures may be found in several texts (Weiner, 1995). The American Psychiatric Association Task Force Report on ECT (1990) is being revised; a new edition should be available in 1997.

Psychotherapies

Most clinicians agree that psychotherapies are indicated to help the patient accept the need for biological treatment; assist with treatment compliance; provide support while the patient awaits treatment response; address psychodynamic, cognitive, or psychosocial causes of symptoms; increase the likelihood of recognizing signs of relapse; and/or mitigate the possibility of remission and improve the quality of life. Specialized (usually cognitive) psychotherapy may be a primary antidepressant treatment in major depression when potentially effective first-line biological therapies are contraindicated for some reason, or are not effective.

Cognitive Therapies. In experienced hands, cognitive therapy or CBT can sometimes produce success comparable to that of antidepressant medications (Hollon *et al.*, 1992; McKnight *et al.*, 1992). One should not assume, however, that every cognitive therapist can accomplish the consistent results one sees with modern medications and ECT. In a meta-analysis of many studies of CBT, Gaffan *et al.* (1995) note that the results of any form of therapy are often highly correlated with the experience and "allegiance" of the therapist.

Although most studies in which CBT is found comparable or superior to antidepressant medication are carried out with less severely depressed patients, this is not always the case. There is some preliminary evidence that CBT may alter the physical correlates of depression (e.g., thyroid axis measures), just as somatic treatments do, in treatment-responsive patients (Joffe *et al.*, 1996). Many reports show CBT to be an effective adjunct to biological treatment. It is associated with decreased depression at follow-up, increased medication compliance, improved quality of life, and several other outcome markers (Wilson *et al.*, 1995; Murphy *et al.*, 1995; Teichman *et al.*, 1995).

Additional discussion of cognitive treatments is found elsewhere in this text. The reader is referred to more detailed descriptions of depression-specific cognitive therapy in works by Beck (1976), Beck *et al.* (1979), and Thase and Wright (1991).

Other Psychotherapies. Several authors and clinicians report successful adjunctive therapy with relaxation training, behavioral therapy, and various brief therapies. Geriatric patients have been especially well studied in this regard in recent years (Hardy *et al.*, 1995; Lichtenberg *et al.*, 1995; Murphy *et al.*, 1995).

Inpatient Milieu and Psychosocial Therapies

Many patients with major depressive episodes require hospitalization for an adequate treatment opportunity, increased efficiency of treatment, and/or protection from suicide. Most patients and families cannot supply the therapeutic structure, treatment monitoring, day-to-day professional attention, or safety that is available in a psychiatric hospital or psychiatric unit of a general hospital.

Medication alone is not sufficient for complete recovery in many severely ill patients. The hospital and professional staff should first provide a specialized setting for evaluation and diagnosis. Then an active milieu, perhaps with depression-specific psychotherapy or psychosocial programs, should promote recovery from the depressive episode and transition to discharge and the next phases of treatment. A number of published models are described in the literature (e.g., Wright *et al.,* 1992; Lichtenberg *et al.,* 1995; Mendelberg, 1995).

The hospital should not be seen merely as an emergency alternative, but rather as a part of the treatment continuum. Inpatient care that is stopped abruptly or arbitrarily, as it might be for an appendectomy or minor medical condition, is often followed by relapse, no matter how effective the medication or other primary treatment. Discharge should be thoughtfully planned and the transition to home and outpatient care made as smooth as possible.

It is important to allow for adequate evaluation procedures and hospital time to assess, and then address, suicide risk. Severely depressed patients may not outwardly show suicidal ideation or behavior until their symptoms have begun to remit, at which time they have more energy and ability to act on self-destructive ruminations and impulses. One should be cautious during the period just after initial response to treatment, and reevaluate suicide risk before allowing passes or discharge.

The physical milieu of the psychiatric unit should be reasonably safe, but, for most patients, not so protective that it becomes sterile and cold. There must be a balance among safety, therapeutic effectiveness, and patient comfort. Hospitals that admit severely depressed patients should be able to provide close staff monitoring and/or safe housing, restraint, or seclusion for patients who require them, although most rarely need such intrusive measures. Clinical judgment and adequate professional staffing are the most important factors, with physical environment taking an important, but secondary, role.

Other Treatments

Sleep deprivation has been recommended for potentiating antidepressant medication, relapse prevention, prediction of medication response, and primary treatment. There is little evidence that it has direct antidepressant action, but recent reviews suggest some utility as an adjunctive treatment and as a way to differentiate depressive pseudodementia from organic dementia (Leibenluft & Wehr, 1992).

Light therapy is discussed on page 235 under "Seasonal Pattern Specifier."

An unusual procedure called repetitive transcranial magnetic stimulation was successful in a small National Institute of Mental Health study of six treatment-resistant inpatients (George *et al.,* 1995). Two had "robust mood improvement," which was sustained with continuing treatment. The study described the technique as well tolerated and apparently free of adverse effects.

Comorbid Disorders

Various mental and general medical disorders may accompany, affect, and be affected by major depression. The mental disorders are discussed elsewhere in this text; their interface with the depressive episode or affective cycle represents an additional facet for understanding and treatment. In general, one should pursue their treatment as recommended for the individual disorder; however, issues of suicide, hopelessness, unrealistic pessimism, cognitive impairment, and treatment interactions must be addressed.

Diagnoses that at first are thought to be comorbid may be part of the depressive syndrome, or at least exaggerated by it. Chronically depressed patients often receive an undeserved DSM-IV Axis II diagnosis, for example, because of dependency, passivity, social failure, or hostility. Since treatment of major depression often produces marked changes within a few weeks, it is prudent to delay other diagnoses in new patients until antidepressant measures have had a chance to work.

Substance abuse is often difficult to separate from primary depression. One school of thought suggests withdrawing all abused substances (sometimes including caffeine) and stabilizing the patient's abstinence before deciding whether or not he or she has a major depression or some other mood disorder. Others treat both at the same time (after initial detoxification and medical evaluation). We suggest the former as a course that may prevent inaccurate diagnosis, with the caveat that although the patient may look better after withdrawal, the clinician should not gloss over the possibility of remaining (or past) depression.

Comorbid general medical conditions (as contrasted with general medical *causes* of depression) are common. Depressed patients have no particular protection against medical illness, and vice versa. One should be alert to the probability that the depression will cloud or complicate the symptoms—and/or worsen the course and prognosis—of the medical condition, make medical treatment more difficult, or even cause the patient to wish for death when his or her condition is not hopeless.

Issues of specific medication interaction and tolerance to treatment in general medical conditions have been briefly addressed above. The reader should consult Sections I and II in this book, as well as more detailed discussions of diagnostic and treatment interactions in the literature.

FOLLOW-UP AND LONG-TERM CARE

After the acute episode, the patient and clinician must address both the possibility of relapse and the possibility of recurrence. The first is related to complete and continuing treatment of the current episode, and the second to long-term care of a chronic disorder. Effective follow-up (and often long-term management) should include medical monitoring, and usually psychotherapy or psychosocial support, in order to provide the best opportunity for lasting remission.

Relapse of the Acute Episode

Prevention of relapse after biological treatment is closely related to continuing medication or maintenance ECT, as already discussed. It is important to continue active treatment well after the major depressive episode. In some cases, medications that were not effective before ECT are useful once the patient is in remission (Lykouras *et al.*, 1995).

Whether from relapse of the index episode or recurrence of a cyclic depressive disorder, 70 to 90% of patients with recurrent depression redevelop severe symptoms if their medication is stopped during the first three years of "maintenance" care, compared with 20% or fewer of those who continue active treatment (Frank *et al.*, 1990). The same principle applies to ECT, in which either medication or maintenance ECT is usually effective in preventing relapse. In severe and/or delusional depressions, particularly, maintenance ECT significantly decreases future hospital admissions and lengths of stay (Petrides *et al.*, 1994; Vanelle *et al.*, 1994).

Several forms of psychotherapy are helpful in preventing relapse and/or enhancing improvement after acute treatment. G. A. Fava *et al.*, (1994) found that CBT decreased residual symptoms and tended to lower relapse rates in successfully treated patients who had had their antidepressant drugs tapered and discontinued some two years earlier. Several other studies cite the effectiveness of CBT in preventing relapse when used with medication (e.g., Wilson *et al.*, 1995)

Long-Term Care

Most major depressive episodes are part of a recurrent cycle with a periodicity of months or years, often gradually becoming more frequent as the patient ages. Over half of patients with a successfully treated major depressive episode will have at least one recurrence of severe symptoms at some point in the future. Thus, chronic treatment in some form should be seriously considered when a recurrent syndrome has been diagnosed.

On the other hand, continuous medication during months or years of remission in which the affective cycle may not require it places the patient at some additional risk, albeit usually small, for adverse effects. The need for chronic treatment may or may not have been sufficiently and individually established. Thus, if the patient has responded well, and especially if there is no history of recurrence, a monitored trial without medication may be considered, but not necessarily pursued, after several months of remission.

All of the major antidepressant medication groups and ECT have been shown to prevent recurrence of depression in a significant proportion of patients. Mood stabilizers also prevent recurrence of both depression and mania, and are preferred in bipolar syndromes (see "Bipolar Disorders," below).

Maintenance treatment should generally be with the same drug or procedure as the successful index treatment, except in cases in which medication is favored after ECT or in bipolar disorder. In the current absence of research support for lower doses, maintenance doses of antidepressant medication or lithium should usually be similar to the acute dose (unlike protocols for antipsychotic drug maintenance in schizophrenia and schizoaffective disorders). When possible, antidepressant maintenance in bipolar disorders should be with a mood stabilizer, rather than an antidepressant alone, since antidepressants do not prevent mania or hypomania and can accelerate cycling. Psychotherapies alone have not been shown effective in altering the recurrent course of cyclic mood disorders, although they may offer episodic relief of intercurrent problems.

300.4 DYSTHYMIC DISORDER

Until 1980, the syndrome now known as dysthymia was considered a depressive personality disorder. The prognosis was pessimistic and treatment was virtually limited to psychotherapy. Since its designation as an Axis I mood disorder, clinicians have been more willing to use antidepressant medication. There have been few studies, almost all quite small, of either medications or psychotherapy in dysthymia; however, modern treatment is much more likely to be helpful than was assumed by most clinicians just a few years ago. Markowitz (1994), particularly, encourages clinicians to pursue vigorous biological and psychotherapeutic treatment for these uncomfortable patients.

Many dysthymic patients eventually develop major depressive episodes. Whether or not active or maintenance treatment prevents them is unclear. Double depression—chronic dysthymia with intermittent major depressive episodes—is often assumed to represent two separate disorders; however, it may be a single, waxing, and waning illness. Antidepressants sometimes, but not always, lead to the remission of both acute and chronic symptoms.

Although good treatment studies are rare, an SSRI, tricyclic, or other modern antidepressant is a logical first choice for most patients. Fluoxetine was effective in 10 of 16 patients who completed a controlled study by Hellerstein *et al.* (1993). Two controlled studies reported good results with desipramine, one in initial treatment (Marin *et al.*, 1994) and one after relapse (Friedman *et al.*, 1995). Adjunctive psychotherapy is helpful in maintaining medication compliance and remission. Nonresponsive patients should be considered for MAOIs, augmentation, and/or focused psychotherapy (see below). Maintenance treatment is likely to be required for the continued remission of this chronic condition, and may delay or prevent the development of major depressive disorder.

Markowitz (1994) found that cognitive, interpersonal, and social-skills psychotherapies have demonstrated some efficacy in small studies of dysthymic patients. He suggests several general principles of psychotherapy for the disorder, including brevity, interpersonal focus, maintenance treatments after remission, and considering combinations of medication and psychotherapy. Thase *et al.* (1994) found that 20 patients with chronic depression in some ways similar to dysthymia (but generally more severe) responded to cognitive psychotherapy more slowly and less completely than did a companion group with uncomplicated major depressive episodes.

Although not the initial treatment of choice, cognitive or interpersonal psychotherapy may be effective as monotherapy or as an adjunct to an antidepressant drug. In spite of common recommendations for psychodynamic or psychoanalytic psychotherapy, even in the American Psychiatric Association Practice Guideline for adult major depressive disorder (Karasu *et al.*, 1993), there is little or no evidence that such treatment is effective in dysthymia.

311 DEPRESSIVE DISORDER NOS

The treatment of clinically significant depression that does not meet the DSM-IV criteria for a specific disorder can often be successfully approached using one or more of the principles outlined above.

296.XX BIPOLAR DISORDERS (I AND II)

We will discuss treatment of bipolar disorder in three phases: manic or hypomanic episodes, depressive episodes (largely covered under "Major Depressive Disorder," above), and interepisode maintenance.

Note: The phrase "mood stabilizer" below refers to drugs that have antimanic properties and also are helpful in preventing the recurrence of major depressive episodes, including lithium compounds, divalproex/valproic acid, and carbamazepine. They do not have acute antidepressant action in most patients. The term "antimanic" refers not only to these drugs but also to antipsychotic medications (both traditional and atypical) and ECT. Some atypical neuroleptics, especially clozapine, show considerable promise as mood stabilizers as well, but further study is needed (see below).

ACUTE MANIC AND HYPOMANIC EPISODES

Acute mania is a medical emergency. Every effort must be made to stop the manic activity at once, whether through temporary sedation or treatment of the disease process. If the diagnosis is unclear (e.g., the syndrome may be caused by something other than a bipolar disorder, such as substance abuse, a toxin, or a general medical condition), it is often safest to sedate the patient with a benign medication, such as a benzodiazepine or barbiturate. Large doses may be needed; close observation of both behavior and vital signs is very important. Antipsychotic drugs should be avoided for patients who are intoxicated with an unknown substance. Diagnostic efforts should continue during and after immediate sedation.

Once the physician is reasonably certain that the mania is related to bipolar (or schizoaffective) illness, sedative antipsychotic drugs may be used. Combinations of an antipsychotic and a benzodiazepine anxiolytic, such as lorazepam, are often effective. Clozapine recently was shown to be effective in a number of treatment-resistant manic patients (Calabrese *et al.*, 1996), and may be a good choice for routine patients as well. After dangers from extreme agitation, exhaustion, or cardiovascular collapse have subsided, attention should focus on a biological means of controlling the manic process.

At this point, there is no significant difference between treatment goals and procedures for mania and those for hypomania, except that a relapse of mania is considerably more serious. Bipolar II patients have no manic episodes, but almost all bipolar I patients experience both mania and hypomania. Prompt and appropriate treatment of early symptoms probably prevents the development of full-blown mania in some patients; however, evidence that interepisode mood stabilization changes the form of eventual episodes (e.g., making them hypomanic rather than manic) is inconclusive.

Some patients require a combination of a mood stabilizer and adjunctive antipsychotics and/or sedative anxiolytics throughout the acute episode. A certain number will need the antipsychotic regimen (or maintenance ECT) during long-term follow-up as well (see below). Clozapine should not be used in patients taking carbamazepine.

Hospital Length of Stay

The resolution of acute manic episodes often takes considerable time. While some patients recover within days, more pessimistic results have been found in a Scandinavian study of "routine" clinical settings, in which about 25% required over 10 weeks of inpatient care (Licht *et al.*, 1994), and in several studies of complex patients (e.g., those with depressive mania [Dilsaver *et al.*, 1993]). More recently, Frye *et al.* (1996) found that either divalproex or a combination of lithium and carbamazepine reduced hospital stay by an average of 40% over carbamazepine or lithium alone. The length of stay is also decreased by ECT, which probably should be considered for routine treatment, as well as for refractory or medication-intolerant patients (Mukherjee *et al.*, 1994).

Lithium is the most studied mood stabilizer for this purpose, and is effective in two to three weeks for about 75% of patients. Blood levels and side effects must be monitored carefully. The drug will not be consistently useful unless the serum lithium level is greater than 0.6 mEq/L (sometimes slightly less in main-tenance treatment), but clinically significant toxicity can arise at or below 1.2 mEq/L.

Prelithium workup includes a general medical review and examination of the renal, cardiovascular, and thyroid systems, as well as pregnancy testing. The adult dose should begin at about 900 mg/day, in t.i.d. or q.i.d. divided doses, titrated upward until the above levels are reached. In some settings, it is com-mon to prescribe ordinary lithium carbonate on a b.i.d. or even q.d. schedule. We do not recommend that practice unless one can establish that the lithium level is stable and within the therapeutic range throughout the day. Controlled-release b.i.d. preparations (e.g., Lithobid and Eskalith CR) are available.

Serum testing should be done 8 to 12 hours after the last dose (e.g., before the first dose in the morning), every two or three days at first, then at longer inter-vals as the level stabilizes and the patient's absorption pattern becomes known. Initial one-dose tests to predict eventual dosing were described in the literature some years ago (Cooper *et al.*, 1973), but are not always reliable. Adjunctive antipsychotic medication is often needed for psychotic patients. Lithium-carbamazepine combinations are often helpful in treatment-refractory mania or hypomania.

Lithium side effects are common, but usually inconvenient rather than severe. The more serious include polyuria and polydipsia, tremor (different from the pseudoparkinsonian tremor of many antipsychotics), gastrointestinal symp-toms, and skin problems, all often related to the dose and/or dosing schedule. One should note that any circumstance that threatens electrolyte balance must be taken seriously, since the lithium maintains an equilibrium with sodium and potassium. Extended diarrhea or vomiting, for example, can quickly increase the lithium level with no change in dose. Patient and family instructions should be clear in this respect. Other side and adverse effects are either discussed below (e.g., long-term considerations) or are beyond the scope of this text. As for all treatment modalities discussed in this text, the physician should be familiar with the relevant medication issues before prescribing.

Divalproex (a compound of valproic acid and valproate, sometimes mistak-enly called valproate) and *valproic acid* alone are also useful in manic episodes. The literature often confuses the two, and may refer to them interchangeably. Fortunately, they are similar in dose, safety, and effectiveness, with differences mainly in the dosage form and perhaps in GI disturbance. Bowden *et al.* (1994) and other investigators have reported this medication group to be as effective as lithium in acute mania, and sometimes found that it is selectively better for "mixed" or dysphoric mania (with lithium slightly more likely to help patients with classic mania) (Hirschfeld *et al.*, 1995; Swann, 1995). Further study is needed.

The medical workup before prescribing divalproex or valproic acid includes a general medical history and examination of relevant systems. Baseline liver function assessment is useful, and should be done if the history is positive for hepatic or bleeding problems. The initial daily adult dosage is about 250 mg t.i.d., to be titrated upward to a serum level of 60 to 125 μg/ml, depending on clinical response. The eventual dose, usually reached over several weeks, is likely to be between 1,000 and 2,500 mg/day. A recent study by Bowden *et al.* (1996) indicates that levels between 45 and 100-125 μg/ml are more likely to be effective than those that are either higher or lower, and "adverse experiences" increase disproportionately above that range.

A rapid, loading dose procedure that prescribes 20 mg/kg/day in divided doses is often used in otherwise healthy manic patients. This approach is commonly used, with few adverse effects, and was recently found effective in a 36-patient controlled comparison with haloperidol. Antimanic and antipsychotic effects were seen in less than three days for most patients (McElroy *et al.*, 1996).

Divalproex and valproic acid do not have the narrow therapeutic window or troublesome therapeutic index (ratio of therapeutic to toxic level) found in lithium. Metabolism is through the liver rather than the kidneys, making the potential for general medical problems or medication interactions different from that of lithium (but hepatotoxicity is a risk). The risk of overdose lethality is lower, although not inconsiderable. Gastrointestinal symptoms, sedation, transient liver enzyme elevations, and occasionally tremor are the most common complaints. These are usually dose related and often improve with time. Other side and adverse effects may rarely occur, including alopecia and leukopenia.

Carbamazepine is probably best seen as a second or third choice in acute mania, although it has been found equal to lithium in at least one study (Small *et al.*, 1991). The precarbamazepine workup should include a history for hepatic problems, bone marrow depression, blood dyscrasia, renal problems, cardiac damage, certain kinds of intolerance to tricyclic antidepressants, and the concurrent taking of drugs that may suppress the bone marrow (e.g., clozapine, which is contraindicated in patients taking carbamazepine). Baseline CBC, renal, and liver function tests are recommended.

The initial daily range is 200 to 600 mg/day, in divided doses, with titration as clinically indicated to a maximum serum level of 6 to 12 μg/ml. Specific serum levels for bipolar patients are not clearly established, but appear to be similar to those for seizure patients. Samples may be drawn before the first dose of the day, and should be checked several days after each dosage change. The adult dose required for therapeutic effect varies within a general range of 400 to 1,600 mg/day. Carbamazepine may be combined with lithium in treatment-refractory patients, often with good results. Additional neuroleptics (e.g., antipsychotic medications) should be added only with caution, because of the increasing chance of delirium (especially in elderly patients). When feasible, carbamazepine should be tapered rather than suddenly discontinued.

Testing for liver damage and bone marrow suppression should be done regularly, about every two weeks for the first two or three months, then at least every three to six months. The serum carbamazepine level may be checked at clinically indicated intervals in order to verify compliance and therapeutic range and/or evaluate for toxicity. Hirschfeld *et al.* (1995) note that unreliable patients should be monitored more closely than those who (or whose families) can report their own clinical conditions. The effect of carbamazepine on divalproex/valproic acid levels, and vice versa, has not been reliably established in bipolar populations. Other side and adverse effects include, but may not be limited to, delirium or confusional states, unsteadiness, sedation, and gastrointestinal symptoms. Many are dose related and decrease with time.

Clozapine may represent a fourth class of mood stabilizer. Zarate *et al.* (1995b) treated 17 patients who were refractory to or intolerant of other mood stabilizers and ECT, and found a significant decrease in rehospitalization. Eleven (61%) continued clozapine alone and had no affective episodes or rehospitalization for an average of 16.1 months after beginning the drug. Calabrese *et al.* (1996) demonstrated impressive clozapine antimanic properties in 25 bipolar and schizoaffective manic patients.

Calcium channel blockers show some promise in the treatment of manic disorders, either alone or as adjunctive agents (Dubowsky, 1995; Lenzi *et al.*, 1995). Further study is needed.

Electroconvulsive therapy rapidly controls acute mania in up to 80% of patients (Mukherjee *et al.*, 1994). It is at least as effective as, and generally safer than, pharmacologic approaches (Milstein *et al.*, 1987; Small *et al.*, 1988; Mukherjee *et al.*, 1988). It does not adversely affect most general medical conditions or medications, and can be used with any of the mood stabilizers, either acutely or in maintenance protocols (see below). Still it is commonly reserved for treatment-refractory patients, for those who are pregnant or prone to untoward medication reactions (e.g., neuroleptic malignant syndrome), and for emergencies, such as manic delirium with hyperthermia.

Induction of mania, a possible adverse effect of ECT and other antidepressant treatments in depressed bipolar patients, should be considered during maintenance (see below). The addition of a mood stabilizer during or soon after treatment of acute symptoms with ECT is a common strategy that is probably effective in many patients; however, various studies suggest that mood stabilizers may, or may not, prevent manic induction if the patient must continue maintenance ECT or antidepressants (Altshuler *et al.*, 1995).

A complete discussion of ECT procedures and guidelines is beyond the scope of this text. See the section on major depressive disorder (above) and any of several specialized texts or textbook chapters (e.g., Weiner, 1995).

ACUTE DEPRESSIVE EPISODES IN BIPOLAR PATIENTS

Major depression in patients with known bipolar disorder should usually be treated with a combination of biological antidepressant therapy (medication or ECT) and a mood stabilizer. In a few cases, the mood stabilizer alone may be sufficient (e.g., when the patient is known to respond to it or when the depression appears to be the result of medication noncompliance); however, none of the three currently available classes (lithium, divalproex/valproic acid, and carbamazepine) has established primary antidepressant properties.

If antidepressant medication or ECT is used alone, the induction of manic symptoms is a significant possibility. Other biological antidepressive treatments, such as light therapy, although not as well studied, probably carry a similar risk. After response and stabilization (noting that some mood stabilizers, such as lithium, take up to four weeks to establish maximal treatment effect), antidepressant medications generally should be tapered and discontinued unless the history indicates a continuing need. Electroconvulsive therapy has both antidepressant and antimanic properties, and is sometimes combined with a mood stabilizer during follow-up and/or maintenance. Although continuing the mood stabilizer through depressive and interepisode periods is a standard treatment, it may not prevent induction of mania if the patient continues to require antidepressant medication or ECT.

Most other antidepressant treatment principles are addressed under "Major Depressive Disorder," above.

INTEREPISODE FOLLOW-UP AND LONG-TERM CARE

Relapse and recurrence are different concepts, but are sometimes hard to differentiate in simple terms, such as time since last mood episode or completeness of past recovery. "Relapse" refers to the return of symptoms of the current episode, and is related to the completeness of acute treatment, adequacy of recovery, and clinically appropriate follow-up. "Recurrence" connotes a new episode in the cyclic disorder.

The American Psychiatric Association *Practice Guideline for Treatment of Patients with Bipolar Disorder* (Hirschfeld *et al.*, 1995) suggests eight goals of psychiatric management: establishing and maintaining the therapeutic alliance, continuing active monitoring, educating patient and family, enhancing treatment compliance, encouraging "regular patterns of activity and wakefulness," addressing psychosocial aspects of the disorder, maintaining vigilance for the recurrence of episodes, and reducing the morbidity and sequelae of the disorder. Some of these are self-explanatory; others are discussed in the remainder of this section.

Encouraging "regular patterns of activity and wakefulness" refers to the likelihood that daily sleep and activity patterns respond to, are related to, and may, in turn, affect manic or hypomanic episodes. For example, some patients (but probably not all) who seem to prefer very late hours and/or sleeping late in the morning may be contributing to their bipolar cycling. At the least, establishing a regular arrangement of sleep and wakefulness helps doctor and patient to watch for changes (e.g., decreased total sleep time) that may herald a manic or hypomanic episode.

Since manic symptoms are not usually dysphoric, patients and those around them must often be trained to recognize signs of relapse or recurrence. One may watch for a decreased need for sleep (especially), unusual sleep patterns, rapid or disjointed speech, markedly increased activity, increased impulsivity, and signs of poor judgment.

Primary follow-up and the prevention of both manic/hypomanic and depressive episodes are biological, usually with one of the mood stabilizers discussed above. Indications that clozapine may be an effective primary mood stabilizer (Zarate *et al.*, 1995b; Calabrese *et al.*, 1996) deserve further study.

Many patients require antipsychotic medication for at least six months after treatment of an acute manic or hypomanic episode. These patients are often those who have compliance problems and/or the most severe manic symptoms (Keck *et al.*, 1996). A comprehensive review by Solomon *et al.* (1995) found that about half of all patients taking lithium, divalproex/valproic acid, or carbamazepine relapse within a year of recovery from a mood episode. They note that unsuccessful patients often have a history of mixed or dysphoric episodes, rapid cycling, a large number of episodes, or comorbid personality disorder. On the other hand, relapse studies select for the more severe and refractory syndromes. Outcome for unselected patients presenting with their first or second manic episode, with adequate biological and psychosocial follow-up and efforts to encourage treatment compliance, is likely to be much better.

Side or Adverse Effects. Medication monitoring is more complex than with most chronically mentally ill patients. Once stable, lithium levels should be checked periodically and the patient followed for conditions or behaviors that might be associated with increase (e.g., GI illness) or toxicity (renal, thyroid). Chronic serum levels of divalproex/valproic acid are important to continuing remission; toxicity (primarily liver) is an issue, but not to the same extent as for lithium. From time to time, patients taking carbamazepine should be evaluated for serum level, bone marrow suppression, and hepatotoxicity, although there is little evidence that this can predict or prevent acute blood dyscrasia. Serum levels of mood stabilizers may be checked at any time to verify treatment compliance. Clozapine monitoring is discussed in Chapter 16, on psychotic disorders.

Some large-agency policies (e.g., in state mental health systems) demand that the patient periodically be given an "opportunity" to reduce or discontinue medication. For many patients with cyclic disorders, this can be unwise, particularly those who have shown brittle remission patterns in the past. The balance between remission and painful recurrence may rest with a few milliequivalents per liter or micrograms per milliliter of medication. Further, there is some evidence that, at least for lithium, once recurrence of symptoms occurs after discontinuing the drug, the patient may not respond to its reinstitution (Maj *et al.*, 1995). Although maintenance levels of lithium, for example, may be slightly less than acute treatment levels, the principle of "lowest effective dose" must be employed differently for mood stabilizers; therapeutic serum level must be maintained regardless of the actual dose, or the treatment is pointless.

Adjunctive treatment may be biological or psychotherapeutic, and includes antipsychotic drugs, maintenance ECT, various forms of psychotherapy, and patient and family education.

Traditional antipsychotic drugs and ECT are often effective in treating and preventing psychosis associated with bipolar disorder (management of recurrent schizoaffective psychosis is more difficult; clozapine is often the treatment of choice). Several recent studies of atypical neuroleptics suggest that risperidone and clozapine have at least an adjunctive role in the prevention of relapse or recurrence. Risperidone was safe and effective at relatively low doses in two small studies of bipolar disorder with psychosis (Madhusoodanan *et al.*, 1995; Jacobsen, 1995). Clozapine, in addition to its apparently good potential for primary mood stabilization (Zarate *et al.*, 1995b), appears to be effective in treating and preventing manic and schizoaffective psychosis (Zarate *et al.*, 1995a).

Psychotherapy, often cognitive or supportive, is associated with increased medication compliance and adjustment to chronic mental illness. Patient and family education can also enhance compliance and early symptom recognition.

Psychosocial factors contribute significantly to overall outcome, perhaps as much as 25 to 30% (Scott, 1995; Werder, 1995). Regular professional staff contact is an important part of community adjustment and the prevention of relapse and recurrence. Many studies that indicate a failure of lithium to prevent cycling, for example, place at least part of the blame on poor compliance, which is, in turn, often related to inadequate outpatient monitoring. Regular clinic appointments are a good first step, but should be enhanced with outreach for those many patients who fail to keep appointments. Assertive community treatment (ACT, PACT) is even better, and more successful. Other psychosocial programs, such as supported housing and supported work, have value in preventing rehospitalization and enhancing quality of life, although they probably do not affect the clinical course of the illness itself.

Suicide risk should not be ignored. Early symptoms of recurrence may escape detection for some time. Seemingly stable patients, when not followed closely by a doctor or clinic, can engage in suicidal behavior before others recognize the symptoms, if indeed symptoms are visible. Other patients are completely lost to follow-up and do not resurface until their psychiatric condition is critical. Although depression is an obvious danger, bipolar patients may attempt suicide during either depressive or manic/hypomanic episodes, particularly those accompanied by psychosis. In addition, patients with poor recovery or rapid cycling often become very frustrated (and sometimes hopeless) with their illness, and with the social, marital, or vocational problems they must endure. Most studies indicate that suicide is a common cause of death in bipolar patients, reaching 11% of the cohort and 17% of all deaths in one study, with no significant difference between unipolar and bipolar disorders (Angst & Preisig, 1995).

Long-Term Studies of Recurrence and Overall Prognosis. Overall prognosis varies greatly with the patient and treatment adequacy. Naturalistic follow-up for three or more years suggests that recurrence risk increases with early age at onset, incomplete or inadequate early treatment, the presence of severe symptoms (e.g. mixed mania, rapid cycling), a history of psychotic symptoms, and psychosocial problems, with over half of such groups experiencing frequent rehospitalization (Strober *et al.,* 1995; Goldberg *et al.,* 1995a, 1995b; Gitlin *et al.,* 1995). (One should note that symptom-severity and social-functioning factors are somewhat self-selecting in studies of relapse or recurrence, and so do not predict outcome for new cases.)

Gitlin *et al.* (1995) found a five-year risk of recurrence of mood episode (either mania or major depression) of 73% for currently diagnosed (not newly presenting) bipolar patients, calculated on a mean follow-up of 4.3 years. Perhaps more important, two-thirds of the recurrence group experienced more than one additional episode. Three-fourths of those who had an additional mood episode did so within two years; mean remission time for the entire group was about 2.9 years. Almost half the group of patients who did *not* meet the criteria for relapse nevertheless had significant mood symptoms at some point; only 17% (12 of the original 82 patients) maintained euthymia (few or only mild symptoms) throughout the follow-up period.

The general rate of recurrence in the Gitlin *et al.* study was not attributed to inadequate medication. Lithium, "valproate," carbamazepine, and combinations were used; however, it appears that no patient received ECT or clozapine, both of which have been associated with long-term remission in several studies (Vanelle *et al.,* 1994; Petrides *et al.,* 1994; Zarate *et al.,* 1995b). On average, the cohort had more education and better follow-up than one would expect in many treatment environments; the average interval between clinic visits was one month. Subjects had an average of 3.5 hospitalizations before the study began; 13% had never been hospitalized.

Recurrence rates are clearly influenced by the serum level of the mood stabilizer. Some of the variance in studies that suggest high recurrence rates in spite of medication compliance may be due to attempts to prescribe the lowest effective dose. Levels of lithium (especially), divalproex/valproic acid, and carbamazepine are not nearly as stable or consistent as those of antipsychotic and antidepressant drugs. We suspect that patients in the lower portion of the therapeutic range who are tested every few weeks or months have significant periods of nontherapeutic levels between clinic visits. Unfortunately, we know of no convincing studies that have evaluated this hypothesis.

301.13 CYCLOTHYMIC DISORDER

Like dysthymia, cyclothymia was viewed as a more or less characterologic disorder for many years. It sometimes escapes clinical attention, since the mood episodes and oscillations do not reach bipolar criteria. Prognosis may be as important an issue as treatment: at least one report indicates that about one-third of cyclothymic patients who present to a psychiatrist eventually develop bipolar disorder (Akiskal *et al.*, 1977). Many bipolar patients have premorbid histories of cyclothymia. Cyclothymic patients are probably more likely to experience the induction of mania with antidepressant treatment, based on their statistical likelihood of developing bipolar symptoms and their frequent family histories of bipolar disorder.

We have found no recent controlled treatment studies for cyclothymia. Lithium is often used with some success. Several authors suggest treating cyclothymia much as one would treat bipolar disorder (Jefferson & Griest, 1994; Jefferson *et al.*, 1987). Jacobsen (1993) found that 15 cyclothymic patients in an open study required lower doses of valproate than did 11 bipolar II patients. We know of no reports regarding carbamazepine, clozapine, or calcium channel blockers in cyclothymia.

Cyclothymic patients with characterologic signs and symptoms, especially antisocial behavior, appear quite refractory to common biological and psychosocial therapies. Many are substance abusers, and often do poorly in rehabilitation programs. Mood stabilizers may be tried empirically in an effort to increase response to substance abuse treatment. A few cases seem consistent with the syndrome of adult attention-deficit hyperactivity disorder (ADHD). There are no controlled studies of cyclothymia in this regard; however, one might consider a carefully monitored trial of methylphenidate or other stimulants (Spencer *et al.*, 1995), with due regard for the possibility of induction of mania (see above). Venlafaxine has been helpful for some adult ADHD patients as well (Wilens *et al.*, 1995).

Psychotherapy is often indicated for spouses and family members, usually to address the effects of the patient's inappropriate behaviors. The patient may be seen as truly "sick," willfully uncontrollable or rebellious, or something in between. For those whose cyclothymia takes on a largely antisocial configuration, one goal is helping the family deal with tendencies to rescue the patient (e.g., making restitution, devoting valuable family energy and resources to treatment programs of questionable usefulness).

296.80 BIPOLAR DISORDER NOS

Treatment of clinically significant cyclic mood syndromes that do not meet the DSM-IV criteria for a specific disorder often can be successfully approached using one or more of the principles outlined above.

SPECIAL SYNDROMES AND CONSIDERATIONS

For treatment considerations related to seasonal, rapid-cycling, and postpartum disorders, see "Treatment of Selected DSM-IV Mood Disorder Specifiers" below.

TREATMENT OF SELECTED DSM-IV MOOD DISORDER SPECIFIERS

Seasonal Pattern Specifier (Seasonal Affective Disorder)

In seasonal affective disorder (SAD) and ordinary depressions with seasonal exacerbations and remissions (e.g., some forms of dysthymia), light therapy has long been advocated to correct abnormal circadian stimuli and resulting neurotransmitter imbalance. Initially, the light spectrum, brightness, and time of day were carefully controlled. Several recent studies, however, suggest that good results can be obtained regardless of the time of light exposure (e.g., morning or evening) (Wirz-Justice *et al.*, 1993), casting doubt on phase-delay theories of SAD etiology and therapy, in which treatment was given in the early morning. This makes light therapy more flexible and practical for some patients.

The light-visor is another recent innovation for patient convenience. Although it is tempting to search for something more practical than large light boxes, and despite good response in some patients, controlled studies have failed to demonstrate superiority of "therapeutic" visor light over other brightness levels or spectra. Teicher *et al.* (1995) found equivalent improvement with both bright white and dim red light, leading them to wonder whether the visors might not really be "an elaborate placebo."

Other biological treatments are also effective for SAD. The SSRIs appear to be assuming a prominent role, perhaps because of seasonal patterns of serotonin metabolism (Lam *et al.*, 1995).

Rapid-Cycling Specifier

Rapid cycling, usually defined as more than four diagnosable mood episodes per year, is seen in up to 20% of patients with bipolar disorder, and is associated with high failure rates for lithium alone (Calabrese & Woyshville, 1995). If the patient is taking antidepressant medication, it should be discontinued if possible (Wehr *et al.*, 1988). Some authors suggests eliminating stimulating medications and foods (e.g., caffeine) as well.

Divalproex/valproic acid and carbamazepine (alone or with lithium) (Bowden, 1995), ECT (Vanelle *et al.*, 1994), and adjunctive verapamil (Lenzi *et al.*, 1995) or antipsychotics are common choices for acute episodes and interepisode treatment, although traditional antipsychotics may increase cycling in some patients. Atypical neuroleptics, such as clozapine (not with carbamazepine) and risperidone, may soon be the adjunctive drugs of choice, and clozapine shows some promise as a primary mood stabilizer in such patients. Thyroid supplementation increases the effectiveness of treatment (Bauer & Whybrow, 1990; Hopkins & Gelenberg, 1994). Carbamazepine is perhaps the most popular primary drug for rapid cycling at present.

Postpartum-Onset Specifier

Women of reproductive years with a history of severe psychiatric problems are often concerned about the possibility of postpartum illness. They may be counseled that up to one-third of those with prior postpartum depression, and a significant number of those with bipolar disorder outside the puerperium, will develop serious problems without preventive measures. They should be encouraged to accept monitoring and treatment immediately after delivery and for at least the following three months.

Postpartum depression is the most common puerperal mood disorder; however, bipolar patients who become pregnant are vulnerable to both mania and depression, and to general worsening of symptoms (e.g., the development of rapid cycling). Both mother and infant are unusually vulnerable at this time. The irritability, impulsivity, poor judgment, and inattention of hypomania make up one set of impairments. Another, the self-absorption and withdrawal associated with severe depression, may be devastating to the early physical and developmental needs of the child (Packer, 1992).

In spite of the cautions expressed below and in the literature regarding the transmission of medication to the fetus or nursing infant, physicians should remember that psychotic and other major mood disorders are serious illnesses, with significant symptoms, morbidity, effect on parenting, and even mortality. Risk-benefit analysis often mitigates in favor of biological treatment, with close monitoring and appropriate awareness of potential adverse effects. Postpartum depression, in particular, must be taken very seriously. Suicidal and combination suicidal-infanticidal impulses, sometimes involving other children, are not common, but neither are they rare in patients whose disorders reach delusional proportions.

Treatment. For the most part, postpartum syndromes respond to the same treatments as do ordinary mood disorders, but late pregnancy and nursing present relative contraindications to some standard therapies. Antidepressants and mood stabilizers pass through the placenta and are found in breast milk. Newborns of mothers taking lithium, in particular, may be toxic, even when the mother's levels are in the therapeutic range. Lithium in breast milk can be 30 to 100% of the mother's serum level (Packer, 1992). If nursing is important to the mother—or if treatment must begin before delivery—ECT is likely be the safest and most effective approach.

Stuart and O'Hara (1995) suggest interpersonal psychotherapy alone in nursing mothers. Some other authors also feel that biological measures should be completely avoided. We believe, however, that serious postpartum disorders generally deserve the rapid and definitive treatment offered by medication or ECT.

For patients who are not nursing, effective treatments include at least the older antidepressants and mood stabilizers described above. Many of the newer drugs have not been well studied in the puerperium, although case reports exist for several (e.g., fluoxetine [Cole *et al.*, 1993]). Hormonal, fluid-volume, and other changes associated with pregnancy and delivery often alter effective dose and expected serum levels. Transdermal estrogen patches have been found effective by Gregoire *et al.* (1996); their study needs replication. Effective estrogen doses have not been established for this indication.

Prevention. Mood stabilizers provide very effective prophylaxis for recurrence of mood episodes in postpartum patients (Cohen *et al.*, 1995). Bipolar patients who have discontinued interepisode prophylaxis during pregnancy should restart it as soon as possible after delivery. The cautions mentioned above should be observed, and serum levels of mood stabilizers closely regulated for the first several months.

Physicians should consider preventive medication for patients with histories of postpartum depression. In a small study of depression-vulnerable women in the puerperium, Wisner and Wheeler (1994) gave one group either nortriptyline or another antidepressant (which had been effective in previous episodes). The other group received monitoring but no preventive medication. The medicated group rarely developed symptoms, but over half of those who were merely monitored became severely depressed.

293.83 MOOD DISORDER DUE TO A GENERAL MEDICAL CONDITION

Treatment of these disorders is discussed in **Part I,** Chapter 8 under "Mood Disorders Due to a General Medical Condition."

SUBSTANCE-INDUCED MOOD DISORDER

Treatment of these disorders is discussed in **Part I,** Chapter 8 under "Substance-Induced Mood Disorders."

296.90 MOOD DISORDER NOS

The treatment of clinically significant mood syndromes that do not meet the DSM-IV criteria for a specific disorder can often be successfully approached using one or more of the principles outlined above.

CHAPTER 18

ANXIETY DISORDERS

Until a few years ago, anxiety disorders were not usually placed among the more serious psychiatric conditions. Today, however, we know that some are serious and disabling for many patients (Rosenberg & Rosenberg, 1994). The DSM-IV diagnostic categories have important treatment and prognostic implications.

PRETREATMENT WORKUP

Like all psychiatric symptoms, severe anxiety can be a manifestation of a number of general medical or substance-related conditions. This chapter assumes that the reader's diagnosis of a "functional" disorder is accurate when discussing panic, phobic, obsessive, or trauma-related syndromes. Nevertheless, we reiterate that physical causes should be thoroughly considered before embarking on treatment, including such simple things as caffeine intake and over-the-counter cold or allergy medications.

PSYCHOTHERAPIES: THE OLD AND THE NEW

It is *de rigueur* to limit psychotherapeutic treatment recommendations for the anxiety disorders to active, short-term approaches, such as cognitive-behavioral, imaginal, and relaxation paradigms, or their combinations and permutations. Patients with anxiety disorders—whether panic, phobic, obsessional, or trauma related—usually respond well to a symptomatic focus, rarely asking the clinician for more. The sophisticated therapist, however, realizes the importance of looking beyond symptoms for those patients who need, or can make use of, a broader approach. We recommend that as one digests the straightforward treatment protocols in this chapter, which are often rewarding for both patient and doctor, one should remember that "clinician" does not always mean "technician." The patient deserves a therapist—medical or nonmedical—who can recognize the need for additional care (e.g., for a comorbid disorder or psychodynamic issue), and then either offer it or make a knowledgeable referral for more complete treatment.

MEDICATIONS

Some of the most exciting progress in the biological treatment of anxiety disorders has been our increasing understanding of the role of serotonergic systems. It is now clear that antidepressants are effective for many anxiety syndromes, separate from any comorbid depressive disease (den Boer, *et al.*, 1995). Selective serotonin reuptake inhibitors (SSRIs) are especially interesting in this regard, and will be mentioned frequently here.

PSYCHOTHERAPY VERSUS MEDICATION

The anxiety disorders are a good example of the (often artificial) dichotomy between psychological and pharmacological therapies. Each is often effective, and combinations are frequently indicated.

On one side of the dichotomy, one can see that in most successful psychotherapies, the patient is asked to experience anxiety in order to overcome or eliminate it. Many such techniques (e.g., those that focus on exposure or response prevention—see below) are difficult for the patient to tolerate. Relief often does not come quickly; support and encouragement from the clinician are crucial to the patient's remaining in the uncomfortable therapeutic situation long enough to benefit from it. In addition, considerable skill is required to maintain the patient's ability to work in therapy while he or she is experiencing psychic and physiological symptoms.

On the other hand, many medications can decrease anxiety or panic almost immediately. Both patients and doctors may see no good reason to prolong discomfort when safe and effective biological means are available to end it. Abuse potential (e.g., of benzodiazepines) and paradoxical reactions are minor concerns in most patient groups, and should generate no more or no less careful consideration than one would have for antibiotics, antihypertensives, or analgesics. Since anxiety is often a self-perpetuating phenomenon, simply interrupting it may be sufficient for lasting relief.

Both dynamic and cognitive therapists recognize the possibility that medications may interfere with definitive resolution of the anxiety disorder. Psychoanalysts and psychodynamic therapists have long known that the very discomfort that drives the patient *to* therapy *also drives the therapy.* When the "pain" is less, so is the patient's motivation to continue difficult therapeutic tasks. A dynamic tension develops between having enough anxiety to motivate treatment and having so much that one runs from therapeutic situations that temporarily increase discomfort.

The traditional solution is to choose a patient who can tolerate anxiety in the service of growth. However, many patients who deserve our attention either lack such ego strength or cannot make the investments needed to work at the fulcrum of the delicate fight-or-flight balance. It is often helpful to prescribe a medication to decrease anxiety, and thus to increase emotional availability for treatment.

Two arguments against such prescribing are (1) that the drug's "artificial" improvement will discourage the patient from continuing difficult psychotherapeutic work, and (2) that at least one class of anxiolytics, the benzodiazepines, sometimes interfere with the learning and memory functions needed in therapy. Both are relative considerations, to be addressed in each patient's individual treatment situation.

It is very important that the clinician be able to offer a broad range of potentially successful treatments and treatment combinations. Although one expects competent psychiatrists and psychotherapists to have an adequate foundation in most or all modern treatments, not every clinician is qualified in every modality. Nonmedical psychotherapists should be aware that many, perhaps most, anxiety-disorder patients need a medical workup and at least a consideration of medication. Psychiatrists and other physicians should either be qualified to provide psychological and psychosocial therapies or, recognizing the need in many patients, be ready and willing to make appropriate referrals.

COMBINED TREATMENTS FOR ANXIETY DISORDERS

Psychotherapies

Most modern psychotherapeutic approaches to anxiety disorders combine various elements of cognitive-behavioral therapy (CBT), relaxation techniques, exposure (*in vivo* or imaginal), and support. Several of the studies cited below purport to separate these and support one therapeutic "school" or another (often either CBT or relaxation-hypnosis techniques). In real clinical situations, the need is not so much to be pure as it is to gain some awareness of what components of one's overall treatment may be contributing most to the overall outcome. Therapists should recall that the superiority of any form of treatment over another in clinical (and, in some cases, research) settings is related to several factors, including the clinician's skill with the particular therapeutic modality and confidence in the potential outcome.

MEDICATION AND PSYCHOTHERAPIES

Treatment-Refractory Syndromes

The treatments described below are effective for a considerable majority of patients with anxiety disorders. Those who do not respond adequately are often being undertreated, a common problem, especially when the patient is treated by primary care physicians (who tend to use lower doses of medication than do specialists) or by clinicians who cannot offer the full range of biological and cognitive-behavioral therapies. In other cases, alternative or comorbid diagnoses should be considered (Hollander & Cohen, 1994).

PANIC SYNDROMES

300.01 PANIC DISORDER WITHOUT AGORAPHOBIA
300.21 PANIC DISORDER WITH AGORAPHOBIA

Most common treatments for panic disorder are effective in either the presence or absence of agoraphobia. Centers for treatment of anxiety disorders often use combinations of drugs and behavioral therapy; however, individual practitioners or clinics in which only biological or only nonbiological therapies are available may focus on one or the other.

Dread of another attack, and/or anticipatory dread whenever one has a slight premonition of anxiety, is an enormous part of panic syndromes. No matter what treatment is eventually chosen, it is important to let the patient know early that one recognizes this phenomenon, and that there will be times during treatment when a symptom returns and the patient will immediately fall into a ruminative, self-fulfilling cycle of "Here it comes again; all my treatment couldn't stop it," or "Oh, God, what if the treatment doesn't work?" Reassuring the patient that brief relapses are a normal part or treatment, and that there may be ups and downs during his or her gradual improvement, is helpful and may keep the patient in therapy. The author has found it helpful to recommend that patients tell themselves, over and over if necessary, "Dr. Reid told me this would probably happen. He reminded me that no matter how bad I think it is, it *will* pass. Nobody ever died of a panic episode, and no matter how long they *seem*, these things never last more than a few minutes."

Biological Treatments

As pharmacologic control is being established, the clinician should also be establishing rapport with the patient and preparing him or her for further treatment.

Drugs that treat panic may or may not address other kinds of anxiety, including the dread that the panic attacks will return. Separate anxiolytic medication may be indicated for such anticipatory anxiety, along with reassurance of the patient's ability to use medication and/or behavioral treatments to establish control over what were once uncontrollable feelings. Later in treatment, many patients who no longer need their medication carry a small vial in pocket or purse as a sort of talisman, as if to say, "It's there if I need it."

Antidepressants. Among the biological approaches, SSRIs have become the initial biological treatment of choice for most patients (Ballenger *et al.*, 1995). Traditional antidepressants, such as tricyclics and monoamine oxidase inhibitors (MAOIs), have long been known to interrupt and/or prevent panic attacks, but may not be a first choice, in part because of their side-effect profiles. Onset of antipanic action takes two to six weeks in any case, with the longer times usually seen with tricyclics and MAOIs. More time is required for amelioration of the entire avoidance syndrome.

The SSRIs are now the most commonly prescribed drugs for panic disorder. Well-controlled studies have been reported that used fluvoxamine (Black *et al.*, 1993; den Boer, Westenberg, *et al.*, 1995) and paroxetine (Oehrberg *et al.*, 1995), although the latter was studied as an adjunct to CBT. The initial activation associated with SSRIs is often disconcerting to anxiety disorder patients; beginning with a low dose (e.g., 5 mg/day of fluoxetine) increases compliance. Some patients respond well before the dose reaches levels commonly assumed to be therapeutic (e.g., 20 to 60 mg/day of fluoxetine) (Schneier *et al.*, 1990). *Venlafaxine*, which inhibits the reuptake of both serotonin and norepinephrine, was reported to be rapidly effective at low doses (50 to 75 mg/day) for four panic-disorder patients in an open-label clinical series by Geracioti (1995).

Imipramine, desipramine, and clomipramine have all shown effectiveness, generally seen as separate from their antidepressant properties (Mavissakalian & Perel, 1995). Clomipramine is sometimes considered the most consistently effective of the tricyclics (Modigh *et al.*, 1992). Effective blood levels are usually attained with doses a bit lower than those associated with treatment of depression, often around 100 mg/day of imipramine equivalent. The therapeutic effect of imipramine rises with increasing blood level until it peaks at about 140 ng/ml. Mavissakalian and Perel found that higher levels are not associated with increased effect. Other cyclic antidepressants (e.g., trazodone, amoxapine) have received mixed reviews. The only common antidepressant that has not shown an antipanic effect in at least one study is bupropion (Lydiard *et al.*, 1988).

The *MAOIs* are not the initial treatments of choice, but have established sufficient efficacy that patients who cannot take, or do not respond to, the tricyclics may be candidates for phenelzine or iproniazid (Solyom *et al.*, 1981; Lydiard & Ballenger, 1987). They should be started at a low dose (e.g., about 15 mg/day of phenelzine), which is then gradually increased while monitoring for undue arousal or insomnia. The selective MAO-A inhibitor moclobemide has not been well studied for this indication, but may be effective.

Anxiolytics. Benzodiazepine anxiolytics, formerly the mainstay of panic syndrome treatment, still have a role in therapy. They usually act more quickly than the antidepressants, although amelioration is not complete for any therapy until the avoidance syndrome is controlled (usually several weeks to two or three months). Benzodiazepines have fewer side effects than the tricyclic antidepressants (TCAs) or MAOIs for most patients, and may be preferred over SSRIs as well.

Alprazolam has been found effective in several studies, the best known perhaps being a multicenter trial by Ballenger and associates (1988) and the Cross-National Collaborative Panic Study (1992). Although the doses in the Ballenger study were sometimes high by today's guidelines (up to 6.0 mg/day), therapeutic effect was seen promptly and side effects, while common, generally were not a serious problem. Later studies suggest that as little as 2.0 mg/day of alprazolam may be as effective as 6.0 mg/day for some patients, although patients who do not respond should be followed up and the dose increased to prevent their dropping out of treatment prematurely (Uhlenhuth *et al.*, 1989; Lydiard *et al.*, 1992). Many other benzodiazepine anxiolytics are also effective for panic, some of which do not have alprazolam's problem of a short half-life. Clonazepam, for example, has a long half-life and fewer withdrawal concerns, and appears to prevent panic at doses that may be lower than those required for anxiolytic effect.

Klosko *et al.* (1990) and others have demonstrated fairly convincingly that alprazolam, and arguably other benzodiazepines, help fewer patients on average than do cognitive approaches (about 50% versus up to 80% after several weeks). However, the drugs act more rapidly than CBT, may keep patients in treatment who would otherwise drop out before it became productive, and are a good choice for many patients who are poor candidates for psychotherapy.

Sustained-release benzodiazepines, such as adinazolam and a sustained-release form of alprazolam, have been studied and found effective for this indication in once-daily doses. In spite of rebound effects, patients taking sustained-release alprazolam were able to tolerate withdrawal without serious adverse effects, at least in the short term (Davidson *et al.*, 1994; Schweizer *et al.*, 1993).

Buspirone has not been well studied for panic disorders. A report by Cottraux *et al.*, (1995) suggests that it may augment the usefulness of CBTs.

Other Drugs. Propranolol, other beta-adrenergic blockers, and clonidine may be useful for selected or atypical patients. Twelve grams per day of inositol, a dietary supplement, reduced panic symptoms in a small Israeli study (21 patients, both with and without agoraphobia), reportedly with very few side effects (Benjamin *et al.*, 1995). Anticonvulsants are not a first-line treatment for panic syndromes, although one or two reports suggest some therapeutic effects of divalproex/valproic acid (Brady *et al.*, 1993; Keck *et al.*, 1993).

The duration of medication treatment is not determined solely by the absence of panic symptoms. One should remember that avoidance of the panic-inducing environment is part of the syndrome. Various authorities recommend prescribing for between several months and one and a half years beyond symptom remission, and then carefully tapering the dose. If rebound anxiety or withdrawal symptoms are encountered, slow the tapering process. If panic symptoms return, the drug can be reinstated, often at a lower dose.

Psychotherapy and Behavioral Therapies

Cognitive-behavioral therapies have been shown to be effective for many patients for whom panic results from a distortion or misperception of common situations (e.g., bodily sensations misinterpreted as heralding a heart attack). The patient learns to identify the distortion early, and thus to prevent the development of the full-blown panic attack (Agras, 1994). Some studies indicate over 80% success, and most show focused CBT of some kind to be superior to other forms of psychotherapy for panic syndromes (Barlow *et al.*, 1989; Klosko *et al.*, 1990; A.T. Beck *et al.*, 1992; Telch *et al.*, 1993). Behavioral adjuncts, such as relaxation or controlled breathing, may aid in defusing the escalating panic (Klosko *et al.*, 1990). Belfer *et al.* (1995) describe a model for group CBT for agoraphobia and panic disorder. Coping skills and avoidance are stressed. No controlled study was made of the results.

One rarely uses pure versions of psychotherapies in real clinical situations. Several "bundled" forms of CBT/psychological treatment for panic disorder have been created by various authors. Although sometimes sounding a bit like a cookbook, they tend to be fairly complete and easily applied to certain kinds of patients, and can be used with groups. One is panic inoculation, which involves education, retraining, cognitive rethinking, and exposure (including purposely taking moderate doses of caffeine) (Telch *et al.*, 1993). Panic control therapy is comparable, having a smaller educational component and no caffeine intake, but with exposure in other ways (eventually finding a cue for actual panic) and special attention to breathing (for recognition and stopping of hyperventilation) (Barlow & Craske, 1989). The reader is referred to the specific references for complete descriptions and treatment protocols.

Two recent controlled trials have reported that specially applied (not generic) relaxation techniques were as effective as CBT in panic disorder (J.G. Beck *et al.*, 1994; Ost & Westling, 1995). In the Ost and Westling study, 65 to 74% of patients in both groups were doing well immediately after 12 weeks of treatment, and both groups improved further during the next 12 months. J.G. Beck *et al.* noted that most psychotherapy treatments contain elements of relaxation, exposure, and cognitive approaches. Their results suggested that either relaxation or cognitive therapies are the primary contributors to treatment success in panic disorders, independent of any use of exposure.

Barlow *et al.* (1989) used *in vivo* exposure to panic-inducing physical sensations followed by cognitive exercises similar to those just described, comparing that paradigm to cued relaxation techniques. The exposure-cognitive approach was significantly more effective than relaxation alone, the latter being not quite statistically superior to the waiting-list control group. Imaginal exposure (for example, during hypnotic trance), with or without biofeedback, may be more efficient (Somer, 1995), but the author has been unable to find well-controlled studies in panic-disorder patients.

Studies of CBT and other psychotherapy approaches suffer from significant patient dropout. Thus, it is difficult to say whether or not a particular patient is likely to respond, since one does not know whether or not he or she will continue the therapy long enough to benefit.

Combination Drug and Psychological Therapy

It seems logical to consider combining the early-response benefits of medication with the promising long-term effects of cognitive therapy, but at least two additional factors should be considered as one proceeds. First, higher doses of such medications as alprazolam may affect the patient's ability to carry out the cognitive task. Anterograde memory effects can occur even at lower doses of benzodiazepines among some patients (Curran *et al.*, 1994). Second, the improvement created with the medication may either help the psychotherapeutic effort (e.g., by keeping patients in therapy or reinforcing the idea that the patient can indeed become panic-free) (cf., de Beurs *et al.*, 1995) or hinder it (e.g., by removing the panic cues and the sense that the *patient,* not the drug, is controlling the symptom. A complex study by Basoglu *et al.* (1994) reported that much-improved patients who had received eight weeks of alprazolam plus either exposure or relaxation, and who believed that their improvement was primarily due to the medication, suffered more relapse several months later and had more difficulty with medication tapering/withdrawal.

Studies that have combined tricyclics, MAOIs, or SSRIs with active (as contrasted with supportive) psychotherapy are uncommon. A well-controlled study by de Beurs *et al.* (1995) found that fluvoxamine prescribed before a trial of therapeutic *in vivo* exposure therapy enhanced treatment results in patients suffering from panic disorder with agoraphobia. Oehrberg *et al.* (1995) found paroxetine (20 to 60 mg/day) significantly more effective than placebo in combination with cognitive therapy.

Follow-up and Long-Term Care

Many, but not all, studies and texts report a good long-term outcome in 85 to 90% of patients successfully treated for panic disorder. Fava *et al.* (1995) followed 81 successful psychotherapy patients (of an initial 110 who had originally come to therapy) for two to nine years. They found very high rates of continuing remission, with patients who had personality disorders or residual agoraphobia not faring as well as the remainder. Six-month to several-year follow-ups have shown consistent remission in patients treated with exposure (Jacobson *et al.*, 1988). Exposure has been cited by Mattick *et al.* (1990) as an important part of any psychological treatment of agoraphobia, with implications for panic disorder as well. Most long-term follow-up studies are on populations who have received psychological treatments, with or without psychoactive medication. The lasting effects of medications *per se* have been reported by Nagy *et al.* 1989 (for alprazolam) and by a few other authors.

Among the studies that have not found such high rates of long-term remission, Brown and Barlow (1995) described a significant return of symptoms in many patients and reported that 27% of 63 patients sought further treatment within two years, often with disappointing results. A "naturalistic" study by Ehlers (1995) reported that 7 of 17 remitted panic-disorder patients relapsed within one year. Thirty-six of 39 untreated panic-disorder patients in the Ehlers (1995) study described continuing panic attacks after one year. A larger group of untreated patients followed by Faravelli *et al.* (1995) showed varying levels of panic symptoms after five years, with almost half describing mild or infrequent symptoms.

J.G. Beck *et al.* (1994) found that some diagnosed panic disorder patients were doing well when followed up a year after *unsuccessful* treatment. These observations, plus the significant placebo response reported in many pharmacologic studies (cf., Shear *et al.*, 1995), should make one cautious about attributing long-term success to a particular form of treatment.

PHOBIC SYNDROMES

Phobias represent one of the success stories of psychiatry and of specialized behavioral therapies, particularly exposure. Sometimes, a strictly behavioral, cookbook approach works for a time. Reliable and lasting results, however, require a preliminary analysis of phobic situations (usually several, ranked in order of the level of fear and avoidance they produce), triggers, consequences of the phobic behavior, and consequences of having the phobia itself. Consequences of the phobic behavior may include both conscious and unconscious reinforcement, in addition to a decrease in immediate anxiety. Consequences of the phobia itself are usually unconscious and related to primary (although sometimes secondary) gain. To understand them is to understand one of the reasons why the phobia persists in the face of illogic, or why temporary success with cookbook operant conditioning or medication is often not maintained over time.

300.22 AGORAPHOBIA WITHOUT HISTORY OF PANIC DISORDER

Almost all of the treatment literature related to agoraphobia is in a context of panic syndromes, not phobia. Goisman *et al.* (1995) note that agoraphobia appears to be on some sort of diagnostic continuum with panic syndromes, and may be better conceptualized as a subsidiary, not separate, diagnosis. With this in mind, the reader should review the behavioral and biological treatment approaches discussed above under "Panic Syndromes."

Psychotherapies

Treatment "packages" often include a number of components, but tend to be based on either exposure or some form of focused relaxation therapy. The sparse literature on agoraphobia without panic attacks includes reviews by Trull *et al.* (1988) and Hoffart (1993), which provide detailed evidence for the effectiveness of exposure-based treatments. Many of the discussions of self-exposure in the section on social phobia, with and without extensive therapist guidance, are relevant to this patient group.

Hoffart (1995) found that a six-week guided mastery paradigm produced good results, but there were few differences from a matched group of patients who received traditional cognitive therapy. The latter group attained somewhat higher "end-state functioning" during treatment.

For a more detailed discussion of cognitive and behavioral therapies in anxiety disorders, see "Social Phobia," below.

Medications

As implied in the section on panic syndromes, combinations of medication and exposure-based treatments may be more effective than either alone. A review by Mavissakalian (1993) found evidence that imipramine and exposure are mutually potentiating. Wardle *et al.* (1994) found no differences in either early improvement or duration of effect in severely agoraphobic patients receiving *in vivo* exposure and either short-term diazepam or placebo. Both groups improved significantly; there were no adverse consequences when the diazepam was discontinued.

300.29 SPECIFIC PHOBIA (SIMPLE PHOBIA)

Psychotherapies

Exposure. The foundation of modern psychotherapy for phobias was Wolpe's "systematic desensitization" (Wolpe, 1973), which combined (usually) imagined, hierarchical exposure to the anxiety-producing situation with accompanying relaxation exercises. Wolpe recommended first establishing the relaxed state, and then imagining the anxiety-producing situation. Other authors and therapists had success with overwhelming exposure (flooding) in a safe setting, often without relaxation.

Today, there are many treatment paradigms in which the patient first learns ways to decrease emotional and physiologic symptoms of anxiety (e.g., using relaxation, hypnosis, or biofeedback). Then, using imagination, light hypnotic trance, or *in vivo* (real) exposure, he or she encounters a mild phobic stimulus and manages the anxiety. Once that level of therapeutic gain is stabilized, the patient moves to a more intense phobic stimulus.

Several authors suggest that *in vivo* exposure is routinely better that any imaginal method; others cite several studies that report little difference in outcome among types of exposure (Schneier *et al.*, 1995). Hypnotic exposure offers safety and convenience with excellent results in experienced hands (Somer, 1995), and can be used both in and outside of the therapist's office. Exposure via virtual reality has been successful in a few small studies (e.g., Rothbaum *et al.*, 1995).

Cognitive-behavioral therapies are often added to exposure and relaxation. Simple education, "disconfirmation" of illogical assumptions (such as those experienced in claustrophobia [Craske *et al.*, 1995]), and more complete cognitive restructuring are examples.

For a more detailed discussion of cognitive and behavioral therapies in anxiety disorders, see "Social Phobia," below.

Other psychotherapies are often indicated for patients who do not respond completely, those with comorbid disorders, or those whose neurotic (e.g., primary gain) characteristics are a barrier to lasting improvement. Natural "self-exposure" may account for some of the improvement in patients who respond to dynamic psychotherapy (Klein *et al.*, 1983).

Medications

Although not a primary treatment of choice, benzodiazepine anxiolytics have a role in treating patients who cannot tolerate unmedicated exposure, and may allow patients to endure phobic situations when they have no choice (e.g., those with morbid fear of flying who must travel long distances in an emergency). Beta-blockers such as propranolol are not specifically anxiolytic, but often alleviate anticipatory anxiety and improve functioning when sympathetic arousal impairs performance (e.g., in stage fright).

300.23 SOCIAL PHOBIA (SOCIAL ANXIETY DISORDER)

"Social anxiety" seems a better term than "social phobia" for this disorder, since it responds to a number of treatment approaches that are successful for generalized anxiety syndromes (including skills training and chronic medication, which would not be expected to affect true phobias). Nevertheless, the anxiety and avoidance behavior may reach phobic proportions, and may respond as well to stimulus-specific treatments such as CBT and exposure. The psychotherapeutic and medication approaches discussed below represent substantial gains in available treatments. They are often used alone, but severely affected patients (or those with comorbid disorders) may benefit from combining the two (Marshall, 1995).

Psychotherapies

Exposure is an important component of treatment. The combination of some form of CBT and exposure is the best established psychotherapy for social phobia, and has been reported as superior to desensitization, exposure, or social skills training alone (Mattick & Peters, 1988; Mattick *et al.*, 1989; Chambless & Gillis, 1993; Marks, 1995). One recent group therapy study, however, suggested that exposure alone produces better results than a combination of exposure and CBT, both initially and at six-month follow-up (Hope *et al.*, 1995). Some experienced clinicians, such as Marks (1995), believe there is "no need to waste time accompanying the patient into the phobic situation," and that the role of the therapist is to teach and monitor the patient as he or she engages in graduated self-exposure "homework" (usually, but not necessarily, *in vivo*); learns to confront panic-evoking social cues; tolerates them until habituation occurs; and records progress in a journal or diary. Several self-help manuals are available.

Turner *et al.* (1995) conducted a small follow-up study of multimodal, skills-based social effectiveness therapy and found good maintenance of gains after two years. Mersch (1995) found that neither rational emotive therapy nor social skills training added significant short- or long-term gains to the therapeutic effect of *in vivo* exposure in a small (34-patient) study. Teaching relaxation skills alone may be helpful for acute situations (e.g., providing a way for the patient to control anxiety in unavoidable phobic situations), but relaxation in this context is better seen as a coping strategy than as a treatment *per se*.

As already noted, CBT lends itself to group approaches. Heimberg *et al.* (1993) describe a three-month program that involves education, skills training, disconfirmation (disputing erroneous thoughts), and exposure, with very good long-term results.

Psychodynamic psychotherapies appear to have more utility in social anxiety than in other phobic syndromes, perhaps because of the apparent roles of shame and humiliation. Nevertheless, we recommend that behavioral and/or psychopharmacological (see below) approaches be employed initially or contemporaneously.

Medications

Within the antidepressant group (although not prescribed for antidepressant qualities), the SSRIs fluoxetine, sertraline, and fluvoxamine are among those associated with very good response in most patients in controlled studies, even without behavioral therapy (van Ameringen *et al.*, 1993; van Vliet *et al.*, 1994; den Boer, van Vliet *et al.*, 1995; Jefferson, 1995; Katzelnick *et al.*, 1995). Fluvoxamine appeared perhaps the least likely to be effective, being associated with substantial improvement in only 7 of 15 patients at doses of 150 mg/day.

Among the MAOIs, phenelzine appears to be effective without additional psychological therapies in 65 to 70% of patients (Liebowitz *et al.*, 1992; Versiani *et al.*, 1992). There have been few recent studies of the irreversible MAOIs, since the reversible MAO-A inhibitors and SSRIs appear at least equally effective, with fewer side and adverse effects. Moclobemide and brofaromine (MAO-A inhibitors) are probably safe and effective for this indication, although they have not been studied to the same extent as SSRIs and are not yet available in the United States (Versiani *et al.*, 1992; den Boer, van Vliet *et al.*, 1995; Jefferson, 1995). Liebowitz *et al.* (1992) found atenolol, a beta-blocker, as effective as phenelzine in a controlled study, although the response was slower (sometimes taking more than eight weeks).

Anxiolytics have long been prescribed for social phobia or anxiety, but have not been associated with lasting improvement. Clonazepam is the most successful benzodiazepine for social phobia. In spite of fairly high rates of inconvenient (but usually not dangerous) side effects, the response rate may be as high as that of phenelzine or the SSRIs (Davidson *et al.*, 1993; Jefferson, 1995). Alprazolam was about as effective as CBT in a study by Gelernter *et al.* (1991), but not as effective as phenelzine, and was not associated with a positive response two months later. This study may not represent a broad clinical view, since, except for phenelzine, neither CBT nor medication fared much better than placebo. Although sometimes tried because of its relative lack of side effects and abuse potential, there is little evidence that buspirone is more than marginally effective. Schneier *et al.* (1993) found it helpful for 9 of 12 patients in an open-label trial, once doses reached at least 45 mg/day.

300.30 OBSESSIVE-COMPULSIVE DISORDER

Obsessive-compulsive disorder (OCD) is arguably the most pervasive and potentially disabling anxiety disorder. It is the only one commonly associated with childhood onset, and the only one for which neurosurgery occasionally may be indicated. It is more often associated with serious comorbid disorders than are other anxiety disorders, increasing the difficulty of treatment. OCD has been met with therapeutic pessimism since the early days of psychoanalysis, but in spite of its treatment-resistant nature, it responds to modern treatments in up to 70% of cases.

Psychotherapies

Exposure and subsequent response prevention are the most effective anti-OCD elements of CBT (Greist, 1994; Munford *et al.*, 1994). Exposure was discussed above. *In vivo* exposure is the preferred format; imaginal techniques are not as effective, and probably do not enhance treatment response even when added to *in vivo* paradigms (Ito *et al.*, 1995).

Response-prevention techniques interrupt the patient's ritual or compulsive behavior while the resulting anxiety dissipates (sometimes requiring 30 minutes or more). In a sense, preventing the patient's usual ritual or behavior extends the pathologic event, increasing exposure time. This is generally therapeutic, but some patients have difficulty tolerating it.

Several studies suggest that cognitive therapy alone is not often successful, nor does it appear to add very much to other psychological or biological treatments (James & Blackburn, 1995). However, van Oppen *et al.* (1995) found that a cognitive approach was comparable to exposure alone. A cognitive theory of obsessive-compulsive behavior has given rise to inference-based therapy, in which erroneous inferences about the *likelihood* of remote and frightening events are addressed, rather than simply taking the common cognitive approach of denying that the events could ever happen (O'Connor & Robillard, 1995).

Remaining in behavioral therapy is a *sine qua non* for success. It is not easy to confront anxiety and compulsions that sometimes reach near-delusional levels, but this is what is asked of the patient. Most unselected patients who do comply are rewarded with significant and sustained improvement (O'Sullivan *et al.*, 1991). Some medications can decrease the compulsion and/or anxiety encountered in behavioral programs. Others, such as benzodiazepines, may interfere with the learning or conditioning process.

There are a few reports of success with psychodynamic psychotherapy (Milrod, 1995), but most authors agree that the role of dynamic and supportive therapies is limited to consolidating gains from other treatments, assisting with compliance, and helping with comorbid conditions.

Medications

The drugs of choice for OCD are the SSRIs and clomipramine (a potent serotonin reuptake inhibitor as well). About 60% of patients will respond favorably to an adequate dose of one or the other within 6 to 10 weeks (Dominguez & Mestre, 1994; Ravizza *et al.*, 1995). Clomipramine was the first OCD-specific drug, and is still the treatment of choice for many patients.

Clomipramine was found more effective than three SSRIs (fluoxetine, fluvoxamine, and sertraline) in an extensive meta-analysis by Greist *et al.* (1995). Nevertheless, fluoxetine (Tollefson *et al.*, 1994), fluvoxamine (Freeman *et al.*, 1994; Dewulf *et al.*, 1995; Piccinelli *et al.*, 1995), paroxetine (Wheadon *et al.*, 1993), and sertraline (Greist *et al.*, 1995) have all been found effective in controlled studies, and in some were comparable to clomipramine. The SSRIs are often the preferred treatment for children and adolescents with OCD (DeVane & Sallee, 1996).

Inadequate dose is a common reason for the lack of response in OCD, particularly with clomipramine (Dominguez & Mestre, 1994). The above studies generally reported success in the range of 200 to 250 mg/day for clomipiramine and 75 mg/day of fluoxetine equivalent for SSRIs. Many physicians (particularly nonpsychiatrists) undertreat with tricyclics; nonphysicians providing CBT may erroneouly suggest that primary-care consultants prescribe "a little medication" for treatment-resistant psychotherapy patients.

There are few controlled drug treatment studies of mentally retarded patients, although obsessive-compulsive syndromes are common in this population. Barak *et al.* (1995) found clomipramine, in relatively low doses (75 mg/day, sustained release), effective in several patients, most of whom suffered from washing rituals.

A few authors have suggested intravenous (IV) clomipramine for refractory patients, followed by oral therapy (Fallon *et al.*, 1992); however, Mundo *et al.* (1995) found acute worsening of obsessions in a controlled study of IV clomipramine infusion in 28 OCD patients (followed by improvement on oral medication).

Several adjunctive drugs have shown some success in treatment-refractory patients. Potent neuroleptics (e.g., low doses of pimozide, risperidone, haloperidol), clonazepam, and MAOIs are common choices (Dominguez & Mestre, 1994; McDougle, Fleischmann, *et al.*, 1995). Phenelzine was comparable to clomipramine in a 12-week controlled study by Vallejo *et al.* (1992). Tranylcypromine had modest positive effects in one open-label trial (Joffe & Swinson, 1990). Risperidone alone may have some efficacy in treatment-resistant patients (Jacobsen, 1995).

Tricyclics other than clomipramine have little effect on OCD in most patients. Benzodiazepines, formerly commonly used in OCD, have largely been replaced by the above drug choices; we know of no controlled study in which a benzodiazepine was found comparable to clomipramine or an SSRI in overall effectiveness. Clozapine had no independent effectiveness in 10 patients treated by McDougle, Barr, *et al.* (1995). Neither lithium nor buspirone appears very effective for this indication (Dominguez & Mestre, 1994), although one small study found buspirone comparable to clomipramine in a six-week trial (Pato *et al.*, 1991).

Neurosurgery and Electroconvulsive Therapy

Severely disabled patients who do not respond to other treatments may be candidates for one of several forms of stereotactic neurosurgery, with acceptable to excellent responses in 30 to 45% of the most difficult-to-treat patients. Baer *et al.* (1995) found that 28% of 18 previously unresponsive patients were virtually symptom-free after more than two years, while another 17% were partial responders. Hodgkiss *et al.* (1995) found comparable results in a review of all stereotactic surgeries performed in a London special affective disorders unit between 1979 and 1991. Serious adverse effects are rare (Cumming *et al.*, 1995; Baer *et al.*, 1995). A controlled neuropsychological study of both treated and untreated patients found no differences in intellectual or memory function, consistent with general clinical experience that stereotactic procedures do not reduce global abilities (Cumming *et al.*, 1995). A recent review by Mindus *et al.* (1994) notes that studies of gamma knife procedures for refractory OCD are underway.

Electroconvulsive therapy is effective in some patients whose comorbid depression causes an obsessive-compulsive syndrome. It may provide relief for a few patients with refractory primary OCD (Mellman & Gorman, 1984).

Prognosis and Outcome

Obsessive-compulsive disorder is a chronic, although sometimes episodic, condition. Severe obsessive-compulsive syndromes in childhood or adolescence predict significant adult problems (Thomsen & Mikkelson, 1995). Seventeen percent of one such pretreatment cohort were receiving psychiatric disability payments as adults, regardless of age of onset or social background (Thomsen, 1995). Age of onset, symptom severity, and symptom duration are correlated with treatment response, however (Keijsers *et al.*, 1994; Ravizza *et al.*, 1995). Vigorous treatment of adolescents with OCD is associated with lack of adult symptoms in over half of patients (Bolton *et al.*, 1995).

The success of biological treatments suggests that neurologic signs may be correlated with treatment response. However, Thienemann and Koran (1995) found no correlation between treatment outcome and either neurologic soft signs or neuropsychological test results.

Behavioral relapse prevention programs, such as that described by Hiss *et al.* (1994), may be helpful.

TRAUMA-RELATED SYNDROMES

Some of the most disabling anxiety syndromes are related to severe trauma. For purposes of this chapter, we will discuss disorders that are related to acutetrauma; we will not consider patients whose adult disorders are believed to be caused by chronic trauma, such as child abuse or spouse abuse.

Most people respond to severe trauma with a variety of effective coping mechanisms. Initial devastation is replaced with healthy repair and emotional growth. The normal stress response typically involves several phases, which occur over weeks or months: immediate emotional reaction, denial and emotional numbing, reexperiencing, and working through (Marmar *et al.*, 1993). When trauma-related symptoms have been present for several months, however, one should assume that they will not diminish spontaneously; treatment is indicated to prevent chronic posttraumatic stress disorder (PTSD).

Even when there are no signs of problems, early intervention may be important to prevent development of acute stress disorder (ASD) or PTSD, or in reorienting the patient before his or her symptoms become ingrained. Victims (e.g., of crimes or disasters) should be handled gently, not immediately debriefed by untrained personnel.

It is important to understand that posttraumatic syndromes are associated with highly individual experiences and premorbid states. The patient's presentation may be one of depression, anxiety, somatoform symptoms, behavioral idiosyncracy, sleep disorder, sexual disorder, or even psychosis. Foa *et al.* (1995) point out that there is no "blanket" approach to trauma-related disorders. Thus, this section will describe various treatments without many overall recommendations. Nevertheless, PTSD and ASD are usually amenable to treatment, even in chronic cases.

309.81 POSTTRAUMATIC STRESS DISORDER
308.3 ACUTE STRESS DISORDER

Since the official recognition of ASD is a recent phenomenon and the symptoms are similar to (or premonitory for) PTSD, the two disorders share many treatment principles.

Treatment goals should be similar to those outlined by Marmar *et al.* (1993), which include promoting normal (not exaggerated or minimized) responses and arousal levels, adaptive coping and functioning, differentiating remembering from reliving the trauma, addressing comorbid conditions, and avoiding development of a "victim" identity.

Many trauma-related syndromes involve transcultural issues. Treatment of torture victims from third-world countries, for example, requires both competence in the clinical approaches below and an understanding of their cultural expectations and idiosyncracies (McIvor & Turner, 1995).

Acute Stress Disorder and Early Posttraumatic Stress Disorder

The handling and prevention of early symptoms often starts with emergency crews or law enforcement officers, not mental health professionals. Curtis (1995) describes several steps of "critical incident debriefing" that can be provided by first-on-the-scene helpers or disaster teams, including identification of need, articulation and expression, ventilation, validation, and acceptance. Armstrong *et al.* (1991) made similar debriefing recommendations a few years ago.

Several authors point out that working with trauma victims is in itself traumatic (Armstrong *et al.*, 1995; Jiggets & Hall, 1995). Support and treatment services should be available to emergency personnel, crisis response teams, and the like, and they should be monitored for signs of damaging stress response. The acute stresses on other caregivers, such as those who work with severely ill patients, should also be considered, particularly when they may be exposed to disease or danger (Armstrong *et al.*, 1995).

Psychotherapies

Brief supportive, expressive, and dynamic therapies are effective for acute traumatic stress and the prevention of later symptoms. The purposes of such approaches include providing support for ego defenses, working toward restabilization, dealing with affects, assisting decision making, and creating an atmosphere of support to prevent regression (Foa, Davidson, & Rothbaum, 1995). Foa, Hearst-Ikeda, and Perry (1995) reported a brief treatment/prevention strategy for female assault victims in which participation in four educational and CBT sessions soon after the assault was associated with a significantly lower incidence of PTSD and fewer PTSD symptoms almost six months after the trauma.

Traditional psychodynamic psychotherapy is successful for many PTSD patients, particularly when the syndrome is not complicated with comorbid disorders or character pathology. It may be less effective than behavioral therapies after the symptoms are entrenched (McFarlane, 1994). The dynamics of both individual and group treatment focus on several kinds of issues related to the trauma (e.g., aberrant self-image, affect, or mood; impaired interpersonal relations; inefficient defensive mechanisms; and inaccurate feelings about the traumatic event). Marmar *et al.* (1993) comment that countertransference can be a significant problem when the therapist has experienced a similar trauma or has other personal issues that generate inappropriate anger at the aggressor, identification with the aggressor, or exaggerated responsibility for the victim.

Traditional group therapies have long been the foundation of PTSD treatment for combat veterans and rape victims. Groups may be peer based, supportive, or dynamically oriented. It is difficult to assess their overall effectiveness. Family therapy may also be useful (Allen & Bloom, 1994); therapists often forget that the patient's family can also represent a supportive group environment (McCubbin & McCubbin 1989).

Individual or group restorative events outside a clinical setting, such as visiting the Vietnam memorial, revisiting a battlefield, or volunteering to help other victims (or even aggressors), are important for many PTSD sufferers (Watson *et al.*, 1995). Many patients describe growth and healing effects with such experiences, which are often undertaken independent of any therapist. Johnson *et al.* (1995) describe the positive effect of special ceremonies and rituals designed to mark such things as return to one's family, forgiveness, acceptance, and release of the dead.

Cognitive-behavioral therapies are often useful. Fairly reliable results have been reported with vivid imaginal exposure to the trauma, anxiety management, and combination strategies, with exposure being the most consistently important element of treatment (Boudewyns, 1996). As for other anxiety syndromes, exposure alone is often difficult for patients, especially combat veterans, to tolerate. Stress inoculation programs have some proponents, particularly for rape victims with chronic PTSD (Foa & Riggs, 1993).

A few therapists worry that successful exposure and habituation for PTSD may be dangerous for some patients. One does not want crime victims, for example, to become complacent about the real dangers of dark streets in bad neighborhoods. The clinical consensus is that this is not a practical problem in therapy; we know of no studies that suggest otherwise.

Eye movement desensitization and reprocessing involve a recently described augmentation of exposure in which the patient imagines or experiences a traumatic event, endures the accompanying feelings, and then focuses his or her attention on the therapist's briskly moving finger while thinking positive thoughts. Scientific support for the technique is limited (Renfrey & Spates, 1994; Rosen, 1995), although several case reports and small controlled studies suggest effectiveness (Lipke & Botkin, 1993; Vaughan *et al.,* 1994; Silver *et al.,* 1995; Spates & Burnette, 1995; Wilson *et al.,* 1995).

Hypnosis is often helpful, not only for simple relaxation or imaginal exposure, but also as a way to enhance psychotherapy or to recover what the mind may interpret as traumatic memories. Both clinician and patient should understand that the purpose of discovering this material is for the therapeutic experience or tool, and not to establish the accuracy of the recovered memory. *Memory-recovery techniques should not be used in cases likely to involve litigation or as a way to try to "prove" the events of a trauma,* although in the hands of forensic subspecialists, it may provide data that can be corroborated independently.

Medications

Anxiolytics or beta-blockers may be used to alleviate acute or catastrophic traumatic stress. Propranolol and clonidine have fewer side effects and less abuse potential. Benzodiazepines are safe and effective, but occasionally interfere with psychological processing.

In more chronic trauma-related disorders, medications are prescribed primarily for symptoms associated with a particular presentation, not for the PTSD itself. Some, such as anxiolytics and serotonergic antidepressants, can alleviate anxiety so that the patient can tolerate an exposure protocol or other psychotherapeutic approach, and can decrease arousal and impulsiveness. Since benzodiazepines may dull response or interfere with learning, SSRIs are commonly used. Fluoxetine (van der Kolk *et al.,* 1994) and sertraline (Brady *et al.,* 1995) have shown promise in both veterans and nonveterans.

Drugs may also be used for specific features, such as anxiety, depression, sleep disorders, or psychosis, whether primarily related to the PTSD or comorbid with it. The dose and duration of treatment depend on the condition and medication, but do not generally differ from those in primary medication indications (although low doses of neuroleptics should be tried before higher ones in nonschizophreniform paranoia or hallucinations). Insufficient dose and premature discontinuation are common reasons for inadequate response (e.g., SSRIs may require up to eight weeks' trial; MAOIs act somewhat more quickly).

Some clinicians recommend neuroleptics for any posttraumatic hallucinatory syndrome; however, the author has treated many patients with nonschizophreniform, PTSD-related hallucinations for whom a supportive, sometimes interpretive, approach is superior. Combat veterans, for example, may experience visual hallucinations that are felt as protective and reassuring as they struggle with flashbacks or new loss.

> A Vietnam combat veteran with no history of mental illness suffered a significant personal and symbolic loss several years after returning to the United States. Living alone, he became depressed and began hearing vague, frightening noises at night, coming from the basement of his empty house.
>
> One night he awoke to see a vision of a former military buddy sitting at the foot of his bed in full combat gear. The image, which returned several times over a few weeks, was that of a man with whom he had "walked point" in the jungle many times, each often saving the other's life. The buddy was eventually killed.
>
> Soon after the "visits" from the buddy began, the patient, intellectually (but not viscerally) aware that he was in no danger, decided on his own to confront the nightly frightening noises in his basement. He walked down the stairs and across a large, dark room, and stood for several minutes before turning on the light. The frightening noises ceased immediately and did not return. Neither did the visual hallucination of his former buddy.
>
> The "buddy" was consistently interpreted as a supportive figure, once again there to "watch his back." Although medication and hospitalization were discussed in therapy, the patient refused and, since progress was apparently being made, the psychiatrist did not feel it necessary to pursue either. No formal behavioral program was ever used, but it is clear that the patient, when he was ready, provided his own exposure paradigm, complete with a protective companion.

300.02 GENERALIZED ANXIETY DISORDER

The primary difference between generalized anxiety disorder (GAD) and the other anxiety syndromes is the frequent absence of a focal symptom or trigger. Thus, specific exposure or desensitizing therapies are less likely to be appropriate. Since symptoms are often continuous and subacute, many treatments are neither episodic nor focal (as they may be in phobias or panic disorder).

A broadly defined disorder, GAD has many different presentations and levels of severity. Most patients who are treated for anxiety, very often by their primary care physicians, do not meet the DSM-IV criteria for GAD, and the differentiation between those who meet the criteria and those who do not is often blurred.

Patients with GAD often have complaints that suggest comorbid disorders. Borkovec *et al.* (1995) found that treatment for primary GAD was correlated with a dramatic decrease in additional diagnoses, a reminder that both patients and clinicians sometimes confuse comorbid conditions with primary ones. A surprising number of patients evaluated for GAD have a high caffeine intake (and thus perhaps not GAD); their symptoms often decrease after withdrawal from caffeine.

Psychotherapies

Psychotherapies work for many patients who are both motivated and able to cooperate with a cognitive or psychodynamic approach. In relatively mild GAD, one may try psychotherapy alone; in more severe cases, medication should be considered as the primary treatment or, more often, as either a treatment adjunct or for symptom relief during definitive treatment.

The most popular form of nonpharmacologic treatment is cognitive or cognitive-behavioral psychotherapies. Some are effective for one-fourth to two-third of patients (Chambless & Gillis, 1993), with the success rate probably depending more on therapist competence and patient confidence than on the particular anxiety syndrome. Cognitive-behavioral therapy has sometimes (but not always) been found superior to nondirective psychotherapy with regard to both short- and long-term gains (Butler *et al.*, 1991; Borkovec & Costello, 1993).

Psychodynamic psychotherapy focuses on the ego's role in communicating emotional danger to the organism. Chronic anxiety is often related to the sense that ego defense mechanisms are faltering, threatening to allow unacceptable unconscious impulses to become conscious. The therapeutic goal, for those who meet the psychological and motivational criteria for this kind of therapy, is to address possible sources of psychic fear in an attempt to eliminate the patient's need for anxiety. Sometimes ego defenses can be strengthened without addressing the unconscious material directly (e.g., without making it conscious). More often, some level of insight is an important part of recovery. Psychodynamic therapy should not be considered "nonspecific" therapy. Simple nondirected group or individual therapy is not particularly associated with improvement of GAD.

Temporary relief from anxiety may be produced in several ways. In progressive muscle relaxation, based on the premise that one cannot be physically tense and relaxed at the same time, muscles and muscle groups are tensed and relaxed according to a training schedule. Meditation and hypnosis-like relaxation are both effective and easily learned. Muscle tension and, especially, alpha-increase biofeedback are often useful (Rice *et al.*, 1993); however, these temporary measures have not been shown to be consistently effective for chronic anxiety over long periods.

For avoidance symptoms, exposure-based approaches are the psychotherapy of choice. These are discussed under the various phobic syndromes, above. Identifying cognitive issues or topics that give rise to anxiety can allow more focused treatment as well.

Medications

For the rapid relief of the *perception* of anxiety, benzodiazepine anxiolytics are still the treatment of choice. They produce the physical concomitants of well-being, such as peripheral muscle relaxation and decreased physiologic arousal. There is some controversy about whether or not these drugs actually address the psychic part of anxiety as well (Rickels *et al.*, 1993). The more quickly absorbed preparations (e.g., diazepam) are often preferred. It is interesting to note in this regard that patients routinely develop tolerance to the soporific and some other physiologic effects of benzodiazepines, but not to their anxiolytic effects. Thus, although abuse or addiction is a concern in some populations, most patients do not exceed prescribed doses, nor do they need to do so to control their anxiety.

When abuse or abuse potential is a significant concern, one may choose a benzodiazepine with slower absorption or a shorter half-life (or elect to prescribe from a different class of drug altogether). Since many different benzodiazepines are available, drug choice can easily be individualized, with attention to hepatic and renal function, the smoother action of longer-acting drugs (balanced against their potential for accumulation), the rapid clearing of shorter-acting benzodiazepines (balanced against their greater possibility of anterograde amnesia), and the remote possibility of disinhibition in predisposed patients.

In the longer-term treatment of anxiety (e.g., beyond three or four weeks), benzodiazepines have been shown to be statistically inferior to at least two other kinds of drug: buspirone and several forms of antidepressants (see below). Nevertheless, they are appropriate for many patients.

Buspirone, a nonbenzodiazepine (azapirone) anxiolytic marketed in part for its lack of abuse potential, interaction with CNS depressants, and side effects, is not rapidly acting. It requires at least two to four weeks to reach maximal effect. Nevertheless, it is often useful for chronic anxiety, particularly in elderly patients.

Although there are few controlled studies that relate directly to GAD patients, buspirone appears to address true anxiety (rather than only physiologic correlates). Its effect on arousal and physiologic symptoms is significantly less than that of benzodiazepines. Hoehn-Saric *et al.* (1995) suggest that buspirone is a less potent anxiolytic in GAD than many antidepressants (see below), an anecdotal finding shared by many clinicians. Cole and Yonkers (1995), on the other hand, write that except for its delay in therapeutic effect, buspirone is "in most ways . . . the ideal antianxiety drug." A French study by Bourin and Melinge

(1995) found 15 to 20 mg. t.i.d. at least as effective as lorazepam (3 to 4 mg t.i.d.), both early and late in a seven-week trial. Delle Chiaie *et al.* (1995) had similar results in Italy.

Buspirone is frequently ineffective in patients who have recently taken benzodiazepines, for reasons that are still unclear but may have to do with its lack of sedative or muscle-relaxant effects. Nevertheless, a well-monitored combination of early benzodiazepine with a gradual shift to buspirone (or an antidepressant; see below) is often an effective strategy in chronic anxiety. One should note that buspirone is not cross-tolerant with CNS depressants, including benzodiazepines. It will thus not attenuate withdrawal from benzodiazepines and should not be rapidly substituted for them in patients likely to experience such symptoms.

Other drugs of the azapirone class have not come to the U.S. market, and few studies appear in the literature. Gepirone has received more attention than most (e.g., Yamashita *et al.*, 1995).

Antidepressants. Several drugs usually considered antidepressants are sometimes effective for chronic anxiety, such as that seen in GAD. The response time is relatively slow (two to four weeks, much like their response time for antidepressant effect), and they do not impart the same physical sensation of relaxation one feels with the benzodiazepines (e.g., muscle relaxation). The SSRIs have not been well studied for GAD *per se,* but both anecdotal and research evidence suggests that they are effective once the dose has stabilized for two or three weeks (Hoehn-Saric *et al.,* 1990; Brown *et al.,* 1994; Baldwin & Rudge, 1995). They are among the most recommended drugs for anxiety in Scandinavia (Drug Administration Office, 1995). Tropisetron, not available in the United States, was very effective in a fairly large study of French outpatients with GAD (LeCrubier *et al.,* 1993). Like buspirone, SSRIs are not a good choice for acute or temporary symptoms.

Other antidepressants that have found a role in treating chronic (but not acute) uncomplicated general anxiety include trazodone and imipramine (Rickels *et al.,* 1993), at about the same doses as those used for depression. They have more adverse effects, including overdose danger, but are on average at least as effective as the benzodiazepines and are fairly well tolerated. Both appear, in some studies, to be more potent than buspirone for this indication. The MAOIs, including moclobemide, are useful in several other anxiety disorders, but do not have very much support in studies of GAD.

A brief word should be added concerning meprobamate and several over-the-counter medications and substances that are sometimes taken for anxiety. Meprobamate is a poorly effective, highly addictive drug that probably has no role in the modern treatment of GAD. Antihistaminics, such as hydroxyzine or diphenhydramine, are rapid acting, somewhat sedating, and produce a pleasant feeling in most people; however, there is little evidence that they affect anxiety *per se.* Alcohol and nicotine are common self-soothing substances, neither of which should be recommended in lieu of medical or psychological treatment for diagnosed GAD.

293.89 ANXIETY DISORDER DUE TO A GENERAL MEDICAL CONDITION

Treatment of these disorders is discussed in **Part I,** under "Disorders Due to a General Medical Condition."

SUBSTANCE-INDUCED ANXIETY DISORDER

Treatment of these disorders is discussed in **Part I** under "Specific Substance-Related Disorders."

300.00 ANXIETY DISORDER NOS

The treatment of clinically significant anxiety that does not meet the DSM-IV criteria for a specific disorder can often be successfully approached using one or more of the principles outlined above.

CHAPTER 19

SOMATOFORM DISORDERS

GENERAL PRINCIPLES

Before embarking on treatment, the physician or therapist must understand several straightforward, but often misunderstood, principles of diagnosis. Without this understanding, both treatment goals and doctor-patient communication may become hopelessly confused. It is often therapeutic to discuss the somatoform diagnosis openly with the patient as well (McCahill, 1995).

Psychosomatic symptoms are very real. They may either be physically real (as in the case of some asthma, heart palpitations, or gastrointestinal complaints such as irritable bowel syndrome), or emotionally and behaviorally real but without physiologic signs (e.g., in hysterical blindness or paralysis).

The latter kind of reality is consistent with conversion symptoms, in which a psychological concern is unconsciously transferred to a sensory or voluntary motor system without physiologic changes. For example, a patient may truly believe he or she is blind, but careful testing reveals that the eyes, optic tract, and occipital area are functioning normally. Conversion symptoms can appear alone, in conversion disorder, or as part of a more complex psychosomatic presentation.

In somatization disorder and undifferentiated somatoform disorder, also associated with displacement and other psychodynamic phenomena, a patient may have conversion symptoms but also present clinically documentable signs or symptoms. For example, emotionally related "palpitations" may be recorded during Holter monitoring, amenorrhea documented in an otherwise healthy woman after psychological trauma, or vomiting (not self-induced) observed to be limited to certain social situations.

Psychosomatic symptoms can create acute or chronic physical damage, such as bowel pathology related to some forms of irritable bowel syndrome, esophagitis or hemorrhage from involuntary vomiting, or respiratory damage from psychogenic asthma. Even patients who sense that their symptoms may be emotionally based are often (appropriately) concerned that their somatoform condition may eventually cause significant health problems if not alleviated.

In this group of disorders more than any other, the treating clinician must accept the fact that unconscious motivation is very powerful, and is indeed unconscious. These diagnoses do not respond to conscious control or "will," even though it is often helpful to have the patient take responsibility for controlling his or her illness behavior (e.g., in hypochondria). This means that criticizing or punishing the patient is unlikely to be effective in primary somatoform syndromes. Accordingly, these disorders must be separated from factitious disorders (in which the patient knowingly feigns illness for unconscious internal—or primary—gain) and from malingering (in which a person feigns illness for conscious—and secondary—gain, such as money).

300.81 SOMATIZATION DISORDER
300.81 UNDIFFERENTIATED SOMATOFORM DISORDER

Note: Although differing greatly in quantitative severity, these two disorders have essentially similar treatment recommendations. For purposes of this section, somatization disorder treatments will refer to undifferentiated somatoform disorder as well.

The first tenet of treatment is the understanding that patients with somatization disorder (Briquet's syndrome) are not immune from physical illness. It is a serious mistake for any physician, especially a psychiatrist, to underestimate the patient's symptoms and the discomfort they are causing, or to label them in discriminatory terms. On the other hand, diagnosis does not usually require invasive techniques. Excessive medical care is expensive, sometimes dangerous, and usually can be avoided.

Many authors speak more of patient "management" than treatment *per se* (Smith *et al.,* 1995). The primary physician can manage many of these patients by developing a good physician-patient relationship, applying rudimentary techniques of behavior modification, expanding the patient's care to include attention to life stresses, treating symptoms conservatively, watching for depression, and understanding the importance of ongoing contact with the patient despite his or her symptoms. Regular, but brief, primary care appointments every few weeks, regardless of the presence or absence of symptoms, as described below for hypochondriasis, is often useful. The patient thus does not have to try to control the doctor, and the doctor can set fairly rigid rules to prevent additional, extraneous visits. Treatment/management becomes, at the least, less confusing.

Consultation-liaison psychiatrists can help the nonpsychiatric treatment team understand the patient's complaints and, perhaps more important, the concept that because these patients cling to their symptoms for emotional reasons, care rather than cure is the cornerstone of management (Lichstein, 1986). Smith *et al.* (1995) found both decreased somatic complaints and decreased health care costs in a small study of somatization disorder patients whose primary care physicians received a psychiatric "consultation letter." Meeuwesen *et al.* (1994) had similar results in a larger cohort of 106 patients with abdominal pain. Koopmans *et al.* (1995) demonstrated the utility of collaboration between the psychiatrist and the primary care physician, particularly for patients in whom comorbid psychiatric disorder could be demonstrated. Such joint efforts are useful, but the patient should understand that the primary care physician is his main "doctor."

Psychotherapy

Some patients treated in the Smith *et al.* consultation-liaison cohort (above) participated in eight sessions of specialized group therapy. Their self-reports suggested some improvement in physical and mental condition after one year (Kashner *et al.*, 1995). The groups focused on "physical needs coping," assertiveness, taking control of one's own life, problem solving, risk taking, and recognizing and continuing positive changes.

Definitive psychotherapeutic treatment involves the removal of the emotional precursors of multiple medical complaints and/or the channeling of coping mechanisms for those precursors into behaviors or emotions that are more effective for the patient than are the symptoms of somatization disorder. While no controlled comparative studies are available, some older papers report success with short-term anxiety-provoking psychotherapy (Sifneos, 1984), relaxation therapy (Johnson *et al.*, 1981), and reality- and insight-oriented group psychotherapies (Schreter, 1980). Each should provide support and tolerable confrontation. The clinician should be alert for nonsomatic symptoms of underlying conflict or depression.

Medication

In the absence of comorbid psychiatric symptoms or illness, the use of medications to treat this and similar somatoform disorders is not generally recommended.

Prognosis

Somatization disorder is quite chronic, with most patients still qualifying for the diagnosis many years after their first presentation (Kent *et al.*, 1995). The prognosis is closely associated with comorbid disorders, especially diagnosable depression and anxiety (Rief *et al.*, 1995), with nondepressed somatizing patients having more chronic syndromes and poorer outcome (Shorter *et al.*, 1992).

This and similar intractable somatoform disorders are often associated with apparent vocational (and other) disability. Clinicians and disability evaluators should be very cautious with designations of disability, however, since such labels are very strong reinforcers of psychosomatic illness and illness behavior, and serve to solidify the symptoms with "official" sanction. Whether or not the symptoms are under direct voluntary control, it is clear that patients who are *not* awarded disability status (e.g., Social Security disability payments), not given doctors' certificates to modify or miss work, and expected to function adequately in society are much more likely to return to work and other routine life activities with time.

300.11 CONVERSION DISORDER

Although most patients with conversion symptoms are diagnosed and treated by emergency or primary care physicians, psychiatric involvement (through consultation, referral, or physician and nurse training) is important to patient care. As for other somatoform disorders, physiologic or traumatic causes for symptoms must be ruled out. The psychiatrist (or sometimes an experienced psychologist or psychotherapist) may recognize unusual clinical presentations and may need to suggest further medical workup after a primary care physician has decided—too quickly—that the symptoms are "psychogenic."

With some exceptions, conversion disorder has a somewhat better prognosis than somatization disorder, and is less likely to have a chronic or disabling course (Kent *et al.*, 1995). It—or conversion symptoms that may not meet criteria for the full disorder—is often described in the clinical literature in terms of single psychogenic symptoms, such as cough, aphonia, or, rarely, a more serious limitation such as paralysis. Conversion reactions often disappear of their own accord over hours or days, either gradually or, less common in natural settings, suddenly. The loss of symptom may be related to abatement of some underlying anxiety-provoking trigger, to the adaptation of more psychically-efficient ways to deal with the source of the symptom, or to the loss of opportunity for secondary but unconscious gain, such as occurs when others ignore the person's "sick role" and continue their social or family expectations of him or her. The rapid loss of symptoms should not be misunderstood as connoting malingering.

More chronic or disabling psychogenic syndromes, such as asthma, pseudoseizures, pseudocyesis (false pregnancy), and psychogenic dystonia, can be discussed as either conversion syndromes or Somatoform Disorders Not Otherwise Specified (NOS). Some patients' asthma, for example, while not involving voluntary musculature, may be entirely psychogenic, and many patients have significant emotional overlay. Appropriate psychological treatment or management can prevent long-term physiologic changes and significant disability. Psychogenic dystonia, on the other hand, is much less common and much less responsive to either biological treatment (e.g., thalamotomy) or psychotherapy (Lang, 1995). There have been no studies of cognitive or behavioral treatments for the disorder. Pseudocyesis is discussed under "Somatoform Disorder NOS," since that is where it is described in DSM-IV.

Conversion symptoms suddenly appearing in groups of people, sometimes called mass psychogenic illness or mass hysteria, is common in some cultures. They are often described as "contagious," following some sort of environmental trigger or sensational media story. When the group is evaluated, treated, or even interviewed together, the symptoms tend to increase. Removal of the trigger and/or dispersal of the group leads to improvement in most "victims" (Selden, 1989; Ford, 1995). Decreasing opportunities for contagion, separating the most affected people from the rest of the group, and promoting calm rather than an expectation of danger were found effective by Gamino *et al.* (1989).

Those patients with more chronic or disabling psychogenic syndromes are often found to have significant comorbid mental illness unrelated to the trigger event. If the comorbid disorder is amenable to treatment, improvement should follow. Patients whose underlying problems are characterologic (e.g., borderline personality) or involve chronic psychosis are more difficult to treat. The presence of litigation (e.g., lawsuits after a toxic spill in which the persons concerned were not physical victims) increases the duration of symptoms. In such situations, the conversion diagnosis should be questioned in light of the possibility of malingering.

If symptom removal is the only goal of treatment, then short-term hypnosis or behavior therapy should be considered, with an expectation of good results. Simple suggestion or "magical" symptom removal through amobarbital interview or clinical trickery should usually be avoided, however, and treatment provided in a broader context. Particular attention should be given to making the improvement permanent, and generalizing it to the patient's other maladaptive ways of handling emotional conflict.

Hypnosis or amobarbital (or lorazepam) interviews are often used for diagnosis (and sometimes for treatment). One should remember, however, that the mere finding that symptoms can disappear under light anesthesia or certain conditions of trance does not limit the differential diagnosis to conversion, or even to somatoform or factitious disorders (or malingering). Suggestion under such circumstances can be extremely powerful, eliminating, for example, movement limitations caused by pain (e.g., thoracic splinting). In addition, the rapid improvement that often comes with such techniques may leave the patient without anything to replace this manner of dealing with his or her underlying problem or trigger. Thus, the "cure" may be short-lived or, less commonly, may precipitate a more serious problem.[1] Nevertheless, hypnosis and amobarbital/

---

[1]Very occasionally, conversion symptoms represent a fragile defense against murderous or suicidal impulses that the patient cannot otherwise keep in check. Some atypical presentations of paralysis or catatonia may be examples. A careful history may suggest which

lorazepam interviews are useful strategies in experienced hands, and the clinician who works in consultation-liaison settings is encouraged to become familiar with both.[2]

Other Psychotherapies

Ford (1995) has stated that many patients with conversion symptoms are resistant to psychodynamic explanations, since their unconscious choice of somatoform defenses suggests limited ego resources and a number are less sophisticated than most candidates for insight-oriented psychotherapy. However, we have found that many patients are quite receptive to brief therapy and interpretation. In most cases, the patient's conversion reaction is the result of a temporarily overwhelming situation, unusual in the patient's life, and thus may not be indicative of inability to develop insight. Patients who develop the disorder late in life, for example, as well as those who have sustained extraordinary trauma and the terminally ill, are often eventually receptive to psychological explanations for otherwise baffling symptoms.

> A patient complained of terrible itching during a protracted stay in the hospital for severe, but not debilitating, medical problems. She had no visible dermatologic changes except those from her scratching. Physiologic causes, including medication reactions, were generally ruled out. Antihistamines were prescribed, but had only a sedating effect.
>
> During an interview with a psychiatric consultant, the patient expressed her frustration with having to stay in the hospital, wasting weeks of what might be her last months on earth. The psychiatrist mentioned, in a more supportive than interpretive manner, that she must be truly "itching to get out of here." The patient immediately grasped the connection and began to talk of not wanting others to know of her terminal illness, not wanting to be reminded that she was likely to return to the hospital in much more serious condition in the future, and being angry at her fate and the impotence of her doctors (who were trying to calibrate her treatment to be "just right" before she went home to a small town some distance away).
>
> The psychiatrist conferred with her oncologist, who agreed that titration of her medication could continue outside the hospital. Her itching decreased almost immediately (before she learned that she would be discharged), and disappeared entirely over a few days.

---

patients deserve referral to special treatment settings, such as a psychiatric hospital, before attempting to remove the psychogenic symptom.

[2]Although simple suggestion often affects the immediate symptom, and may be helpful in diagnosis, we recommend that the clinician be familiar with more sophisticated hypnotic techniques when treating these patients.

Other psychotherapeutic approaches include relaxation and biofeedback, described in a number of case reports for psychogenic cough (Riegel *et al.*, 1995).

Lasting benefit from any therapy is associated with what Ford (1995) describes as the "three Ps": predisposition, precipitating stresses, and perpetuating factors. Predisposition includes personality and ego characteristics, as well as existing Axis I or general medical conditions. Precipitating stresses may come from virtually any part of the patient's life, but are often related to interpersonal (e.g., family) issues, denial, and anger-related conflict. Perpetuating factors, in our view, are always founded in primary gain, such as calming of internal conflict and, to paraphrase Ford, the degree to which the conversion solves the patient's internal problem. Once again, the reader must not confuse primary gain with external gain, such as financial compensation. Ford also mentions social expectations that may mitigate strongly against the outward expression of certain feelings in some cultures.

Medication and other biological treatments are generally not indicated except to address comorbid or underlying disorders, such as depression.

Symptom "Pseudotreatment"

Some clinicians suggest that the conversion symptom receive specific treatments that resemble those for similarly appearing physiologic conditions. That is, a patient with psychogenic weakness may be referred for physical therapy or faradic stimulation, or one with aphonia for speech therapy or laryngeal biofeedback. This is assumed to allow an opportunity for the patient to give up the symptom gradually, as his or her psyche, and pride, will allow. Such face-saving measures may be effective or supportive for some patients; however, one should remember that external or "official" validation of a purported physical cause for somatoform symptoms may also solidify them, legitimize them in a physiological sense, or, arguably, lay a foundation for their return in the future. We recommend that the clinician be gentle but honest with the patient.

Prognosis

Patients with good premorbid adjustment, absence of major psychiatric syndromes, and the presence of a stressful event associated with acute onset of the conversion symptoms are associated with a good prognosis. Most patients without severe underlying psychopathology continue to be significantly improved several years after treatment, although for some the conversion reaction is an indicator of ongoing emotional problems or, as mentioned above, developing physical disease.

Hysterical seizures or convulsions are among the most disturbing presentations of conversion disorder. Diagnosis is difficult, since although conversion symptoms are usually associated with voluntary musculature or sensory perception, patients with conversion seizures may (like many normal people) also have nonspecific electroencephalogram findings, and some truly physiologic seizure disorders improve with specialized hypnosis. Some conversion patients respond to anticonvulsant medication; others do not. Neither response to biological treatment nor response to specialized hypnotherapy absolutely establishes the presence or absence of a neurological etiology.

307.xx Pain Disorder

The treatment of pain disorder may be designed to relieve acute or chronic pain, decrease disability or "pain behavior," increase the quality of life, decrease reliance on analgesics, or any combination of these. In some cases, good pain management can ameliorate hopelessness and suicidal ideation in disabled or terminal patients. We will focus on psychological aspects of pain, pain behavior, and disability, mentioning some medications and management techniques common to psychiatry. Choice of analgesia *per se,* specific medical topics (e.g., managing cancer pain), and treatment of addiction or withdrawal are beyond the purview of this chapter.

The treatment of acute pain disorder is fairly straightforward, focusing on the pain itself and comorbid disorders. Chronic pain syndromes are much more complex, involving not only the pain, but also its underlying emotional and psychosocial antecedents, pain-related dysfunction or disability, comorbid disorders, and pain-sustaining factors.

The clinician's belief that the patient actually feels pain and requires treatment is an important part of treatment. This—and the corollary belief that the patient is being honest with the physician—may be lacking in many of the person's previous doctor-patient interactions. This does not preclude the psychiatrist's expressing his or her belief that even very considerable pain can begin in, and/or be mediated by, the human mind. Anxiety, in particular, is clearly associated with the perception of illness-related pain (cf., Velikova *et al.,* 1995); much of the effectiveness of common narcotic analgesics is probably related to relief of that anxiety.

Specialized pain disorder treatment is sometimes criticized for its emphasis on simply decreasing pain behavior, hospital visits, and demands on the physician's time. Such goals should, however, be seen as being attained because the patient no longer finds the pain behavior necessary. Reassurance that the doctor and other means of alleviating pain are available is a large part of showing the patient that he or she does not need to *use* medical facilities to prove that they are there.

Multidimensional View

This disorder should be viewed multidimensionally, placing the psychiatrist in a multidisciplinary group of physicians and others who have a common goal of alleviating and preventing the patient's pain. One important aspect of this approach is that it may allow the patient to accept psychiatric intervention more readily, in a situation that the patient perceives as not related to mental illness. The psychiatrist should be one who works well within medical settings and is comfortable discussing and evaluating medical illness in his or her patients. The dual orientations of medicine and psychology offer reassurance that the patient continues to be medically monitored.

PAIN CONTROL PROGRAMS

One view of pain disorder compares it to illness- and trauma-related chronic pain, and recommends treatment along similar lines. Pain clinics, usually found in larger medical institutions, use clear guidelines for evaluation, treatment goals, and the attaining of those goals. This structuring activity, which often requires a residential setting, transforms a confusing and/or overwhelming pain experience into one with manageable parts. The patient participates in the program and gains some measure of mastery over feelings and sensations toward which he or she was formerly passive.

Such programs are primarily multidisciplinary and multimodal, with reinforcement for decreasing pain behavior as well as for the more obvious goals of decreased use of medication and lessened perception of pain. Biofeedback and group therapy are often used. Since the chronic pain takes place in, and is part of, the patient's family and social life, attention is paid to family education and counseling and preparation for activities of daily living. Programs generally last for several weeks or months, and frequently have high success rates among patients who have not done well with previous (usually drug-oriented) regimens (Flor *et al.*, 1992).

Most successful programs for the control of chronic and severe pain are inpatient or residential; however, Sullivan (1993) and a few others describe multidisciplinary ambulatory pain clinics with psychiatric consultation, but which are not primarily psychosomatic in orientation. They offer good patient acceptance and lower system cost, but their comparative effectiveness is yet to be established.

Many clinicians believe that it is very difficult to change severe, often personality-related chronic pain behavior, usually associated with primary and secondary gains, in an outpatient setting. Many of the techniques below may be applied to either ambulatory or residential patients.

PSYCHOTHERAPY FOR PAIN CONTROL AND PAIN BEHAVIOR

Insight-oriented psychodynamic psychotherapy is not often a treatment of choice, although it may be indicated when the sustaining factor for the pain is accessible internal/neurotic conflict. When this approach is chosen, it is useful to isolate the pain symptom carefully from the bulk of the verbal therapy (see "Hypochondriasis," below). *Supportive therapy* may serve to keep the patient functioning in his or her social environment, but generally has little more than superficial value. The association of some patients' chronic pain with childhood antecedents, such as physical or sexual abuse (Walling *et al.*, 1994), suggests certain kinds of "victim" groups and psychotherapies; however, such relationships are usually tenuous and treatment results are inconsistent. *Meditation-based stress reduction* was reportedly helpful in a medium-sized study of fibromyalgia patients (Kaplan *et al.*, 1993). *Relaxation* is a useful adjunct to biological treatments for acute pain, and may be part of treatment programs for chronic pain as well. *Hypnosis* has its proponents, alone or as part of an overall pain control program. It should be applied in a medical context, or with the understanding that the patient's medical needs are being addressed elsewhere as appropriate.

Although *biofeedback* has many advocates, its use has recently centered largely on relaxation or specific syndromes, such as those related to muscle tension (e.g., muscle pain, headache). *Cognitive-behavioral approaches* are recommended as part of overall treatment programs (see above). These and *operant conditioning* address parts of the complex matrix of chronic pain syndromes (e.g., regaining physical and social functioning, overuse of narcotics).

BIOLOGICAL THERAPIES

We will briefly discuss drugs commonly used in psychiatry; however, a detailed discussion of specific analgesic and combination regimens is beyond the purview of this chapter. The reader is referred to medical and surgical texts, as well as specific references such as the report of the Acute Pain Management Guideline Panel (Agency for Health Care Policy and Research, 1992).

Antidepressants

Although chronic pain is often associated with depression, and vice versa, several antidepressants have established analgesic properties independent of their psychotropic qualities (Magni, 1991; King & Stoudemire, 1995). Many tricyclics (TCAs) have been reported to be effective—notably amitriptyline (which may be too sedating for some patients), clomipramine, imipramine, and nortriptyline. The dose is often, but not always, below those used for antidepressant effect (as low as 25 mg/day in some patients). TCAs may be especially effective for neuropathies. Monamine oxidose inhibitors (MAOIs) and trazodone may also be useful. Magni especially cited evidence of their relieving intractable headache, fibromyalgia, arthritis, and neuropathies. Selective serotonin reuptake inhibitors (SSRIs) are slowly developing a reputation for some syndromes (Sindrup *et al.*, 1990), but other reports dispute their effectiveness (Max *et al.*, 1992; Saper *et al.*, 1994). Doses studied thus far are in the antidepressant range.

Neuroleptics

Low doses of neuroleptics, such as haloperidol, are often used as adjuncts to analgesics, separate from their antipsychotic indications. We are unaware of studies of atypical neuroleptics (e.g., clozapine, risperidone) for chronic or intractable pain. Lithium is sometimes used to prevent cluster headache (Solomon *et al.*, 1991).

Other

Transcutaneous electrical nerve stimulation (TENS) is a benign, patient-administered technique that has shown good patient acceptance but inconsistent research results. Acupuncture is well accepted in some clinics, but physiologically based results are very difficult to separate from those of suggestion and placebo effect. The results of treatments that contribute to relaxation, such as massage and diathermy, are similarly difficult to quantify. All physical measures for pain control have considerable placebo value and are known to produce relief in some patients whose pain is largely psychogenic, as well as in those whose pain is known to be primarily physiologic.

Chiropractic manipulation has good patient acceptance; however, virtually all studies since 1988 that have reported it to be effective are in one journal (the *Journal of Manipulative Physiological Therapeutics*) and were carried out by chiropractic schools or practitioners without allopathic (M.D.) or osteopathic participation. Outside that journal, we found only two reports (from one British study of low back pain) that suggested chiropractic referral (Meade *et al.*, 1990, 1995), and one other (on fibromyalgia) that described a need for objective, controlled trials of chiropractic manipulation and other alternative approaches (Simms, 1994). The Meade *et al.* methodology was criticized by Assendelft *et al.* (1991). A few case reports suggest risks associated with misdiagnosis and aggressive manipulation in some chiropractic techniques (Svartzman & Abelson, 1988; Haldeman & Rubinstein, 1993; Powell *et al.*, 1993).

LEGAL CONSIDERATIONS

Although most patients seeking help from legitimate clinicians are not malingering, many do have lawsuits or employment actions pending. It is a truism that the litigation process, in a variety of ways, encourages the continuation of symptoms and removes motivation—conscious and unconscious—for improvement. It may be impossible to unravel the associations among pain, its causes and sustaining factors, and legal issues (Weintraub, 1995); however, the clinician should be alert to their effects on the patient, and to the possibility of being manipulated by parties to a lawsuit. In some cases, it may be prudent to delay definitive treatment until all legal matters are settled.

300.7 HYPOCHONDRIASIS

Before treating a patient for primary hypochondria, one must address two issues. First, physical illness must be adequately ruled out (including brain disease that manifests as delusions of bodily symptoms or dysmorphia). One should realize that hypochondriacal patients and those with dysmorphic convictions are not immune to serious physical illness. Second, other psychiatric disorders that may be causing or exacerbating anxiety, obsessions, or delusions of bodily disease should be treated. The symptomatic therapies for hypochondria are not helpful for illness behavior based on, for example, guilt-ridden depression or paranoid psychosis.

One frequent obstruction to a successful doctor-patient relationship is the physician's anger at being manipulated. One should simply accept the fact that the patient can force medical attention by escalating the seriousness of his or her complaints, and that if this occurs, the physician has no choice but to increase medical attention or to rebuff the patient. Neither solves very many problems.

Several clinicians suggest that a single physician have a clear role as the primary caregiver (Smith, 1992). Specialists and therapists should defer to, and refer back to, that person. Simple psychiatric consultation with communication of treatment suggestions directly to the primary care physician, rather than referral for psychiatric treatment, allows the main doctor to control the patient's care, consolidates information about progress and medical condition, prevents splitting and confusion of care, and prevents the patient from feeling abandoned.

Psychiatric Referral

Lipsitt (1995) makes some practical suggestions for increasing patient acceptance of psychiatric referral, but believes that they are usually unsuccessful. This has not been our experience, so long as the referring general physician expresses confidence in both the psychiatrist and the referral itself, not treating it as something that "might help" or as "last resort." Referring physicians should become aware of psychiatrists in their areas who are experienced in somatoform disorders, and then help the patient to understand that the psychiatrist is a medical specialist with knowledge and treatment options outside usual primary care boundaries. The general physician should not, however, imply that he or she is abandoning the patient to another doctor; both physicians will participate in the patient's care.

We have focused thus far on psychiatric consultation or referral. Nonmedical psychotherapists are often at a disadvantage in the therapy of hypochondria (but perhaps not in body dysmorphism), since they do not usually have either the medical knowledge or the patient's confidence to deal with general medical complaints. The seemingly logical treatment team of primary care physician and psychologist or clinical social worker often does not work in this disorder. The patient may continue to require medical referral due to the therapist's appropriate caution about physical complaints. On the other hand, a serious physical problem may become worse if the nonmedical therapist is too cavalier about ignoring illness behavior.

When a nonmedical psychotherapist is used, there should be frequent communication between physician and therapist (but not between patient and physician); the patient must not feel that he or she has been referred and forgotten. It is often a good idea to continue regular, short visits to the primary care physician, for the reasons already discussed above, and to allow the therapist to defer medical issues to that routine medical contact.

Kellner (1992) described his experience with a cohort of patients treated over many years, often successfully, suggesting practical ways for the primary physician to treat hypochondriasis and several other somatoform disorders. He noted that reassurance is an underestimated tool in decreasing illness behavior, and suggested that (1) the benign nature of the somatoform disorder be emphasized, (2) patients be given accurate information about the interaction between their emotions and possible physical symptoms, (3) the fact that there is a good medical prognosis be celebrated by the physician, and (4) *the patient be reassured that he or she will not lose the doctor-patient relationship.* Instead, the patient is allowed to have regular, but brief, physician visits, at which focused clinical examinations take place. The patient is not allowed to expand his or her visits into frequent, as-needed medical calls, but is reassured that he or she has a consistent place on the physician's appointment schedule.

Some authors agree; others do not. A recent paper by Barsky (1996) echoes the general view that, whatever the approach, physician discussion must support the doctor-patient relationship, avoid perceptions of abandonment, and shift from the feared illness to illness behavior and coping with hypochondriacal anxiety. It seems likely that success will often be associated with both the severity of the patient's disorder and the attitude (and tolerance) of the physician.

Medication

Psychotropic medications have not been shown to be useful in primary hypochondria, although they may be indicated in secondary illness behavior related to another disorder. An uncontrolled study by Fallon *et al.* (1994) suggested that moderate doses of fluoxetine (up to 80 mg/day) may be helpful in hypochondriacal patients without diagnosable major depression. Low doses of high-potency neuroleptics have been advocated for some patients, but with mixed results. Kellner *et al.* (1989) suggested benzodiazepines to interrupt anxiety-related illness behavior patterns and ameliorate anxiety as the patient anticipates change.

Psychotherapies

In any psychotherapy, recognition of underlying depression, anxiety, or another Axis I disorder that causes or exacerbates the illness behavior greatly improves the prognosis (Kellner, 1992). If such a primary syndrome is found, the patient often then fails to meet criteria for a somatoform disorder. The following discussion refers to therapies for hypochondria *per se*. The approach to be employed should be influenced by both the patient's psychopathology and the therapist's area of expertise.

Insight-oriented therapies, in experienced hands, are sometimes effective. One technique we have found useful in both brief psychotherapy and long-term intensive work is to limit firmly the patient's talk about the hypochondriacal symptoms, with the idea that this topic is a resistance and prevents the surfacing of other important material. At times, and perhaps throughout some forms of brief therapy, the patient's discussion of physical symptoms may be strictly limited to, for example, one session per month or 10 minutes at the end of each session. Patients often test this, use their special "medical" time enthusiastically for awhile, and then forget about it in favor of other therapeutic work. When they say "I forgot to mention my (pain, dizziness, etc.) when I was supposed to, so let me just say . . .," the therapist should interrupt and be quite rigid about limiting such topics to the special "medical" time.

Cognitive-behavioral therapies have been tested for this and other indications. They are sometimes successful, largely to the extent that the hypochondriasis presents as a disease phobia or anxiety syndrome. Primary hypochondria, however, is a more complex disorder. Studies generally have been small and uncontrolled. *Educational therapies* alone usually fail, since the patient's reason for illness behavior is not related to actual knowledge about symptoms or disease. It is generally more useful to try to educate physicians and nurses regarding their hypochondriacal patients (see above). *Behavior replacement,* in which illness behavior is extinguished and replaced with another gratifying (but more productive) activity, often with insight, is helpful for some patients.

Monosymptomatic Hypochondriasis

Obsession with a particular nonexistent serious physical disorder or symptom, such as a true delusion of aberrant body image, body smell, internal parasite, or malformation, is frequently associated with severe personality disorder, psychosis, or intracranial disease or injury. Evaluation should be vigorous, particularly if one of the senses (e.g., smell, taste, touch) is involved. Treatment often requires antipsychotic medication, even if a brain lesion is present.

300.7 BODY DYSMORPHIC DISORDER

Body dysmorphic disorder differs from hypochondriasis in the degree and focus of the symptom(s), but otherwise has much in common with it. The clinician may use many of the same principles just reviewed, but the dynamics of fear of abandonment or loss of the doctor-patient relationship are not a prominent feature.

A few clinicians still recommend cosmetic surgery for some presentations of body dysmorphic disorder, with the view that removing the immediate complaint will permanently resolve the patient's concern. There have been no convincing reports of success, however, and patients whose symptoms reach near-delusional intensity are unlikely to receive lasting satisfaction with this approach (Phillips *et al.*, 1993) (cf., the intractability of aberrant body image in such disorders as anorexia nervosa or delusional disorder, somatic type).

Phillips *et al.* (1993) reported that half of 30 patients with delusional and nondelusional body dysmorphic disorder responded well to fluoxetine or clomipramine. They noted that almost all of their patients had had a mood disorder diagnosis at some time, well over half an anxiety disorder (often obsessive-compulsive), and one third a psychotic disorder. The MAOIs have also been suggested, but their role in treatment, if any, is unclear.

Reference to psychotic disorders, and many similarities to delusional disorder, is the basis for the antipsychotic treatment of patients with delusional symptoms. Pimozide is the drug most often mentioned in the literature, but the absence of recent studies would suggest trials of other, perhaps atypical neuroleptics as well. Lipsitt (1995) believes that neuroleptics are not effective for this indication.

Older case reports describe various forms of psychotherapy. None has been extensively studied, but both psychodynamic and cognitive-behavioral approaches probably deserve consideration for selected patients.

300.81 SOMATOFORM DISORDER NOS

Pseudocyesis (false pregnancy), although quite rare in the United States, is commonly mentioned as an example of somatoform disorder NOS. It should not be confused with factitious pregnancy, in which the patient knows she is not pregnant and feigns the condition. As in the case of other somatoform disorders, physiologic causes for the patient's symptoms, some of which are quite serious, must be ruled out.

Treatment consists of first attempting to show the patient clearly that she is not pregnant, with results of pregnancy tests, sonograms, and the like. This should be done in a supportive environment, with follow-up counseling easily available. A few authors suggest inducing menses (perhaps calling it a "miscarriage" to allow the patient to "save face"); however, we recommend that clinicians or therapists be scrupulously open and honest with patients, and deal with emotional reactions as they arise. Addressing the patient's personal and situational needs for the pregnancy is often helpful, although not immediately curative.

When pseudocyesis occurs in modern Western culture, the underlying psychopathology is usually significant and relapse is not uncommon. Frank delusional false pregnancy should be treated as a delusional disorder, somatic type. In occasional cases, the patient's reaction to not having a baby creates a danger of her kidnapping or harming other women's infants (e.g., through feelings of entitlement or a delusion that someone has taken her baby).

Other Disorders

Other clinically significant somatoform disorders not meeting specific DSM-IV criteria may respond to one or more of the treatment principles outlined above.

CHAPTER 20

FACTITIOUS DISORDERS

300.xx Factitious Disorder

The treatment of patients with factitious disorder is clouded by the lack of established approaches to which the disorder will respond, the absence of controlled studies of its treatment, the frequent presence of Axis II psychopatholgy, and the assumption, sometimes well founded, that the patient will leave medical care soon after the disorder is discovered. Such measures as "blacklisting" patients and denial of hospitalization are repugnant to most physicians, and could have disastrous consequences. Extensive behavior modification programs may be helpful (Hyler & Sussman, 1981); however, these are almost never feasible.

Since most patients present as inpatients or in emergency rooms, the psychiatrist or psychologist is often called as a consultant and may be given the job of confronting the patient. Although confrontation may be recommended at some point, it is the primary or attending physician who usually should carry it out, perhaps with the psychiatrist. The confrontation should be unambivalent, but also kind and therapeutic. Factitious symptoms are motivated by unconscious factors that are not amenable to superficial conversation or entreaty. The psychiatrist may also help by communicating with medical and nursing staff about the nature of the disorder and the inadvisability of punitive approaches.

Because of the danger that the patient often represents to himself or herself (or, rarely, to a proxy patient), the possibility of risk from unneeded diagnostic procedures, and financial risk for the health care system, most authors feel that searching the patient and the patient's belongings for evidence or instruments of self-harm is justified.

PSYCHOTHERAPY

The intelligence and presence of a professional background that often characterize these patients imply that one should at least consider psychotherapeutic options. Folks and Freeman (1985) suggest that the best treatment may simply be rapport, with continuation of necessary medical treatment and the setting of limits on the illness behavior. Personality-disordered patients usually have a poor prognosis. Those with obvious depression often fare much better; antidepressant treatment (e.g., medication) may eliminate factitious behavior or clear the way for psychotherapy (Earle & Folks, 1986).

For those occasional patients who are successfully encouraged to pursue psychotherapy, the uncovering, in a supportive surrounding, of reasons for the masochistic or substitutive behavior may bring marked improvement. Psychotherapy may also address the patient's need for attention and caring, and his anger against objects who withhold this from him. One dynamic issue that has been discussed in this context, as well as with regard to other self-mutilating patients, concerns an apparent need to sacrifice one part of the body (e.g., through surgery) in order to protect the whole from suicide or decompensation into psychosis. Plassman (1994) reviewed intensive psychotherapy of factitious disorders and describes 24 personal cases in Germany. Twelve accepted initial clinical psychotherapy followed by long-term analytic therapy. Ten continued treatment and improved significantly.

Eisendrath (1989) eschews confrontation and has described several psychotherapeutic techniques with a goal of allowing the patient to give up his or her factitious symptoms and behaviors without "losing face." Hypnosis, for example, can let the patient believe that *others* believe that trance work has found some special avenue of healing. Eisendrath also discusses the therapeutic use of double binds.

Behavior therapy has been described (Klonoff *et al.*, 1983), with the recommendation that psychodynamic considerations be addressed in a combined format. Solyom and Solyom (1990) reported success in a patient with factitious paraplegia using a somewhat deceptive form of aversive conditioning. They avoided confronting the patient, agreed that he needed treatment, and prescribed uncomfortable electrical stimulation to his leg muscles. After learning that the length of treatments would increase if they were not effective at the original level, the patient soon began to walk again. In addition to the conditioning and deceptive nature of this approach, there may have been an element of face saving (see Eisendrath, 1989), in which the patient could say that the treatments healed him.

A kind of paradoxical hospitalization was described in a 1993 report of a fairly successful case (Schwartz *et al.*, 1993). A frequently admitted patient with severe factitious behavior was allowed unlimited access to an inpatient bed for one year. At the end of the year, she had spent only about half as much time in the hospital as in the year before (130 versus 235 days), without the expense of repeated admissions and discharges.

MEDICATION

Except for the use of neuroleptics in comorbid severe personality disorders, antidepressants are the only medications routinely associated with the amelioration of factitious disorder. They are not known to be effective for factitious impulses or behaviors *per se*, but there are a number of reports of remission after treatment of a comorbid depressive disorder. It is not clear how many of the improved patients had illness-producing behavior as a result of their depression, as a result of some other (e.g., Axis II) disorder that responded to the antidepressant drug, or coincidentally. Brodaty (1993) notes that elderly patients and those with known chronic illness in addition to their factitious symptoms may be particularly prone to atypical depressive presentations. Although one might expect the newer antidepressants, such as the selective serotonin reuptake inhibitors, to displace tricyclics in treatment efforts, the author knows of no published reports that test this hypothesis.

Sometimes the most reasonable treatment is merely a coordinated discharge and defusing of the staff's anger and other feelings. A number of cases are reported in which patients with no incentive for emotional change responded to humane behavioral approaches while in the general hospital, leading to at least a temporary reversal of deceptive, self-destructive behavior. (Simmons *et al.*, 1987).

FACTITIOUS DISORDER WITH PREDOMINANTLY PSYCHOLOGICAL SYMPTOMS

Psychiatric or psychological presentations of factitious disorder are quite rare. They should be treated with the same general methods as described for physical presentations, and may afford a greater opportunity for psychiatric intervention. Unfortunately, few treatment reports, and no controlled studies, are available.

This diagnostic group is sometimes erroneously substituted for the older concept of Ganser's syndrome. Ganser's syndrome, however, is not under voluntary control and should be treated with a combination of environmental change (when possible—its presentation is often in prisoners), support, and the temporary use of antipsychotic medication. Antipsychotic medication or other biological treatment for factitious disorders, except insofar as some patients have significant depression, has not been effective.

FACTITIOUS DISORDER BY PROXY

The clinician should be suspicious when considering a diagnosis of so-called factitious (Munchausen's) disorder by proxy, in which an adult induces physical symptoms in a child or other vulnerable person. Roesler and colleagues (1994) describe a number of cases in which a child's reported food allergy or intolerance was actually a product of bizarre parental beliefs. Many "proxy" presentations actually represent the willful abuse of a child or disabled person, and not true factitious disorder (which also can be characterized as abuse). Meadow (1984), for example, found that factitious epilepsy in children was sometimes related to anoxic episodes caused by parental abuse. In either event—factitious disorder or straightforward abuse—recognition and prompt action to protect the victim are imperative.

SPECIAL CONSIDERATIONS

Staff Reactions

The psychiatrist should take the time to observe the patient and to communicate with the unit's medical and nursing staff (including psychiatric nursing staff) about the patient. Factitious disorders are easily misunderstood, and can generate harmful countertransference and other reactions in caregivers, even when they understand the situation intellectually.

Potential Dangers

One should not forget that the patient has a psychiatric disorder, even though he or she appears merely to be squandering treatment resources and frustrating busy staff members. The factitious symptoms have a very important purpose in the disorder. Completely obstructing symptom expression, such as by too-vigorous confrontation or hospital blacklisting, can lead to the escalation of the factitious behavior, concomitant increases in danger to the patient (or to a victim-by-proxy), and/or the emergence of severe nonfactitious symptoms (including psychosis or suicide [Spivak *et al.*, 1994]).

300.19 FACTITIOUS DISORDER NOS

The treatment of patients who fall into this residual category should be based on the control of patient-induced illness or injury and the underlying psychopathology, using the guidelines just described. It should be noted particularly that patients who are malingering or who have somatoform disorders should not be treated as if they have a factitious disorder.

CHAPTER 21

DISSOCIATIVE DISORDERS

GENERAL PRINCIPLES

The dissociative disorders are frequently discussed together, since there is considerable overlap in presentation, many of the concepts have much in common with posttraumatic syndromes, and some symptoms appear in more than one disorder (e.g., amnesia, depersonalization). We will attempt to separate the disorders, in part because of the style of this text, but will refer the reader to other sections from time to time.

Today's most popular school of thought with regard to understanding and treating the dissociative disorders conceptualizes them as posttraumatic syndromes. Whether the trauma is physical or emotional, in childhood or in the recent past, chronic or singular, the principles of treatment are roughly the same: creating a safe and stable environment, establishing a strong therapeutic alliance and reassuring the patient about that safety, working through traumatic and psychodynamic issues, and stabilizing gains so that the patient reintegrates his or her psychic and social lives. For a comprehensive discussion of these treatment principles, in a context of traumatic disorders, see J. L. Herman (1992).

300.12 DISSOCIATIVE AMNESIA

Crisis Management and Acute Treatment

In patients whose amnesia is associated with a recent internal or external trauma, memory may return spontaneously once a safe environment is established. For others, simple reassurance that this form of amnesia is a logical and self-limited response to trauma often leads to memory recovery within a short time. The therapist must engender confidence in himself or herself, which sets the stage for the patient's faith that memory will return when the time is right. This suggestion of permission to recover may be conveyed in a number of ways, including the use of a light hypnotic trance.

If the amnesia continues, psychotherapy is indicated. The environment should be well removed from the traumatic event (e.g., site of an auto accident, natural disaster, or combat). A solid therapeutic alliance should be established and the psychodynamic meaning(s) of the patient's unique response to the event(s) explored and resolved. When the amnesia is related to chronic and/or long-past trauma, such as child abuse, the therapy is more complex, return of entire memory more difficult, and accuracy often questionable.

In some cases, such as when working with dissociative identity disorder (multiple personality), recovering particular areas of recall may require careful planning in order to avoid creating previously nonexistent "memories" (see "Special Considerations" below), interfering with ongoing therapy, recurrence of the trauma syndrome, or other decompensation. Caution should also be exercised when recovering potentially distressing memories in patients with severe exacerbations of physical or mental illness, inadequate ego strength, or current personal crisis. It is often important that the therapist be available to help manage and work through memory recovery and, when necessary, reintegrate the memories into the patient's current life. Abreaction can be prevented and affects contained in a number of ways, including Spiegel's "screen" technique (in which the patient "replays" the memory as if on a television screen, with controls for picture and volume) (Spiegel, 1994; Grame, 1993).

Information about the patient that is supplied by friends or relatives (or other sources, such as the contents of a wallet or purse) usually helps to begin recall. Competence in hypnosis is useful; most patients are readily hypnotizable. Many patients respond to simple relaxation techniques. If there is no source of collateral information, several hypnotic techniques, such as automatic writing, fantasied scripts or pictures, or even nontrance free association, may start the recovery process.

Lowenstein (1995) advises against "abreaction," or the very rapid release of images and affects, in an effort to bypass the need for more lengthy therapy. Basic dynamically informed psychotherapy, with an understanding of trauma principles, is preferred, and usually successful.

Resolution and Follow-up

When memories return during therapy, the patient should be encouraged to explore and assimilate them as parts of the therapeutic work, and discouraged from immediately taking them at face value (e.g., for confrontation of people apparently involved in a past trauma). When working with recollections from the distant past, the patient should not despair if they begin to fade again. Repression and suppression are normal ways of dealing with the huge number and variety of memories in one's past. Neither integration nor therapeutic work (nor future functioning) requires that they remain completely conscious.

Occasionally, clinicians in busy emergency rooms help patients recover their memories (or, in the case of fugue, their identities) and then discharge them with a few words of support. As already mentioned, many patients commonly considered hysterical or psychosomatic respond positively to placebo or hypnosis given by authoritative doctors. It is sometimes tempting to send the patient on his or her way and move on to more serious disorders. We encourage more attention than this to the patient's problem, and at least the offering of an opportunity for working through and resolution with a therapist.

Special Considerations

Amytal Interviews and Similar Drug Techniques. Near-anesthetic sedation is often associated by laypersons with memory recovery and the revealing of unconscious (or purposely concealed) material. In fact, the concept of "truth serum" is an elusive one, with little place in modern psychiatry. Narcosynthesis is sometimes useful for eliciting material to be explored at a later time or facilitating later verbal process; but it should not be understood as producing true memories. It should only be undertaken by experienced physicians, with appropriate anesthetic precautions.

Forensic Presentations. Remote memory is a delicate and subjective phenomenon. There are great differences among the purposes and techniques of memory recovery for relief of amnesia, for psychotherapeutic work, and for documentation of one's true past. This section is concerned with the patient's *relief* and the recovery of memory that is personally useful and eventually reassuring. Ordinary clinical methods should not be construed as producing legally accurate recall.

There are several circumstances under which the clinician should use particular care in memory recovery, especially when hypnosis is involved. (Note that "suggestion" or "trance" is not always limited to formal "hypnosis"; indirect trance and suggestive processes are common in many forms of interview and psychotherapy.) One should exercise great caution if asked to "enhance" the memory of a civil or criminal defendant or potential court witness. "Recovered" memory, although it usually sounds quite logical, is likely to be altered (sometimes subtly, sometimes significantly) to fit the needs and expectations of the patient (Frankel, 1993). Interested readers may wish to consult the American Psychiatric Association's *Statement on Memories of Sexual Abuse* (American Psychiatric Association, 1994). Finally, dissociative amnesia often occurs in a context of other psychiatric disorders that may affect the form and impact of the memories eventually recalled.

300.13 DISSOCIATIVE FUGUE

Dissociative fugue implies and includes amnestic symptoms, which are addressed in the foregoing section. The patient may or may not be outwardly distressed, but generally recognizes his or her unusual condition and cooperates with treatment efforts.

Treatment techniques for the fugue itself are similar to those for amnesia, with most causative trauma being singular and recent (and thus fairly uncomplicated, albeit symbolically associated with past conflict or trauma). The principles of safety, processing, and resolution apply here as well. Hypnosis is a common form of nontraumatic intervention and, in some cases, of regressing to past memories that can be used as a starting point for recovery.

Definitive psychotherapy is indicated for most patients, both for reintegration after recovery of their identity and memory, and to address underlying psychopathology and conflict. Sometimes the past trauma is complex, but it may also be quite straightforward, such as in aberrant grief.

> A young woman presented to the emergency room disoriented and unaware of her identity. She was quiet, and superficially appeared catatonic. After physical examination, she was admitted to the psychiatric service where a psychiatrist was able to attempt a complete history under conditions more relaxed than those in the emergency room. The patient was cooperative, but could supply little information. When he asked about her parents, her affect changed slightly. A few days later, under hypnosis, she was asked about her family once again and described events that were apparently from her adolescence. When gently pressed about where her parents might be, she recalled that her father was deceased.
>
> Further exploration in trance produced a disturbing recollection of coming home one day to find her father dead in a closet. She was given the choice of remembering or not remembering the event upon leaving trance, chose to remember it, and experienced considerable catharsis and grief. She recovered her memory and identity completely, her mother was contacted, and she recuperated without incident. In retrospect, she had been "protected" from the facts surrounding her father's death by other family members, who sent her to stay with friends until well after the funeral. The current fugue had been precipitated by finding her pet bird dead in his cage.

300.14 DISSOCIATIVE IDENTITY DISORDER (MULTIPLE PERSONALITY DISORDER)

The treatment of multiple personality disorder (MPD) is far more complex and lengthy than that of any of the other, relatively encapsulated, dissociative disorders. This rare disorder is not synonymous with schizophreniform disorders, and should not be treated with antipsychotic medication unless indicated by the symptoms presented. The traditional approach, popularized by Thigpen and Cleckley (1957), is intensely psychodynamic or psychoanalytic, often aided by hypnosis. Integrating the various separated parts is the goal of treatment.

The large number of cases reported during the past several years appears to be related in part to the "popularity" of the disorder among certain therapists who specialize in its treatment. Diagnosis and treatment should be approached with considerable caution, in part because:

1. Focus on the possibility of "multiple personality" for a borderline or similarly primitive patient creates a setting in which a highly suggestible person may unconsciously create (or worsen by adding additional parts) the very disease being treated. This is especially likely with hypnotic treatment by relatively inexperienced clinicians.
2. The therapist may be seduced by the professional notoriety of treating these sometimes-exotic individuals.
3. The patient's responsibility for his or her actions, including legal responsibility, may be questioned or avoided altogether. Even if MPD is present, exoneration is often inappropriate, and almost always countertherapeutic.
4. Serious countertransference reactions, including anger, exasperation, exhaustion, and even sexual seduction or violence, are common (Coons, 1986).

Treatment begins with agreement between patient and therapist that integration (fusion) of the parts of the patient's personality is the goal. Later, each alter will have to agree to fusion as well. This can be very frightening for the patient (often expressed through fear in the alters). The integration that slowly follows includes the patient's memory, identity, perception, and consciousness (Spiegel, 1994).

Psychotherapy

The psychotherapeutic treatment of MPD requires sufficient subspecialization that the clinician should either be experienced in this area or be supervised. The patient, with his or her various often uncooperative parts, will often be demanding and frustrating. Psychoanalytically oriented therapy, with or without adjunctive hypnosis, has been favored for many years by most clinicians. Cognitive techniques are finding a place in many practices as well, although not as the primary approach. No matter what the psychotherapeutic treatment choice, resistances related to repression, denial, secrecy, and crises will threaten the treatment process.

Individual Therapy. Kluft (1991, 1995) describes several generic stages and specific principles of treatment that are compatible with both hypnotic and nonhypnotic approaches. The principles rely on a posttraumatic view of MPD, with a need to reinstitute shattered boundaries, understand MPD as truly involuntary and the result of others' irresponsibility (and thus requiring extraordinary trust and therapeutic alliance), and recognize cognitive errors.

Hypnosis. It is a truism that virtually any treatment effect that can be produced with hypnosis can be produced without it. Indeed, MPD patients often respond to their therapists in very similar ways whether or not they are in an intentional trance. Nevertheless, hypnosis is an important foundation for many psychotherapeutic treatments for MPD.

Techniques described by Smith (1993) and used at the Menninger Foundation include developing "self-soothing" techniques, mapping the system of alters, facilitating communication (both between alters and with the therapist), managing abreaction, and aiding integration (fusion). Almost all patients are easily hypnotizable; in some ways, the dissociative process itself can be conceptualized as an autohypnotic phenomenon.

Nevertheless, one should be aware of the possibility that using hypnosis to address the parts of the patient's personality (which should be clearly understood as *parts,* and not separate personalities) will actually create new parts or "personalities" in response to the highly suggestible emotional milieu. The danger is exacerbated by the strong implication that the therapist expects, and will be gratified by, the uncovering of additional personalities.

The process of uncovering or communicating with parts of the personality in trance and then suggesting that they will be integrated with the dominant personality is simplistic and incomplete. The patient must see his or her parts as parts of an already existing whole, and perhaps even encouraged not to refer to each part by a separate name. The therapist should not accept any inference that the patient actually contains more than one "person."

Treatment should proceed slowly and methodically, with a focus on assuring a safe environment without initial disruptions or too-rapid regression. One common obstruction is the hidden alter, which may be accessible only under hypnosis at first and then will respond on demand by the patient or therapist. The range of specific techniques that may be used is too complex to be described here.

Group Therapy. There are few recent reports on group therapy for MPD. Buchele (1993) described three kinds of groups that may be useful, provided the therapist has specific training in the treatment of dissociative disorders and MPD: incest survivors, general groups, and those specifically targeted for MPD patients.

Containment. The concept of containment has been addressed in discussions of the therapy of severe personality disorders and some dissociative conditions. Containment may refer to both the condition and the assurance of safety within the therapeutic process, and to the maintenance of firm borders around strong affects and impulses. Sometimes physical containment, implied or real, is helpful in that assurance and allows progress to be made. Hospitalization is one form of physical containment; medication can be another.

A word should be added about the therapeutic use of physical restraint as a containment, as suggested by a few authors (Young, 1986). This technique suggests voluntary, intermittent use of restraints to work through "dangerous" situations of abreaction and the treatment of angry or aggressive parts of the personality, with the aim of providing a physically and emotionally safe environment for both patient and therapist. One should exercise caution with this and other abreactive techniques, and seek experienced supervision. There is considerable danger of creating an inappropriately "special" and potentially gratifying treatment environment, as well as a potential for sensationalism and patient abuse.

Hospitalization

It is not unusual for some parts of treatment to require support and containment not available in the outpatient clinic. Unless admission is solely for crisis resolution or some comorbid condition, inpatient or day hospital programs specifically designed for MPD are best, given the specificity (and sometimes controversy) associated with the disorder and its most effective treatments. The staff should be well trained and therapeutic procedures carefully followed. Stabilization may be accomplished in a day or two, but when specialized inpatient or residential care is to be used for progress in fusion, several weeks may be required. Much longer stays are occasionally necessary.

Biological Treatments

The use of narcosynthesis, such as amytal interviews, has not been explored recently. A chapter by de Vito (1993) describes a case report. Other biological treatments generally should be reserved for symptomatic use.

Follow-up and Prognosis

Integration of an alter implies that it no longer exists by itself. It can no longer be found by the clinician or patient, even under hypnosis. Further, *the features of the alter are now found within the patient (and his or her perception of) himself or herself, rather than associated with some separate part.* Related memories are no longer disjointed or discontinuous, and the patient notices a more consolidated feeling. Kluft (1995) suggests that a good definition of fusion requires at least three months of these characteristics, and that the phrase "stable fusion" may be used after an additional two years. Integration *per se* should not signal the end of treatment, since there invariably are other problems in the patient's life, many of which predispose her (most patients are female) to relapse.

Kluft (1993, 1995) believes that patients who enter treatment have a good prognosis. Some other authors are less optimistic, particularly in the presence of primitive character pathology. A 1986 series (Coons, 1986) in which many patients were treated by relatively inexperienced therapists reported treatment lasting up to over three years with only a 25% rate of full integration. Patients who receive no treatment may experience less dissociation late in life.

Special Considerations

Recorded Sessions. Recording hypnotic sessions or amytal interviews may allow the patient to observe otherwise unconscious material; however, there is little evidence that it is helpful in MPD and other dissociative disorders. If the patient is ready to recall the material, he or she will do so with (and often without) simple prompting by the therapist. Taping for forensic use or even for risk management (e.g., to defend against accusations of therapist impropriety) should be approached carefully with consideration as well, since considerable expectation and sensation are associated with being "on television."

Comorbidity. Severe comorbid disorders are common in MPD; it probably does not occur without accompanying psychopathology. It is often unclear which disorders are a result of MPD, which are causatively associated with it (or with its presentation), and which are coincidental. It is interesting to see symptoms—sometimes even major behaviors such as substance abuse—sometimes fall away with integration. More often, the comorbid disorder(s) complicate treatment, sometimes causing its termination.

Forensic Issues. We have already discussed the great potential for inaccuracy of repressed memories (Frankel, 1993; Spiegel, 1994), and the need to use such patient productions as treatment tools rather than as statements of fact. The apparently very high incidence of child abuse in the background of MPD patients, and suggestions that such abuse indeed causes the disorder, does not mean that the patient should be encouraged to pursue action against parents or others. When legal issues do arise, the clinician is often asked to become involved as a forensic expert. This is inappropriate; the two roles—therapist and forensic expert—are ethically incompatible.

The treatment setting should be one that focuses on contemplation and restructuring, not acting out related to past injustice (even in the name of healing). Therapists who do choose to state emphatically that abuse by a particular person occurred in the past, or who encourage confrontations or legal action in their patients, are vulnerable to legal action themselves.

300.6 DEPERSONALIZATION DISORDER

The experience of depersonalization can herald a number of organic disorders, as well as functional depersonalization disorder. A careful medical workup is necessary for any new patient with severe depersonalization, especially those presenting in middle or late life. Depersonalization that is clearly part of anxiety or panic attacks does not require as much physical assessment. As for other dissociative disorders, an understanding of both symbolic and physical trauma and posttraumatic treatment concepts is important.

Psychotherapy

The principles of establishing and assuring physical and emotional safety, mentioned earlier in this chapter, are part of the foundation for treatment of depersonalization as well. Simple education and reassurance that one is not "going crazy" decrease barriers to exploration and allow a search for possible triggers, which is especially important in recurrent depersonalization. Triggers may not appear extremely stressful, but are symbolic and powerfully associated with past trauma or early conflict.

Hypnosis. Hypnosis (including self-hypnosis) is useful for controlling symptoms, creating/visualizing a safe environment for psychotherapeutic work, and doing the work itself. It has also been described as useful for the self-injurious behaviors that are often a part of depersonalization in patients with more primitive presentations (or, perhaps, that the depersonalization process allows to occur) (Simeon *et al.,* 1995).

Psychodynamic/Psychoanalytic Therapies. These therapies usually highlight the treatment of patients with comorbid borderline-like syndromes using object relations theory. Little has been written about them *vis à vis* depersonalization *per se* in recent years, but the concepts are important for the many patients whose disorders involve much more than dissociative symptoms. The reader is referred to the general literature on psychoanalytic treatment of Axis II disorders.

Group Therapies. These therapies have been discussed by Buchele (1993) and others. Treatment may be directed toward the specific dissociative symptom or toward simple normalizing of the patient's view of himself.

Behavioral Therapies. These therapies may be useful if clear triggers can be defined. There is little evidence that any behavioral or cognitive-behavioral therapy is a treatment of choice.

Biological Treatments

In addition to the treatment of commonly comorbid disorders, such as depression and anxiety disorders, several drugs appear to have a positive effect on depersonalization symptoms themselves. None addresses the underlying disorder; conflict resolution and posttraumatic integration require psychic restructuring. However, patients who wish simply to decrease the discomfort and inconvenience of their depersonalization symptoms may choose medication alone (or with "self-help," below).

The antidepressants are the most commonly effective medications. Until the advent of the selective serotonin reuptake inhibitors (SSRIs), monoamine oxidase inhibitors, such as phenelzine, were slightly preferred over alprazolam and trazodone, with tricyclics generally a third or fourth choice (Shader & Sharfman, 1989). More recently, SSRIs such as fluoxetine and fluvoxamine have taken over the field (Hollander *et al.*, 1990). It is not clear whether they are more effective for the depersonalization or for underlying depression, or simply are better tolerated. There is one report of depersonalization apparently *induced by* fluoxetine (Black & Wojcieszek, 1991).

In spite of the severe disorganization reported by many patients and the presence of primitive Axis II disorders, neuroleptics have received little study (virtually none for the newer "atypical" antipsychotic drugs). There is little reason to use them as a first or second choice. Anxiolytics probably have only a small role in the specific treatment of depersonalization, in spite of their usefulness for anxiety and panic symptoms. There is little indication that commonly prescribed mood stabilizers are effective.

SELF-HELP

There are several things that healthier patients can be taught to do to control or contain their own symptoms. Many are discovered by patients on their own but perhaps are not effectively applied without professional guidance. The simplest is merely to touch some stable object firmly, perhaps closing one's eyes and reassuring oneself. Picturing oneself in a pleasant fantasy environment, commonly used in hypnosis, is another technique. Briere (1992) describes several others in work with adult victims of child abuse. All of these could be construed as forms of containment. None is a treatment for the depersonalization disorder itself.

300.15 DISSOCIATIVE DISORDER NOS

The treatment of patients with dissociative symptoms that do not fit any of the above DSM-IV categories should focus on the symptoms and syndromes as they present, and on the apparent underlying psychopathology. As implied in the preceding pages, the presence of dissociation suggests a massive defensive effort in the patient. This, in turn, suggests a relatively acute trauma that has rekindled earlier conflicts by virtue of either the strength of the conflicts or the strength of the trauma.

For those patients with relatively good premorbid functioning and/or well-encapsulated symptoms, a symptomatic approach is likely to be helpful. One example is the treatment of some forms of sleepwalking (somnambulism). Many such patients, after sleepwalking as children, are free of the symptom until some external stress appears in an otherwise uneventful life (e.g., an important loss). In most cases, symptom removal can occur without psychodynamic complications. For most dissociative disorders, however, it is important to address both the symptoms and their sources.

CHAPTER 22

SEXUAL AND
GENDER IDENTITY DISORDERS

SEXUAL DYSFUNCTIONS

GENERAL TREATMENT PRINCIPLES

Great progress has been made in the treatment of sexual dysfunction during the past two or three decades. Whether generalized or situational, lifelong or acquired, "functional" or biologically related, more and more patients are willing to seek help for their sexual problems, and more and more professionals specialize in their care.

A complete sexual history is a prerequisite for the discovery, diagnosis, and differential diagnosis of dysfunction. Every mental health professional should be familiar with the elements of a sexual history (Risen, 1995), and should be comfortable enough with sexual issues to address them in routine evaluations. The topic should not be reserved only for patients presenting with sexual complaints. The medical history, including information about prescribed and illicit drugs, should provide hints to possible problems or causes (e.g., in diabetics, alcoholics, and patients taking certain antidepressants) (Buffum, 1992; Wise *et al.*, 1992). See **Part I** for treatment of conditions related to substances or general medical conditions.

Differential diagnosis is as important to the treatment of sexual dysfunction as it is to other disorders. Apparent hypoactive sexual desire, for example, may be masking sexual aversion or premature ejaculation (Ponticas, 1992), or dyspareunia may present as an orgasmic disorder.

For treatment to be successful, the therapist must understand the broad variability of normal human sexual function. Different interests, cultural mores, and

293

preferences must be taken into consideration when setting treatment goals and evaluating treatment response. The clinician should carefully explain treatment procedures, which are usually quite explicit sexually, and determine the patient's (and partner's) level of acceptance of them. Similarly, therapeutic objectives may be unrealistic unless one is certain the patient will be comfortable with his or her new sexual functioning.

Sex therapy is usually provided on an outpatient basis, often about once a week, for 12 to 15 weeks. Related couple, family, or psychodynamic issues may require a different, often longer, schedule.

The sexual issues being treated almost always involve a close relationship with a spouse. One should be suspicious of the patient who wants only to be "cured," without discussing the marital or conjugal relationship. The partner often even becomes a "therapist," as he or she participates in "homework assignments." Relationship issues may be situational or deep-seated, and often should be addressed in specific conjoint or group counseling (Metz & Dwyer, 1993).

Relapse prevention, a concept well known in the treatment of the paraphilias, is also important in sex therapy. The couple should be encouraged to continue therapeutic and relationship-building activities after the dysfunction has been alleviated. Realistic goals and the likelihood of occasional lapses should be discussed before discharge, and clinical follow-up arranged when possible (McCarthy, 1993).

Finally, the sex therapist must be mature, comfortable with his or her own sexuality, accepting of a variety of sexual behaviors that others may find stimulating, and able to articulate the issues and instructions necessary to accomplish whatever interventions may help the patient. Those who are overly inhibited, coldly "clinical," poorly educated in sexual matters, or not in control of their own libidinal issues should refer sexual dysfunctions to another professional. Since this field is fraught with countertransference issues and lay misunderstandings, many therapists—even very experienced ones—arrange for periodic supervision from a colleague.

SEXUAL DESIRE DISORDERS

302.71 HYPOACTIVE SEXUAL DESIRE DISORDER

Education, cognitive therapy to address psychological reservations, and counseling for relationship issues (e.g., using sex to control the partner) are frequently the most productive clinical avenues (Rosen & Leiblum, 1995). Hurlburt (1993) found group therapy with orgasmic training more effective than group therapy alone. Medications are rarely useful as primary treatment, although comorbid Axis I disorders should be treated, and the temporary relief of anxiety may be indicated in some patients.

Helen Singer Kaplan (1995) described a therapeutic technique that is highly individualized to each patient/couple and draws upon a rich panoply of interventions and homework assignments to enhance desire and, often, to address emotional and relationship issues. Practical interventions include self-exploration, sex education, sexual skills training, use of erotic materials, sensate focus and self-stimulation, social or courting exercises, and "permission" to experience freely a range of fantasies and behaviors that the patient or couple find stimulating. The last item, permission, is often important when the patient's view of himself or herself conflicts with stimulating fantasies (e.g., a male patient reluctant to "sully" a wife whom he sees as "pure"; a patient of either sex who eschews violence but is aroused by sadistic or masochistic images).

It must be emphasized that these techniques are not applied in a rote manner. Rather, the patient must become convinced, in a nonjudgmental context, that the paucity of desire stems from within himself or herself. Kaplan described this as accentuating the negatives, and deaccentuating the positives, of sex. The patient comes to understand that sexual desire is generally within his or her control and responsibility, and begins to use those tools for enhancement that are available through educational, cognitive, and/or experiential means.

302.79 SEXUAL AVERSION DISORDER

Ponticas (1992) and other authors note that the phobic avoidance that characterizes sexual aversion suggests treatment techniques different from those of hypoactive desire.

Most authors recommend a behavioral approach, usually systematic desensitization (imaginal and, primarily, *in vivo*), coupled with counseling related to the psychological source of the aversion (Becker & Kavoussi 1994). Kaplan (1986) emphasizes the distinction between the comparatively open behavioral and experiential procedures for hypoactive desire and the careful successive approximation necessary in sexual aversion, although some of the assignments may be similar (e.g., genital examination). The desensitization process is highly individualized, but works toward, and usually includes, genital penetration by patient and partner.

Accompanying psychotherapy should be insight oriented and empathic, but focus on sexually related issues. The patient's progress in the behavioral exercises and general motivation for success usually allow early clarification of resistances and rapid psychodynamic gain.

Although the desensitization process can usually begin at once, Kaplan (1995) recognizes the special vulnerability of patients whose aversions are caused by severe sexual trauma. Posttraumatic issues should be addressed and resolved, when feasible, before commencing behavioral treatment (especially that involving a partner).

Medications

In some patients, confronting the aversion produces panic symptoms. Single doses of such drugs as alprazolam (0.25 to 1.5 mg) or trazodone (50 to 100 mg) (Kaplan, 1986) may be required for *in vivo* desensitization. The medication should be considered ancillary rather than a primary treatment.

SEXUAL AROUSAL DISORDERS

302.72 FEMALE SEXUAL AROUSAL DISORDER

In spite of the DSM-IV focus on physiologic signs (swelling and lubrication), the arousal phase of sexual response is a "total body phenomenon" (Rosenbaum, 1995) necessary for orgasm. Difficulty may arise due to physical (see **Part I**), situational, or more lasting psychological issues (e.g., from past sexual trauma).

Most treatment approaches depend on sensate focus or "pleasuring" principles similar to those commonly effective for erectile disorder (see below) and attention to the issues addressed in hypoactive sexual desire disorder (above). Genital stimulation, while very important, is comparatively less an issue for women than for men, as women are more likely to experience sex as intertwined with intimacy and/or reproduction. Therapy itself often begins with many of the elements discussed under hypoactive desire and sexual aversion, including reassurance, permission, education, partner training and participation, and skills training. Pleasuring exercises proceed in a hierarchy, with intercourse prohibited until both clinician and patient feel that genital insertion is the next step. Sometimes, penile insertion without thrusting ("vaginal containment") is a useful intermediary between manual or oral stimulation and coitus.

Stimulation that is physically and mentally uninterrupted (and not likely to be interrupted, such as by a child's knocking on the bedroom door) is important for most women. Anticipation of orgasm, or anxiety about it (e.g., wondering if neighbors will overhear, reluctance to abandon oneself to the pleasure and release of sex), may interrupt arousal as well. Thus, approaches that enhance stimulation should also address lessening the probability of interruption.

Physical Aids

A number of artificial lubricants are available to allow comfortable intercourse; however, they do not specifically increase sexual arousal (unless lack of lubrication and accompanying discomfort have prevented arousal in the first place). The most effective are water-soluble and tasteless, and may be applied or inserted some time before intercourse.

Medications

Estrogen is the primary hormone responsible for maintaining the vaginal mucosa, including the lubrication response to arousal. Postmenopausal women and others with dry or atrophic vaginal mucosa should be evaluated for estrogen therapy.

302.72 MALE ERECTILE DISORDER

When not related to a substance or general medical condition, erectile disorder is often characterized, and perpetuated by performance anxiety. Reassurance that most males experience erectile difficulty at some point is helpful.

The most common treatment is simply assigning homework in which the couple engages in nondemanding, intimate, but initially nonsexual pleasuring (Masters & Johnson, 1970). Manual and/or oral genital stimulation assignments follow eventually, but intercourse is specifically prohibited until the erection can be easily and consistently sustained.

Erectile failure during or after otherwise successful treatment must be discussed with the patient (and partner, when possible). Occasional loss of erection must not be allowed to connote a loss of overall progress or the failure of treatment.

Psychotherapy

Psychotherapy is often unnecessary, but some patients benefit from individual, couple, or group counseling. Common therapeutic issues are sexual anxiety (including anxiety about fantasies or impulses), performance expectations, intimacy, relationships, guilt or shame (e.g., over adultery or past relationships), fear (e.g., of giving or receiving HIV), resistance to cure, and cognitive dissonance (e.g., feeling that one's new wife is too special to use as an object of sexual desire) (Leiblum & Rosen, 1992; LoPiccolo, 1992; LoPiccolo & Daiss, 1988).

Physical Treatments

These treatments include medications, devices, and prostheses. Unless there is a specific testosterone deficiency, hormonal approaches are usually ineffective. Yohimbine may be helpful for a few patients felt to have an erectile dysfunction (particularly age-related or mild neurogenic dysfunction). Bromocriptine may be tried as well.

Vacuum pump devices are effective for producing erections, although a constricting ring at the base of the penis is often needed to maintain it. They are commonly used in neurogenic erectile dysfunction and are popular for masturbation in some social subgroups. They are useful for augmenting partial erections. Improper use (e.g., overpumping, leaving the constricting band on the penis too long) can cause discomfort, although the principle is simple and side effects are few.

Intracavernosa injections of papaverine combinations and other preparations are effective, but their risks suggest reserving them for refractory and neurogenic disorders. They are discussed in more detail in **Part I**, on sexual dysfunction related to general medical conditions. Penile prostheses are discussed in **Part I**. They are not indicated for psychogenic impotence.

ORGASMIC DISORDERS

302.73 FEMALE ORGASMIC DISORDER (INHIBITED FEMALE ORGASM)

Many of the principles outlined in the above sections apply to the encouragement of orgasm, including permission for sexual fantasies and behaviors, the importance of sexual traumata in anorgasmia, and a frequent need for uninterrupted stimulation in order to kindle orgasm. In addition, performance anxiety, situational factors (e.g., marital issues, fatigue, stress), and neurotic factors (e.g., fears of one's out-of-control impulses, of vulnerability to one's partner, or even of death) often play a significant role.

Husbands are an important part of the therapy, especially when coital orgasm is the primary goal. Men sometimes feel threatened by not being able to "give" their wives orgasms, and by the possibility that sex therapy for the wife will uncover some flaw in their own masculinity. Sometimes, male sexual dysfunction or inadequate sexual behavior does surface; it must then be addressed just as would any other barrier to therapeutic success. No matter what the object of treatment (in this case, female orgasm), one should try to create a blameless alliance of therapist, wife, and husband against the common problem.

Unmitigated fantasy is encouraged. Acting out erotic roles and/or using erotic paraphernalia should be mentioned (and in some cases recommended) by the therapist, since the patient may need permission even to bring up the subject. As stepwise body, then genital, pleasuring proceeds, the therapist adds instruction for masturbation (directed masturbation) by oneself or one's partner, with or without a vibrator or other device. Masturbation during vaginal containment may be helpful as well.

The well-known Kegel exercises, which stimulate and strengthen the pubococcygeus, may be physically useful, and in addition allow the patient to gain additional familiarity with, and control of, this part of her body. Familiarity may also be encouraged by unabashed self-exploration, or merely visual scanning (Rosenbaum, 1995) of one's own body.

The man's sensitivity to the woman's pleasure must not be omitted from any discussion of female orgasm. Even those husbands who have been married for some time may lack a basic understanding of female orgasm, such as the importance of clitoral stimulation and uninterrupted arousal. Pointers on physical techniques, such as caressing and manual or oral stimulation, should be offered (by wife or therapist) and accepted. The husband should also either initiate or accept sexual positions that stimulate the clitoris if this gives his wife pleasure.

Women usually continue to be receptive and enjoy intercourse well after orgasm (and may be able to have additional orgasms if stimulation continues). Men, on the other hand, are genitally, and usually erotically, spent after ejaculation. It is thus logical that the man try to control his own orgasm until his wife has had at least one. Unless the woman indicates that she does not wish more thrusting or other stimulation, the man should usually consider the rule to be "Ladies first."

While a cognitive and experiential approach, with permission, education, training, and graduated experience, is often effective by itself, psychodynamic issues are almost always important to complete and lasting relief. Anorgasmia and other sexual dysfunctions, in men or women, are rarely sole symptoms. Although the primary focus is on a particular complaint, the therapist should be both willing and competent to explore beyond specific sexual function when clinically indicated.

302.74 MALE ORGASMIC DISORDER (INHIBITED MALE ORGASM)

When not related to a general medical condition, this is far less common than female orgasmic disorder; there is little about it in the sex therapy literature. Some of the techniques used by women may be applied to men (e.g., giving permission to engage in whatever fantasies produce orgasm) (LoPiccolo, 1994). If the man is able to masturbate to orgasm, guided fantasies about coitus itself may be helpful. Masturbating with one's wife and quickly inserting the penis just before ejaculation is a common approach (usually discovered by the couple themselves). Successive approximation of intercourse itself, rather than moving to insertion on the first try, may be necessary.

302.75 PREMATURE EJACULATION

This is the sexual dysfunction most associated with complete, successful treatment by behavioral means. The "squeeze" technique is an effective, hierarchical desensitization method. The female partner stimulates the penis almost to orgasm, then prevents orgasm and ejaculation with a few seconds of firm (but not painful) pressure just below the ventral glans. It is now widely accepted that squeezing is not always necessary. The man can merely tell the woman when he is near orgasm, at which point she stops stimulating him, the sexual feelings are allowed to dissipate, and the process is repeated five or six times before ejaculation is allowed. Men may practice a similar technique during private masturbation.

Once consistent control is attained, the penis is inserted into the vagina with no thrusting, merely being contained. When this can be done without ejaculation, a thrust-then-pause exercise is done inside the vagina, with the woman controlling the movements and stopping when ejaculation is near. As the hierarchy progresses, male thrusting is allowed until a sensation of loss of control is felt. The similarity to other desensitization techniques, in which failure is not allowed, is obvious, and is extremely important to treatment success.

Medications

Although unnecessary for most patients, several drugs have been used in a few cases, and there are a handful of controlled studies of orgasm-retarding and/or libido-reducing effects. Fluoxetine is a recent choice of many clinicians, usually at about half the antidepressant dose (Nitenson & Cole, 1993). Waldinger *et al.* (1994) reported significant effects in a small study using paroxetine. Segraves *et al.* (1993) reported some success with clomipramine.

If premature ejaculation and the resulting loss of erection are intractable, some patients may consider the injection and prosthetic alternatives discussed in the section on male erectile disorder.

SEXUAL PAIN DISORDERS

GENERAL TREATMENT PRINCIPLES

Sexual pain, particularly dyspareunia, should be medically evaluated before a diagnosis of functional disorder is accepted and treatment begun. Once this is accomplished, the therapist should gently but thoroughly seek both fear-based and neurotic (i.e., defensive, conflictual) sources for the pain and for the relationship problems that it either causes or perpetuates. The possibility of past significant sexual trauma should always be considered, although, if found, it may not be etiologic. Behavioral and desensitization approaches are often useful, as is reasserting anatomic comfort and control in women (e.g., with self-examination or Kegel exercises).

302.76 DYSPAREUNIA (NOT DUE TO A GENERAL MEDICAL CONDITION)

Functional dyspareunia may be approached in a manner similar to that of somatization disorder and some other somatoform disorders, in that it is a physiologic manifestation of emotional conflict. As with the somatoform disorders, the pain is—for the patient—a means of dealing with an unacceptable fear or impulse. With this in mind, approaches to treatment should consider psychodynamic issues, and may include insight-oriented psychotherapy. The probability of primary and/or secondary gain associated with the avoidance of intercourse or manipulation of the sexual or marital relationship should be addressed. In men, nonorganic postejaculatory pain may be related to guilt or other neurotic issues, which should be explored in psychotherapy (Kaplan, 1993).

Behavioral approaches, such as systematic desensitization, that employ gentle, nonpressured, graduated attempts at stimulation, orgasm, and intercourse are recommended. If such approaches have already been tried informally by the couple, they may be told that it is important for behavioral methods to take place in a professional, structured context, accompanied by individual or conjoint psychotherapy.

306.51 VAGINISMUS (NOT DUE TO A GENERAL MEDICAL CONDITION)

As in the case of functional dyspareunia, functional vaginismus is likely to reflect emotional characteristics similar to those found among the somatoform disorders. Psychodynamic exploration and understanding of potential manipulation, secondary gain, and primary gain are highly recommended, with either conjoint or concomitant counseling of the spouse, since this condition involves and threatens the couple's relationship.

Physical deconditioning of the vaginal musculature using graduated dilation is an effective treatment but should be accompanied by psychotherapy, at least to the extent of supportive counseling. Most behavioral approaches are similar to the desensitization of phobias, beginning with exposure (i.e., visual inspection and touching) and proceeding through the insertion of one, then more, fingers (or lubricated graduated dilators), first by the patient herself, and then by her husband. When the penis is finally used, initial control of the speed and depth of penetration, as well as of coital position, should rest with patient.

Shaw (1994) recently proposed an alternative view of the meaning and treatment of vaginismus, suggesting therapy that addresses issues of mastery, autonomy, boundaries, and differentiation.

625.8, 608.89 SEXUAL DYSFUNCTIONS DUE TO A GENERAL MEDICAL CONDITION -.-SUBSTANCE-INDUCED SEXUAL DYSFUNCTION

The treatment of these disorders is discussed in **Part I.**

PARAPHILIAS

GENERAL TREATMENT PRINCIPLES

Treatment of paraphilia is often, although not always, complicated by a lack of dysphoria associated with the paraphilic behavior, great physical gratification from the behavior, legal and ethical dilemmas (such as whether to call a behavior a psychiatric disorder or a social issue, use of controversial treatments, or office management of patients who are sometimes dangerous to others), and/or frequently associated personality disorders. Nevertheless, patients often come to professional attention in one way or another. The clinician should be prepared either to treat the patient or talk with him or her about treatment before referral to a subspecialist.

It is practical, but not always psychodynamically accurate, to draw distinctions among those paraphilias that do not intrude upon the wishes of others (e.g., fetishism, transvestic fetishism), those that intrude but are nonviolent (e.g., exhibitionism, voyeurism), and those that are both intrusive and aggressive or injurious to others (e.g., pedophilia, sexual sadism). Patients with primarily aggressive disorders that sometimes become manifest in sexual terms (e.g., many rapists) are addressed to some extent in this section; however, their conditions are often more properly seen as disorders of impulse control, direct aggression, and/or antisocial behavior.

The patient may come to treatment in a variety of ways. One should be suspicious of the individual who requests treatment simply because he or she "wants to change." Far more often, some sort of family, social, or legal crisis is the motivating factor. This issue should be carefully clarified before deciding whether or not to accept the patient for treatment, and whether or not to consider the paraphilia as the primary treatment issue. Patients anticipating criminal or civil trial, or otherwise being coerced into treatment, are unlikely to make the necessary commitment to the rigors of serious treatment, and are not in a position to make long-term treatment decisions. Patients who seek (or remain in) treatment after the case has been resolved may have a good prognosis.

On the other hand, lack of initial motivation is not an absolute contraindication to beginning treatment. If, for example, a marital crisis or condition of probation brings the patient to the clinic for a few visits, one can discuss treatment motivation and coercion and work to motivate the patient further (e.g., "I know you don't want to be here, but perhaps we can use this time to explore some ways to make your life go more smoothly"). The paraphilias may also be associated with forced treatment. This usually occurs in correctional settings, although courts may order outpatient medication or other treatment.

The clinician who treats these patients must have a therapeutic orientation rather than a punitive one, and must be comfortable with his or her own feelings regarding these sometimes outcast and/or criminal patients. This is particularly important when the patient's behavior is exploitive, aggressive, or pedophilic. Serious manifestations of countertransference will almost certainly arise, and must be understood and managed.

Patients with paraphilias are prone to other kinds of problems as well, including marital and family difficulty, social and legal crises that may give rise to psychiatric symptoms or diagnosable disorders, anxiety or depression during times of guilt or shame, and medical illness related to sexual indiscretion. Substance abuse is commonly comorbid, although it should not be blamed for the paraphilia. Dementias, on the other hand, often have an etiologic role in perpetrators who have no early history of inappropriate sexual behavior; they are discussed in **Part I.**

Contrary to some conventional psychiatric opinion, paraphilia *per se* should not be equated with antisocial syndromes such as psychopathy or predatory behavior. In some cases, there is considerable guilt after (and sometimes before) the deviant behavior. Often, the behavior is quite circumscribed, occurring within an otherwise normal life but causing personal, family, or social difficulty. In many syndromes, however, the perversion either exerts inordinate disabling influence over the patient's life or is dangerous.

Patients—and some clinicians—often inappropriately associate paraphiliac behavior with transient stress. Indeed, various situational conditions may increase the frequency or strength of paraphiliac impulses. Nevertheless, if a disorder is clearly chronic, the therapist should not allow the patient to rationalize or devalue the syndrome with such statements as, "My job pressures were just too much," or "The whole thing happened because my wife was pregnant." Spouses (or patients) may also use the paraphilia as an excuse, or scapegoat, for other problems. In such cases, complete treatment should include a serious attempt to uncover other, often nonsexual issues.

Risk of Suicide

After the discovery of significant paraphiliac behavior, particularly pedophilia, the risk of suicide may be significant, particularly in professional people or those highly visible in the community. Men recently discovered or arrested for embarrassing or humiliating activities should be closely observed.

Legal and Ethical Issues

The treatment of paraphilia, especially pedophilia, is often affected, or constrained, by legal conditions such as probation, incarceration, or loss of custody of one's children. Some of these can be used as motivating factors and barriers to denial. Others, such as society's legitimate need to protect its children, necessarily interfere with treatment voluntariness and confidentiality.

The therapist must be aware of the laws, employment conditions, and ethical guidelines under which he or she treats (particularly aggressive or predatory) paraphiles, and should clarify them to the patient at the beginning of treatment. Those working in correctional settings have separate duties of "agency" to the institution (or court) and the patient that are not always clinically compatible. When patients are referred as a condition of parole, probation, or civil commitment, one's responsibility to the court (e.g., to report progress, request permission for passes, notify someone of relapse, etc.) must not be ignored.

Even in purely clinical referrals, legal and ethical decisions regarding breach of confidentiality to protect potential victims must sometimes be made. In pedophilia, for example, many states have reporting criteria that are so strict that should an active pedophile come voluntarily for treatment, the clinician must report him or her to a law enforcement or child protective agency.

TREATMENT MODALITIES

Since many of the biological and behavioral treatments for the paraphilias are similar from one disorder to another, each of these general treatment principles can be applied to several of the specific disorders discussed later. We will describe three primary kinds of treatment for many paraphiliac disorders and a fourth, combination approach.

Insight-Oriented or Psychoanalytic Psychotherapy

Such therapy is helpful for many patients who meet the usual criteria of motivation, ego strength, and intelligence. Patients in insight-oriented psychotherapy should view their behavior as a symptom of internal conflict. In that context, it is worthy of exploration and not solely a heinous and irreversible part of the personality. There are many anecdotal reports of success with patients, but no controlled outcome studies. This form of treatment probably should not be the sole approach for the intrusive and aggressive paraphilias described above.

Behavioral and Cognitive-Behavioral Paradigms

These paradigms vary considerably in their effectiveness. Various success rates are reported, usually with optimistic results for the first few months (especially while the patient is either in active treatment or under legal scrutiny). Some of the techniques include negative reinforcers, such as electric shock, or apomorphine injections. Conditioning to milder shocks or the use of the "rubber band" technique (in which the therapist or patient snaps a rubber band against the patient's skin as a reminder) have largely replaced the more severe reinforcers. Generalization of conditioned responses to nonclinical settings and the lasting success of measured (e.g., plethysmographic) responses are not well established.

During the past two decades, behavioral therapy of many sex offenders has moved from passive aversion therapy to self-management programs (including the self-administration of aversion) and sexual skills training. In experienced hands, cognitive-behavioral paradigms are among the most successful kinds of treatment for many paraphilias (Abel *et al.*, 1993; Marshall *et al.*, 1991). Three highly specific techniques for cognitive restructuring have been established:

- *Fading,* in which fantasies are gradually shifted from deviant to conventional sexual contact during periods of sexual arousal. The patient may focus on visual stimuli (such as photographic slides that fade from a deviant scene to an appropriate one) or fantasy while masturbating.
- *Masturbatory satiation*, in which the patient receives specific instructions to masturbate to orgasm with conventional fantasy or stimuli, but then to continue masturbating for up to an hour while visualizing the deviant situations or object(s).
- *Covert sensitization*, in which fantasies of deviant arousal (or, more effectively, prearousal scenes) are paired with immediate switching of the fantasy to terrible consequences (e.g., getting caught, being sent to prison, losing one's job and family, hurting an innocent child).

Abel *et al.* (1993) describe a process of listing alternative interpretations for the patient's distorted thinking about paraphililac behavior, applying the interpretations to patient behavior, and helping the patient to examine the illogic of the distorted thinking.

Purely cognitive therapies are helpful in relapse prevention, part of which focuses on the patient's awareness, and avoidance, of situations likely to precipitate paraphiliac behavior (see below). Inadequate sex education, erroneous beliefs about sex and victim behavior, perpetrator attitudes, secrecy, and specific cognitive distortions may also respond (McCarthy, 1994; Berlin *et al.*, 1995). Cognitive therapy alone should not be the primary mode of therapy in aggressive or predatory syndromes.

Biological Treatments

Biological treatments, particularly antiandrogenic, serotonergic, and luteinizing hormone releasing hormone (LHRH) antagonistic medications, show great clinical promise. Some have been used and studied for many years; others have only recently been tried for paraphiliacs. They will be discussed in more detail below.

Combinations of behavioral, psychotherapeutic, psychosocial, and/or biological approaches are the best overall strategy for most patients. Blends of biological treatments, behavioral paradigms, and environmental shaping (usually by the patient, such as avoiding tempting settings) hold the most promise for sex offenders. For example, Meyer *et al.* (1992) found a combination of depot medroxyprogesterone acetate (MPA) and psychotherapy effective in decreasing aberrant behaviors in 40 pedophiles, rapists, and exhibitionists of various ages, some with histories of head trauma.

Abel *et al.* (1984) were the first to report a combination treatment system for severe paraphiles (including child molesters) that involves the intensive use of covert sensitization, masturbatory satiation, sex education, social skills training, and other psychosocial concepts in a group setting. The program provides roughly 40 hours of therapist and group contact and another 40 to 50 hours of homework. The patient receives instructions for specific masturbatory and covert sensitization techniques, records the practice sessions, and discusses them with the therapist and group. The outcome for patients who complete this program and remain in follow-up is good. Specific outcome comparisons with antiandrogenic and more recent medications have not been made; however, the Abel *et al.* program can be set up with little social or legal interference, does not require exclusively psychiatric therapists, and, particularly when provided in a group setting, is relatively inexpensive.

Family Involvement

No matter what form of treatment is chosen, many authors recommend some level of participation by the patient's family whenever possible. Spouses may work in conjoint therapy or act as cotherapists in some treatment programs. This helps the patient, allays family anxiety, and increases the spouse's acceptance of the patient and treatment. Treatment is often severely compromised if the patient insists that the family not be informed of the disorder. The therapist should at least encourage disclosure to the patient's spouse (perhaps in the therapist's office), and promote the same honesty in the patient's life as is expected in the treatment.

MEDICATIONS IN THE TREATMENT OF PARAPHILIA

The goals and types of medication treatment are generic to many different paraphilias, although the acceptable risks, benefits, and end points of treatment are considered differently for different disorders (e.g., intrusive and aggressive versus nonintrusive syndromes).

Antiandrogens

These drugs are an excellent method of sex-drive reduction. The best studied agents currently in use are medroxyprogesterone acetate (MPA) and cyproterone acetate (CPA). Both are effective in controlling deviant hypersexuality and paraphilia by reducing serum testosterone. Cooper *et al.* (1992) found them equally effective in a small, placebo-controlled study, and both are available in oral and intramuscular (IM) preparations (MPA in a depot form). Leuprolide acetate (LPA, luteinizing hormone releasing hormone, LHRH, GHRH), now available in depot injections, also eventually lowers circulating testosterone, but LPA actually increases testosterone during the first six to eight weeks (Bradford, 1985). An adjunctive antiandrogen (e.g., flutamide, sometimes used in prostatic carcinoma) and/or close supervision is necessary during this period.

Both behavioral and physiologic results with MPA and CPA have been confirmed in several controlled studies and numerous open-label trials (Bradford & Pawlak, 1993; Hucker *et al.*, 1989; Wincze *et al.*, 1986). Most U.S. experience with MPA is with the IM depot form, in which measurable blood levels may persist for up to two months. The disadvantages of oral preparations for this particular patient population (e.g., those with problems with compliance and convenience) generally outweigh the advantages (e.g., ability to stop the drug quickly if adverse reactions occur), at least after dosage stabilization.

The depot use of MPA begins with frequent injections (e.g., two to three times a week) of 100 to 200 mg, and progresses to a maintenance amount every one to four weeks as circulating testosterone levels indicate. Although CPA may be given orally at up to 200 mg a day, lower, often widely spaced, doses are usually sufficient. Both drugs require several weeks for their full effects to materialize. Specific individual dosing and monitoring guidelines are beyond the scope of this discussion.

Adverse effects are relatively few, particularly at the low doses used for paraphilias (compared with gynecological use in women). Potential side effects of MPA that should be considered include weight gain, gallbladder problems, alteration of glucose metabolism, hypertension, and, for those patients wishing to father children in the future, altered spermatogenesis. Although CPA may cause weight gain, feminization, fatigue, or depression in some patients, most feel that the benefits greatly outweigh its potential for adverse effects. Finally, LPA appears to have fewer side effects for most patients than MPA or CPA, although comparative studies are lacking. Doses of the antiandrogens can often be titrated to allow normal (i.e., conjugal) sexual performance, and it is not unusual for patients to father children while taking an antiandrogen.

Although some therapeutic effect may remain after the medication has been discontinued, one should assume that the beneficial effects of these drugs last only as long as the patient continues to take them. Some clinicians are tempted to titrate the dose to very low levels, or even to discontinue the medication; however, this should be done only with great caution. When relapse occurs, it is almost always associated, at least in part, with medication noncompliance.

Serotonin Reuptake Inhibitors

The apparently obsessional quality of some paraphiliac behaviors (Bradford, 1994), as well as complaints of decreased libido in depressed patients treated with serotonin reuptake inhibitors (SSRIs), has been linked with at least partial treatment success using fluoxetine, sertraline, fluvoxamine, and others in paraphilias (Emmanuel, 1991; Greenberg *et al.*, 1996; Kafka, 1991, 1994; Kafka & Prentky, 1992; Perilstein *et al.*, 1991). In very recent studies, Bradford and colleagues (Bradford *et al.*, 1995; Bradford & Greenberg, 1996) found that sertraline decreased both self-reports and physiologic measurement of pedophilic impulses at mean doses of 131 mg/day, often without affecting normal sexual response.

The same group found that three SSRIs (fluoxetine, fluvoxamine, and sertraline) were equally effective in decreasing the reported number and severity of paraphilic fantasies from about 76% to 31% over 12 weeks (Bradford & Greenberg, 1996).

The SSRIs and other psychotropic drugs sometimes suggested for the treatment of paraphilias (e.g., buspirone, lithium) do not have a specific antiandrogen effect, and do not directly lower testosterone levels. Thus, although they show some promise, patients likely to harm others (e.g., pedophiles) should be carefully monitored for reoffense. Nevertheless, the SSRIs are both more familiar and less socially controversial than antiandrogens and generally have fewer side effects. They may be a particularly good choice for adolescent sex offenders, for whom the hormonal agents are more likely to be (relatively) contraindicated (Bradford, 1994). Fedoroff (1993) has reviewed a number of favorable case reports and clinical trials of serotonergic agents.

Other Medications

No other drugs have yet shown great promise in the treatment of paraphilia, although definitive studies have not been carried out. Because of its antiobsessional effects, clomipramine has been prescribed in a few case reports and small comparison studies, with hints of therapeutic effect but no striking results to date (Stein *et al.*, 1992; Kruesi *et al.*, 1992). Fedoroff (1988, 1992) has used buspirone with some success in a few cases of transvestic fetishism. Kafka (1991) and Coleman *et al.* (1992) have reported limited effectiveness of lithium, often combined with other psychotropic drugs, in several paraphiliac syndromes.

RELAPSE PREVENTION

Once testosterone levels and libido are lowered, it is tempting to believe that the paraphilia has been successfully treated. Drugs must not be given in a therapeutic vacuum, however; psychotherapy and psychosocial measures are imperative. Treatment dropout is common, particularly when medication is given without appropriate relapse-prevention strategies.

Several measures can decrease the probability of relapse beyond that associated with simple drug treatment. Relapse prevention for outpatients (sometimes called maintenance of therapeutic gains) may include surveillance groups (family, friends, or parole/probation officers who know of the problem and monitor the patient's behavior and antecedent symptoms), training and lifestyle modification to avoid triggering situations and tempting environments, therapy for denial of the paraphilia's chronicity, acknowledgment of its highly gratifying nature, stress and crisis management, and monitoring for severe depression (Abel & Osborn, 1995; George & Marlatt, 1990; Laws, 1989).

SURGICAL TREATMENTS FOR INTRACTABLE PARAPHILIA

There is no doubt that surgical interruption of sexual physiology affects sex drive and paraphiliac behavior. Physical castration has been practiced in various cultures for centuries, and sometimes is considered in modern societies frustrated and frightened by the intractability of (especially predatory) sex offenders. Offenders themselves often ask for castration (surgical or "chemical") so that they can have a chance to get out of prison and lead more normal lives.

Although the testes are not man's only source of predatory obsessive or antisocial behavior (cf., the effectiveness of SSRIs, above), their removal is very effective in preventing reoffense in sexual sadists, nondemented pedophiles, and paraphiliac rapists (Stürup, 1968a, 1968b; Heim & Hursch, 1979). Nevertheless, surgical castration is not so simple an answer that it can be widely recommended, since it is irreversible, destroys the possibility of retaining some appropriate sexual and reproductive function, and is repugnant to many social groups.

Stereotactic neurosurgery to ablate small areas of the brain associated with aberrant sex drive appeared promising during the 1970s (Cullington 1976; Freund, 1980); however, we are unaware of further studies of its use in the Western literature.

302.4 EXHIBITIONISM

Exhibitionism is among the most common paraphilias presenting to the psychiatrist's office. Resistance of the symptoms to change, either with treatment or with time, approaches that of pedophilia, although it is far less intrusive or exploitive for its victims. A number of treatment methods have had limited success, including the behavioral and psychosocial combinations discussed under "General Treatment Principles," above. Lamontagne and Lesage (1986) describe a case of covert sensitization with success at two-year follow-up. Relapse prevention should include a search for, then avoidance of, exposure-prone conditions and situations.

Exhibitionism would appear to be ideal for a trial of SSRI therapy (c.f., Richer & Crismon, 1993), since these drugs are easier for the general psychiatrist to prescribe and monitor than MPA or CPA, and therapeutic failure is not associated with real danger to others. The frequent intractability and association of exhibitionism with humiliation and/or arrest may lead one to consider antiandrogenic medication (Meyer *et al.*, 1992).

Individual psychotherapy can be useful for those patients who fit the usual criteria, provided motivation continues and denial is not allowed to exert too great a resistive influence. Group psychotherapy has been a common approach, with a number of anecdotal reports of success. Participation or cotreatment of spouses is advocated by many (Bastani & Kentsmith, 1980). Treatment approaches that focus on the situational components of exhibitionism and other impulsive paraphiliac behaviors, which often appear strikingly obsessive and anxiety related, may be helpful (Snaith & Collins, 1981).

302.81 FETISHISM

Presenting complaints of fetishism generally focus on guilt or difficulty with one's spouse. Involving the partner in treatment is important if marital difficulty is part of the presentation, or if the spouse has rejected the fetishistic behavior. If the complaint is mild, education about the condition and its benign course may alleviate anxiety about, for example, whether the symptom indicates deep-seated mental illness. In situations in which guilt is more significant, if the patient recognizes the fetishistic symptom as only one of a constellation of neurotic symptoms or if the fetishism interferes with desired or necessary activities in other spheres, more intensive treatment is needed.

The recent treatment literature on simple (not transvestic) fetishism is sparse. There is disagreement about both the need for treatment of what is usually a harmless sexual preference and the usefulness of various psychotherapeutic, behavioral, biological, and hypnotherapeutic strategies. When treatment is required or requested, we prefer therapies aimed either at the resolution of underlying conflicts or at the development of more efficient ego defenses. It is important that the therapist not ally himself or herself with the symptom-producing portion of the patient's ego; it must be confronted as something that the patient has labeled undesirable. This is particularly true if the disorder has led to inappropriate behavior, such as stealing women's underclothing.

Wise (1985) and others have noted the potential usefulness of such behavioral paradigms as aversive conditioning (electric shock, apomorphine injections), covert sensitization, or snapping rubber bands attached to the wrist, although generalization and their lasting effectiveness are questionable. Masturbatory satiation, useful in many paraphilias, can be helpful in fetishism as well (see above). Lorefice (1991) has described a patient treated with fluoxetine.

302.89 FROTTEURISM

Frotteurism is often seen as similar to exhibitionism and voyeurism. We found no controlled treatment studies in the literature. The fact that frotteurism (or *toucherism*) involves physical contact with a victim implies more inappropriate intrusion than other minor paraphilias, and perhaps a greater potential for escalation to more aggressive behavior (although this has not been well studied). A case report by Perilstein *et al.* (1991) described success with fluoxetine. Intractable or particularly aggressive patients may require antiandrogenic medication.

302.2 PEDOPHILIA

A famous philosopher, upon his second arrest and lengthy sentence for pedophilia, was asked why he had returned so quickly to the behavior when he knew his punishment would be severe. He replied, in effect, "because it is worth it." This statement seems to reflect an intractability that is common in the other paraphilias, but for a variety of reasons, seems even more prominent in those who molest children. This section assumes that most patients who come to treatment are male; the female pedophile will be only briefly addressed.

Careful initial evaluation, with experienced penile plethysmography, if possible, is imperative to clarify treatment objectives and—as a beginning for treatment—to breach the denial that is almost always present. Pedophiles often describe their behavior as limited to one form of offense (the one for which they were caught, a posture often voiced by other paraphiles as well). Thus, the patient discovered in incest may say that he has no interest in other children, or one caught with an adolescent boy may deny any interest in prepubescent ones. In most cases, however, standardized penile plethysmography produces graphic evidence of arousal by several ages and both sexes of children. The results can be shown to the patient and used as a foundation for therapy. Similarly, patients routinely say that they have only molested children a few times (again, the times they were caught). The therapist must not accept such a statement, and should openly assume (to himself and to the patient) that the behavior has occurred far more times and is extremely hard to control.

Psychodynamic psychotherapy of pedophilia assumes an immature or improperly fixated choice of sexual objects, whether because of basic defects in development *per se* or because of regression based on more recent psychopathology. The insight-oriented psychotherapies are not well accepted for this disorder, however. Once the symptoms have become visible, society demands more rapid, observable modes of treatment, which can be given under at least a semblance of social control (see "General Treatment Principles" above). The social magnitude of the pedophilic activity being greater than that for any of the other paraphilias, the opportunity for denial, guilt, self-castigation, marital problems, and the like is greater as well.

Development of empathy for the victim is an important part of relapse prevention and some aspects of covert sensitization. Pithers (1994) reported some success with group therapy focusing on empathy in a correctional setting; long-term effects of this approach are unknown. Group and individual therapy may also be helpful in correcting cognitive distortions about victims, victim behaviors, and impact on victims, as well as other aspects of sexual feelings and their appropriateness.

Pedophiliac incest involves all of the above treatment considerations, with greater attention to the family dynamics involved. Although many pedophiles categorically deny that they are attracted to their own children, the probability cannot be ignored and children in the family should be carefully protected.

Conversely, the incestuous offender is virtually always aroused by other children as well, his or her own children being more readily available and less likely to tell others. There are a number of therapy approaches for families; it is likely that each member requires treatment. Unfortunately, reporting laws for the protection of victims have a chilling effect on some families' seeking treatment. There are apparently no studies that differentiate treatment of incestuous pedophiles from that of other pedophiliac offenders.

302.83 SEXUAL MASOCHISM

We found no reports or studies specific to the treatment of sexual masochism in the recent treatment literature. Those discussions that do appear often describe patients who do not meet DSM-IV criteria.

Superficial symptomatic treatment with assertiveness training, bolstering self-image and self-worth, and the like may be helpful for some patients (e.g., those who have in the past accepted a "victim" role but are no longer satisfied with it). If evaluation reveals roots of the masochism in depression or existential apathy, then specific psychotherapeutic or pharmacologic treatment may be helpful. More intensive psychotherapy to discover and resolve causative conflicts, and develop more efficient, less destructive defense mechanisms, is indicated for those patients who can tolerate and utilize this treatment approach. The paraphiliac behavior will retain its gratifying value for a long time, and will probably be used during periods of regression.

302.84 SEXUAL SADISM

When the patient does not limit his or her sadism to noninjurious activities with consenting adult partners, physical containment and biological approaches, such as antiandrogen medications, are recommended (Bradford & Pawlak, 1987) (see "Medications in the Treatment of Paraphilia," above). Aggressive and/or predatory sexual sadism is extremely dangerous, may be found in adolescents as well as in adults (Myers, 1994), and should not be treated on an outpatient basis without very close monitoring and, if found effective, control of the patient's hormonal status.

Follow-up studies of surgical castration and stereotactic neurosurgery, primarily completed during the 1960s and 1970s, describe considerable success in sexual sadists, pedophiles, and perpetrators who would today be called paraphiliac rapists (Stürup 1968a; Heim & Hursch, 1979) (see "Surgical Treatments for Intractable Paraphilia," above).

302.3 TRANSVESTIC FETISHISM

One of the most important treatment considerations in transvestic fetishism (transvestism) is that its resemblance to transsexualism or homosexuality is only superficial. Treatment principles are related to those for fetishism; however, in transvestism, the clinician often should not give "permission" for the activity. We agree with those who recommend that the therapist ally himself or herself with those parts of the patient that are working toward change, and not with those parts that want to continue a behavior that has been defined as troublesome.

Patients rarely come to psychiatric treatment in the absence of accompanying external problems (e.g., discovery by others, with subsequent marital, social, vocational, or legal problems), shame, depression, or gender dysphoria. Treatment is frequently sought because of age-related changes. In this regard, both transvestism and fetishism are more erotic in adolescence and early adulthood than later in life. Mature and older transvestites generally associate their cross-dressing more with feelings of relaxation than with sexual activity (Frances & Wise, 1987; Croughan *et al.*, 1981).

Reassurance that transvestism *per se* does not imply homosexuality or impotence may be helpful to both patient and spouse. Most authors suggest that transvestites not attempt to keep their impulses or activities a secret from wives or fiancees. Disclosure and discussion may best take place in the company of the therapist, who can provide objective, usually reassuring information about the syndrome.

Treatment of the urge to cross-dress *per se* is difficult; there are no descriptions of lasting success in the few case reports that discuss psychotherapy with such patients. Operant (e.g., aversive) conditioning can extinguish erectile response to female clothing, but there are no studies of generalized or lasting effect. There are only a few reports of drug therapy, but the various medications used for more aggressive paraphilias should be effective in the generic reduction of aberrant sex drive. Antiandrogens should only very rarely be indicated, but buspirone may be considered (Fedoroff, 1988). The SSRIs have not been reported to be successful (Stein *et al.*, 1992). The clinician should not confuse treatment of transvestism with that for transsexualism; feminizing hormones and surgery have no place in the management of this disorder.

Because of treatment refractoriness, or perhaps because they are reluctant to recognize victimless paraphilias, some authors have changed their definition of treatment success to mere acceptance of one's symptoms (Brown, 1995). We would disagree, and prefer simply to acknowledge that there currently is no reliably effective treatment for those who wish to change.

302.82 VOYEURISM

Like transvestism, voyeurism rarely comes to treatment until social or legal problems intervene. Psychotherapy is rarely directly helpful, although analytic uncovering and restructuring of the developmental underpinnings of the patient's looking and peeking can decrease aberrant urges. Treatment with SSRIs has been attempted, with some reports of success (Emmanuel *et al.*, 1991). Antiandrogens are effective, but should be reserved for severe cases in which the benefits are felt to outweigh the risks. As discussed at the beginning of this section, a complete program of monitoring, therapy, and social support should be employed whenever they are prescribed. Relapse prevention measures should be used with any treatment strategy (see "General Treatment Principles").

302.9 PARAPHILIA NOS

The treatment of individuals who fall into this residual category (e.g., telephone scatologia, klismaphilia, necrophilia) should be predicated on their presenting symptoms and underlying psychopathology. The extent to which treatment should be vigorously pursued by the clinician, and to which the more invasive therapies (e.g., antiandrogenic drugs) should be used, depends in large measure on how intrusive or injurious the paraphilia is for persons other than the patient, the depth of dysphoria attached to the symptoms, and the magnitude of the social and legal implications of the paraphiliac behavior.

GENDER IDENTITY DISORDERS

GENERAL TREATMENT PRINCIPLES

This section addresses transsexualism, for which several levels of treatment may be considered: treatment for adjustment syndromes or comorbid disorders; psychological, psychosocial, and medical interventions to determine the appropriateness of sex reassignment; preparation for sex reassignment; sex reassignment procedures themselves; and postreassignment therapy and follow-up.

Gender identity disorders that reach the level of transsexualism, which should be differentiated from transvestism (transvestic fetishism) and homosexuality *per se*, are associated with significant morbidity and comorbidity. Walker *et al.'s* "standard of care"—more appropriately considered a guideline—for decisions about hormonal treatment and sex reassignment surgery (including related cosmetic surgery) was updated in 1990 (Walker *et al.*, 1990), and is referred to in most modern treatment discussions. Professionals wishing further information may consult the Harry Benjamin International Gender Dysphoria Association (P.O. Box 1718, Sonoma, CA 95476; telephone 707/938-2871).

Some reports in the treatment literature refer to patients whose gender identity problem is seen in a context of schizophrenia or other psychotic illness. The sexual syndrome should not be considered primary in such patients; the psychosis should be treated and cleared before assuming that a separate sexual disorder is present. There is also significant comorbidity with other Axis I diagnoses. We will briefly discuss concomitant depression, anxiety, adjustment issues, and other secondary syndromes.

Attempts to change sexual orientation are socially controversial, but may be indicated by a patient's wishes and discomfort. Unfortunately, there is little indication that any behavioral or psychotherapeutic approach is very successful at altering gender preference or orientation (Haldeman, 1994).

Some patients who present for treatment believing they are transsexual (or homosexual) are in reality only reacting to situational stimulation (e.g., in military training, locker rooms, prisons, or even childhood sleepovers), transvestic fetishism, or simply normal variations of human arousal. When this is the case, the diagnosis is not true gender identity disorder, and therapy with reassurance can be very successful. Experienced evaluation to determine whether or not the diagnosis is justified is very important.

302.85 GENDER IDENTITY DISORDER IN ADULTS

Treatment for adjustment syndromes or comorbid disorders requires some understanding of the complexity and differential diagnosis of gender identity disorder; however, most symptoms (e.g., depression, anxiety, panic, ambivalence, personality traits) can be managed in a generic fashion. Comorbid personality disorders, some unstable, are common. The clinician should try to determine which symptoms are related to the gender identity problem and which are separate from it. Many patients believe that all their discomforts stem from their being trapped in a man's (woman's) body. They are likely to have unrealistically negative expectations about psychotherapy outcome, and unrealistically positive hopes that sex reassignment will solve everything.

For a variety of reasons, most patients will never receive sex reassignment surgery. Helping those who choose to lead their lives as a member of the opposite sex without surgical changes is a useful role for the therapist. While supportive therapy is the most common role for the professional in this context, several clinicians who specialize in this field recommend a therapist-patient relationship that is much more active and comprehensive (e.g., encouraging comfort with cross-dressing, specifically approving other-sex identification and activities, helping the patient contact support groups) (Schaefer *et al.*, 1995).

If sex reassignment is the patient's goal, screening is extremely important if the patient is to avoid a dismal result from irreversible surgical procedures. Unlike cosmetic procedures, genital alteration is not simply an elective procedure, to be available on consent. A second opinion and/or peer review should precede referral for sex reassignment, and acceptance of the referral by the surgeon or surgical team (Walker *et al.*, 1990).

Virtually all authors recommend one or two years of actually living as a member of the opposite sex (which many patients will have done already), changing body appearance nonsurgically (e.g., with electrolysis), and engaging in meaningful psychotherapeutic exploration of the disorder and the patient's expectations before surgical measures are undertaken. Some clinicians require hormonal treatment at this point, to determine whether or not the patient will be pleased with biological feminization or masculinization.

Preparation for Sex Reassignment

The patient, who has been living as a member of the opposite sex, must now prepare for an irreversible change in gender. If hormones have not already been started, they should be prescribed. Permanent cross-gender changes should be made in the patient's life, such as officially changing one's name and sex on licenses and other credentials. Second opinions and peer review should be obtained, and the medical risks, benefits, and procedures carefully explained and understood.

Sex reassignment procedures in males consist of removal of the testes and penis, creation of a vagina, and the use of tissue and innervation from the glans penis to create a somewhat functional artificial clitoris. The "neovagina" is often almost indistinguishable (externally) from a natural vagina, can be created to a depth that will accommodate a normal penis, and requires a period of manual dilation after healing (Hage *et al.*, 1994). Procedures to produce feminine secondary sex characteristics, in addition to those discussed above, can include laryngeal surgery (to raise the voice register) and mammoplasty.

Natal females have their breasts removed and may or may not undergo hysterectomy along with their oophorectomy. An artificial penis is created using one of several procedures. There usually must be some compromise between sexual functionality (creating a permanent partial erection) and the ability to urinate (and control urine flow) through the phalloplasty itself. Interestingly, a recent study of patient preference indicated that some 90% of natal female transsexuals place a higher priority on urinary function than on sexual function, commonly expressed as the ability to stand at a urinal (Schaefer *et al.*, 1995). Some female sex reassignment omits the phalloplasty, since male hormones can produce considerable enlargement of the clitoris (up to 6 cm in some cases) (Meyer *et al.*, 1986).

Postreassignment therapy and follow-up help the patient adjust to both surgical and sexual changes (Becker *et al.*, 1994). Transsexuals of either natal sex should have been cautioned that although they will probably be able to function sexually, they often cannot experience orgasm. In a small follow-up study, Lief and Hubschman (1993) found that more natal males than natal females were able to experience orgasm after reassignment surgery. General satisfaction with sexual functioning was high in both groups.

Long-term outcome has been difficult to study in this patient population. In years past, prostitution and exotic dancing were common vocations for patients after sex reassignment. Emotional and lifestyle problems were routine. Today, however, probably due to a combination of better screening and preparation for reassignment and improved surgical procedures, most clinicians report high rates of patient satisfaction. Patient age (under 30) and effective use of vaginal dilators after the procedure appear to be correlated with satisfactory postreassignment sexual functioning in natal males (Rubin, 1993); however, by the time reassignment surgery is undertaken, realistic patients should not equate success with sexual function alone.

Finally, Schaefer *et al.* (1995) recommend encouraging the patient to retain important memories, souvenirs, and legal documents related to his or her previous (natal) life. They can be important to the resolution of emotional issues (e.g., loss and grief) and unexpected legal problems, and can add value to the totality of one's existence.

302.6 GENDER IDENTITY DISORDER IN CHILDREN[1]

Core gender identity is usually established by the age of three years, and gender role behavior by the age of 6. About one in 25 boys and one in 10 girls exhibits gender atypical behavior during latency. About 1% wish to be the opposite sex during that developmental stage. During this period, parents should gently but unambivalently guide the child toward gender-appropriate dress and activities. Some males with gender identity problems have histories of being encouraged by a parent to dress and/or play as a girl, perhaps being shown off to others as "cute".

Except for brief fantasies and play during latency, gender confusion and gender identity problems in children and adolescents should not be considered normal. Children who consistently show many gender-atypical behaviors should be evaluated by an experienced clinician. It is a mistake to believe that an abnormal gender role has been predetermined and thus should be left to develop on its own, or to believe that the child is "different but normal."

Congenital 5-α-reductase and 17-β-hydroxysteroid dehydrogenase deficiencies produce boys with female-appearing genitalia. Almost all of these boys, who are raised as girls, change to a male identity with little difficulty when testosterone produces virilization at puberty. The ease of transition to a male orientation may be related to the genitalia's being different from those of normal girls, or to societal mores regarding maleness.

Intervention for gender dysphoria is most effective before puberty. Parental counseling is essential. Decreasing social conflict and associated psychopathology are the usual therapy goals. The effectiveness of behavior modification is well documented, as is that of individual and group psychotherapy.

---

[1]Primarily contributed by Beverly J. Sutton, M.D.

CHAPTER 23

EATING DISORDERS

The American Psychiatric Association's *Practice Guideline for Eating Disorders* (American Psychiatric Association, 1993) describes a number of biological, psychotherapeutic, educational, and nutritional treatment strategies for anorexia nervosa and bulimia nervosa. This section is generally consistent with the work group's recommendations, but more recent studies presented herein (e.g., of the newer medications) may alter the clinician's treatment decisions. (*Note:* This section refers primarily to the treatment of adults and older adolescents. Younger adolescents and children may require further specialized evaluation and care that are beyond the scope of this text.)

307.1 ANOREXIA NERVOSA

Patients with anorexia nervosa are rarely self-referred for treatment. Their family or friends bring them to the hospital or clinic, often after the eating disorder has become thoroughly ingrained and dangerous malnutrition has developed. It is imperative that the clinician try to form a trusting relationship with the patient and begin to suggest that treatment has advantages over the potentially lethal, but maddeningly seductive, impulse to starve oneself.

Treatment of anorexia nervosa must not be limited to increasing and temporarily stabilizing the patient's weight. Reestablishing normal weight, regulating behaviors (including, but not limited to, eating behaviors), changing body perception and other pathological beliefs, treating comorbid psychiatric symptoms and disorders, and treating physical complications are all required for the prevention of relapse and lasting treatment success.

Reestablishing Weight and Eating Behaviors

Although the patient will eventually choose her own meals, dietary assistance should be part of the treatment plan. For severely emaciated patients, caloric intake and nutritional balance must be carefully calculated, and often does not exceed about 1,600 calories[1]. During weight gain, intake may reach 70 to 100 kcal/kg/day, decreasing up to 40% for weight maintenance. An inability to gain or maintain weight at these rates suggests that the patient is exercising too frequently, vomiting, or not actually eating. A few patients may simply have an elevated metabolic rate. One should resist the temptation to rely on special high-calorie preparations, such as liquid supplements, after severe malnutrition has been alleviated, since the objective is to have the patient eat, and enjoy, a balanced diet of normal foods.

Hospitalization

The American Psychiatric Association's *Practice Guideline for Eating Disorders* (American Psychiatric Association, 1993) underscores the seriousness of anorexia nervosa and recommends hospitalization for initial treatment, against the patient's will if necessary, unless weight loss is not rapid, body weight is greater than 70% of that recommended for height and build, outpatient social support and close monitoring are "guaranteed," and the patient is metabolically stable. Halmi (1994) notes that bingeing and vomiting are also indications for inpatient treatment, for both safety and effectiveness.

The goals of inpatient programs are to regain and stabilize weight and establish patients' control over their eating patterns. A reasonable schedule for weight gain, with behavioral reinforcement for both gain (e.g., allowing exercise or other privileges) and loss (e.g., restricting exercise or activity), is essential. In addition to careful monitoring of diet, fluids, intake, and output, medical observation may include electrolyte, cardiovascular, and gastrointestinal status.

Staff members should be supportive but firm in their encouragement, and develop reasonable, credible relationships with the patient and family. All staff members should understand that the symptoms of anorexia nervosa are largely ego-syntonic, and that patients often attempt to manipulate the staff and conceal purging. In adolescents (and some adults), the patient's family should thoroughly understand the principles and process of treatment, and may participate as appropriate.

Inpatient care should continue until normal weight is stable and additional behavioral goals are reached. Inpatient psychological gains should be sufficiently robust that outpatient therapy is likely to continue without setback or

---

[1]"Calories" in this section refers to the commonly used lay term. Quantities actually describe kilocalories.

relapse. A detailed ambulatory treatment plan should be established that focuses on all aspects of the disorder (not just maintenance of weight).

The transition to outpatient care is particularly notable. The outpatient therapist should establish both the therapeutic alliance and the therapy itself while the patient is still in the hospital. Family understanding, participation, and support are very important. In some cases, patients who comply with treatment completely and voluntarily may be discharged a bit earlier, provided good aftercare and weight gain after discharge can be assured.

Other Residential Settings. Intensely nurturing group home environments for severely anoretic women have been described, largely on television and in lay publications. Striking successes with individual patients who were near death have been reported in a few media descriptions, but the author was unable to find reports in the professional literature. These appear to be highly specialized settings, with staff members who are very experienced in the care of both anorexia and its medical complications. They should not be confused with ordinary group homes or residential care facilities.

Outpatient Care. Failure to achieve outpatient weight gain and other signs of treatment progress, even fairly briefly, should cause the clinician to consider hospitalization for more definitive management. This is particularly true early in treatment, and whenever there is doubt about the adequacy of outpatient support and monitoring. Although expectations for weight gain in outpatient programs are lower than those for hospital-based care (1.5 to 2 pounds/week versus 2.5 to 3 pounds/week), one must be certain that the gains do occur. Allowing the patient merely to "try harder next week" is insufficient when weight gain is not consistent. When a few pounds are critical, weighing should be done in an almost ritualistic protocol (e.g., first thing in the morning, after voiding, wearing the same pajamas or gown as before). Be aware that the patient can temporarily increase her weight by drinking fluids (a pint of water weighs one pound).

Behavioral Therapy

Behavioral therapy can be used in both outpatient and inpatient settings, and is most useful for restoring nutrition and promoting consistent weight gain (as contrasted with changing psychological characteristics). It is seen both in special treatment units for anorexia and, after competent behavioral analysis, in individualized treatment programs. Halmi (1994) reminds us that the timing of reinforcement is important: An adolescent needs at least daily reinforcement for weight increase. She also recommends that bingeing and purging patients be closely observed for several hours after every meal, noting that "very few patients vomit in front of other people." Cognitive-behavioral therapy (CBT), which examines chronic distortions in processing and interpretation, is well accepted in the treatment of anorexia.

Psychotherapy/Psychosocial Interventions

Psychotherapy is very important to the stabilization of behavioral gains and long-term survival and success. True change requires psychic change, most often brought about by a combination of psychotherapy, corrective experience, maturation and adapting to new reinforcers, decreased reliance on pathological reinforcers, and alleviation of comorbid psychopathology.

The physical condition of most patients brought for treatment makes early psychotherapy almost impossible, but education and support should begin early in care. Problem-solving and insight-oriented approaches should follow as the patient's nutritional status improves and she can attend to the therapeutic work. Individual, group, and family settings may be used at various times in treatment, depending on the patient's needs and progress.

As in the case of other disorders at the interface of psychiatry and the rest of medicine, such as the somatoform disorders, it is often desirable to separate the roles of physical health management and psychotherapy. For example, the psychiatrist or other therapist may wish to give full responsibility for medical management and nutritional monitoring to a primary care physician—with good communication between clinicians—so that psychotherapeutic issues can be pursued more freely.

Medications

Psychoactive medication is not usually a part of the acute treatment of severe weight loss, but may be important after malnutrition has been alleviated. Special caution is necessary when prescribing any medication for nutritionally deficient patients.

Neuroleptics may decrease the obsessional, even delusional, distortions of self-image associated with anorexia nervosa. *Antidepressants* are often useful for commonly associated depressive symptoms but should not be the sole treatment.

Cyproheptadine, an antihistamine, has been used to increase weight gain, but recent reports and controlled studies are lacking. It has a mild euphoric effect.

Medical Complications. The management of malnutrition requires more than dietary and behavioral measures; appropriate medical consultation is imperative. Tube or parenteral feedings may be necessary, and must be prescribed and overseen by competent medical staff. Invasive feeding usually should be reserved for times of marked nutritional need, and not used as a routine negative reinforcer in behavioral programs (although the patient certainly may be reminded that it will be used as her weight or metabolic status dictates). One exception to this general recommendation is the patient early in treatment who is so morbidly passive that temporarily taking over her eating responsibility (e.g., by using a nasogastric tube) is clinically indicated. Patients who vomit persistently should have ongoing electrolyte monitoring.

Follow-up and Long-Term Care

Course and prognosis are guarded for most patients with anorexia nervosa. Completion of a comprehensive treatment program is associated with much higher rates of survival and eventual success, but patients should be followed for several years before one can relax the vigil for relapse. Controlling dysphoric moods and managing the severe personality disorders that are commonly comorbid should be included in overall treatment. Psychodynamically oriented psychotherapy is useful for those who are candidates for it.

Follow-up should include, or at least consider, psychiatric monitoring (frequent at first); specialized case management; individual, family, or group psychotherapy; provisions for residential care, rehospitalization, or partial hospitalization; and general medical consultation. Patients with a long history of anorexia may engender less ambitious goals, such as fewer relapses and maintenance of a "safe" weight rather than a "healthful" one (American Psychiatric Association, 1993).

Family Involvement and Support. For patients still living with their parents (and those few who are married), the program should attend to family participation and support from the beginning of care, including reasonable involvement in treatment planning when feasible. Russell *et al.* (1987) suggest that formally including family therapy in treatment is statistically associated with improved outcome in adolescents under the age of 18, but not in older patients. Nevertheless, the family may be inaccessible or unable/unwilling to understand the patient's complex disorder and needs. Therapists must be alert for parents or siblings who are overly critical of the patient, and for those whose own issues or psychopathology interferes with treatment. Preliminary treatment of one or more family members without the index patient may enhance later therapy.

Exercise Compulsions. Many patients feel strongly compelled to engage in extraordinary aerobic exercise, although those in end-stage anorexia nervosa are too weak to engage in almost any activity. This makes the availability of exercise a powerful reinforcer for behavioral programs. The form and extent of exercise must be carefully planned, however, so that the "reward" does not undermine the principles of treatment (i.e., one should exercise for overall fitness rather than to burn calories) or significantly decrease weight gain. Mild exercise, within the limits of food intake and impaired physical condition (e.g., decreased bone density or anorexia-related cardiac dysfunction), may be part of the program to promote health and healthful habits.

Lay Treatment Efforts. Women's groups and publications often describe lay programs, such as generic support groups for "women's issues," self-help manuals, or 12-step programs. Some of these mention eating behaviors in general, and not specifically anorexia or bulimia; others may be touted as easy or inexpensive cures for very complex disorders. While some may be helpful adjuncts to a definitive treatment program, none should be used as a primary treatment modality.

307.51 BULIMIA NERVOSA

Bulimia nervosa is not so ominous or life-threatening as anorexia nervosa, but it causes significant disability and marked medical and psychosocial problems in a sizable minority of patients. Most patients eventually respond to one or more outpatient treatment approaches, usually a combination of education, traditional psychotherapy, behavioral therapy or CBT, and/or medication. Some will require hospital care, either for definitive treatment of their bulimia or because of significant related psychopathology or medical complications.

Behavioral Therapy

Several studies have found that cognitive-behavioral, interpersonal, and behavior therapies are all effective in reducing both bingeing and depression, although CBT is sometimes considered better for changing *attitudes* toward body appearance, dieting, and vomiting (Fairburn *et al.*, 1991). A review by Yager (1994) states that nonbiological treatment approaches are "at least equivalent to medication approaches" for bulimia.

Behavioral and cognitive-behavioral therapies are the most commonly reported in the recent literature. Treatment initially focuses on controlling bingeing and purging, using diaries and regular eating schedules, controlling the likelihood of encountering a stimulus (e.g., not buying foods associated with binges), and substituting more healthful behaviors when tempted to eat. Education related to nutrition, adverse effects of purging, etc., is included. Cognitive restructuring of attitudes toward the self, body and weight, and problem solving follows, then termination and transition to life without strict behavioral controls. Programs usually last five to seven weeks. In many reports, success is positively correlated with hours of direct treatment and with the number of adjunctive treatments offered (e.g., individual psychotherapy, diet counseling). Several treatment manuals describe specific techniques (Agras, 1991; Mitchell *et al.*, 1991).

Noncognitive behavioral treatments either address anxiety and stress or focus directly on eating habits. The anxiety-reduction paradigm assumes that bingeing (and even ordinary eating) causes anxiety, which is soothed by purging. Exposure (eating binge-prone foods) and then prevention of vomiting during sessions is part of most such treatments. Stress-reduction models attempt to define idiosyncratic stresses that cause distressing emotions and for which the binge-purge cycle is assumed to be a regulating mechanism. Eating-habit-control programs try to educate the patient to her cycle of unnecessary dieting, decreased weight, and compensatory bingeing.

Response prevention is a controversial topic. Several studies of treatments that add exposure to stimuli followed by prevention of vomiting, to comprehensive treatment programs suggest that it adds efficacy (Leitenberg *et al.,* 1988; Wilson *et al.,* 1986). Agras *et al.* (1989), however, reported a decrease in effect when exposure and response prevention were added to the treatment program.

Psychodynamic and Interpersonal Therapies

Psychodynamic and interpersonal therapies compare favorably to behavioral and CBT techniques on most measures of acute treatment success (Fairburn *et al.,* 1991; Garfinkle & Goldbloom, 1993). In the Fairburn study, both CBT and interpersonal therapy groups diminished binge eating by more than 90%, with comparable success in attaining abstinence. Both groups improved greatly on measures of depression, psychopathology, and social function. Interpersonal therapy tended to be less effective in reducing dieting and vomiting behavior and in changing attitudes about body weight and shape. Psychodynamic, psychoanalytic, and interpersonal therapies are also useful for treating underlying causes of behavior and dysfunction, and for addressing the residual features of Axis I and II psychopathology that are often found in bulimic patients.

Group Therapy

Psychodynamic group therapy, either alone or with other techniques, has been reported to be helpful, although recent and controlled studies are lacking (Frommer *et al.,* 1987). Oesterheld *et al.* (1987) analyzed 40 group treatment studies and found moderate efficacy and good maintenance of improvement after one year.

Group CBT is roughly as successful as individual treatment, provided the patient completes the therapy. Significant reductions of bingeing and purging are seen in about 75% of patients, with abstinence achieved by half as many. Completion of therapy is a problem, however; Garner *et al.* (1987) reported twice as many dropouts as for individual therapies.

Early uncontrolled reports of feminist-oriented group therapy implied limited success (Boskind-Lodahl & White, 1978; White & Boskind-White, 1981). The studies have not been replicated.

Medications

Medications are best seen as one component of a comprehensive treatment program. Most medications associated with positive results in bulimia are antidepressants, although they may address specific bulimic, depressive, obsessive, or impulse-control components of the bulimic syndrome. Other categories of drugs may be useful for comorbid disorders, such as borderline or schizotypal personality, but are not generally prescribed for eating disorders. Doses tend to be in the antidepressant range or above. Of course vomiting soon after ingestion of the drug prevents its absorption.

Most studies suggest that combination therapies (e.g., medication and CBT) are better than single-focus programs. Agras *et al.* (1994) compared desipramine and CBT, both alone and in combination, in 61 patients. They found that combinations had the best results, both acutely and after one year. A 16-week course of desipramine was poorly effective, although 24 weeks produced good results for many patients. Leitenberg *et al.* (1994) reported that desipramine alone was insufficient for patients in a very small study, and that combining desipramine with CBT did not increase the benefits from the latter.

Mitchell *et al.* (1990) compared imipramine, intensive group psychotherapy, combined treatment, and placebo. All active treatments were superior to placebo. Group psychotherapy was considerably better than imipramine alone. Imipramine did not enhance the antibulimic effect of group psychotherapy, but further reduced anxiety and depression.

A number of studies of tricyclic antidepressants during the 1980s indicated that imipramine and desipramine can reduce bulimic symptoms and behaviors (Pope *et al.*, 1983; Hughes *et al.*, 1986; Agras *et al.*, 1987). The Hughes study was limited to bulimic patients with no indications of significant depression.

It is surprising that only a few studies of SSRIs and other atypical antidepressants have been reported. Early accounts are largely positive. The Fluoxetine Bulimia Nervosa Collaborative Study Group (1992) found fluoxetine effective in double-blind, controlled studies. A large multicenter study by Goldbloom and Olmsted (1993) showed short-term effectiveness with fluoxetine at 20 and 60 mg/day. Both behavior change and psychological change were demonstrated, with improvement not related to the initial presence of depression. Ayuso-Gutierrez *et al.* (1994) reported some success in a small, short-term study of fluvoxamine, 50 to 150 mg/day. Pope *et al.* (1989) found trazedone effective for bulimic symptoms in a double-blind study.

With regard to MAOIs, phenelzine was superior to imipramine in a well-controlled study of bulimia and atypical depression by Rothschild *et al.* (1994). While acknowledging the usefulness of antidepressants in bulimia, they attributed the difference between phenelzine and imipramine to the superiority of MAOIs over tricyclics in atypical depression. Phenelzine was shown to reduce bulimic symptoms by Walsh *et al.* (1984) as well. Isocarboxazid has also been successful (Kennedy *et al.*, 1988). Some authors suggest caution with MAOIs in bulimic patients because of difficulty maintaining a low-tyramine diet.

Fenfluramine, an appetite suppressant with serotonin agonist properties, was used in an eight-week trial of CBT (Fahy *et al.*, 1993). Although effective in suppressing overeating and snacking, it failed to show any antibulimic advantage over CBT alone. Lithium and carbamazepine have not proved useful in controlled trials.

Other Biological Treatments

An interesting series reported by Lam *et al.* (1994) suggested that light therapy similar to that which is useful in seasonal affective disorder has positive short-term effects in some bulimic patients. Seventeen patients were randomly selected (not according to any seasonal variation in symptoms) and given two weeks of 30-minute, early-morning treatment of 10,000 lux of white light or 500 lux of dim red light in a crossover design. The bright white light condition was superior on all mood and eating measures, for all patients. The seven patients with seasonal bulimic symptoms improved more.

Hospitalization

Hospitalization is rarely necessary in uncomplicated bulimia. However, patients who have not responded to conservative treatment should have an opportunity for inpatient care that offers close observation, intensive behavioral and psycho-therapeutic intervention, and appropriate medication to break the binge-purge cycle (American Psychiatric Association, 1993). Such hospitalizations should not be considered "short term," since several weeks are required to accomplish their goal and stabilize improvement sufficiently to allow consistent outpatient progress. Hospitalization should also be considered when comorbid disorders, such as severe depression, esophageal damage, or substance abuse, threaten the patient. Residential or day programs may take the place of hospitalization, provided medical complications are not severe.

Conservative Treatment

There is some indication that the initial treatment for mildly dysfunctional patients can be as conservative as intensive education or therapist-guided self-help. Cooper *et al.* (1994) treated 18 patients by merely supervising them in the use of a self-help manual based on cognitive-behavioral treatment for the disorder. Many improved, and half were said to have stopped their bingeing and purging. Treasure *et al.* (1994) compared use of a self-help manual to CBT and waiting list patients, with short-term success reported in equal numbers (24% and 22%) of the small CBT and self-help groups. Olmsted *et al.* (1991) found that five sessions of structured education alone were sufficient for a minority of mildly bulimic patients. It should be noted that these studies involved professional supervision. They should not be confused with lay groups (see below).

Long-Term Response and Follow-up

Many bulimic patients, like those with anorexia, have other psychiatric disorders. After the goal-oriented techniques already described have decreased or eliminated bulimic behaviors and attitudes, psychotherapy or biological treatment is often needed to address symptoms of, for example, borderline personality or depression. Such continuing clinical attention is important to maintaining initial improvement and providing maximum symptom relief and social function.

Well over half of patients with access to competent treatment programs decrease their bingeing and purging behaviors significantly, and that improvement tends to persist. A smaller, but still considerable, number also eliminate their inappropriate and dysfunctional attitudes about self and eating. Many patients continue to improve after active treatment has stopped, although stopping treatment prematurely (e.g., before the end of a structured program or before improvements in behavior and attitude have stabilized) is associated with much higher failure rates.

Patients with milder presenting symptoms and fewer years of illness tend to do better, as do those who are functioning well in other parts of their lives (i.e., activities and relationships not related to eating). Patients with comorbid primitive personality characteristics, with accompanying severe personal and social dysfunction, are at a concomitantly greater risk of failure.

Olmsted *et al.* (1994) studied 48 women two years after successful treatment in a specialized day hospital program. Thirty-one percent had relapsed, most during the first six months. Relapse was predicted by younger age, greater use of vomiting, and higher scores on specialized attitude (before treatment) and personality (after treatment) tests. Interestingly, binge frequency, depression, and social adjustment were not good predictors. Fahy and Russell (1993) assessed 39 patients during treatment and one year after CBT. Duration of illness before treatment, greater pretreatment symptom severity, and presence of a personality disorder were associated with poor outcome. Wonderlich *et al.* (1994) found that, except for borderline personality, four- to five-year follow-ups of 30 patients did not support an association of SCID-II personality disorder diagnosis with bulimia outcome, although other indicators of psychiatric problems were increased. Blouin *et al.* (1994) found only family discord (conflictual, controlling, and "over-organized" family environments) to be associated with relapse in their series of 69 bulimic women.

Studies of inpatient treatment appear superficially to show fewer lasting gains; in one study (Swift *et al.*, 1987), roughly half those of many outpatient series. One must remember, however, that only the most severely ill patients, including those who have already failed at outpatient care, are treated in hospitals.

Some patients will get better without treatment. The relatively low rate of spontaneous improvement, however, and the significant potential for serious complications both suggest that neither patient nor clinician should take this disorder lightly.

Family Involvement and Support. Family involvement, including family therapy, is recommended for patients currently living with parents or spouse. Its usefulness for adults living independently is much less clear, and there is some indication that it may impede behavioral treatment.

Substance Abuse. The American Psychiatric Association (1993) guidelines recommend that, in the absence of severe malnutrition or other medical problems, concurrent substance abuse disorders be treated before the bulimia is addressed. Most treatment programs are not staffed and equipped to treat both eating disorders and substance abuse comprehensively.

Lay Treatment Efforts. Some patients benefit from such groups as Overeaters Anonymous; however, they should not take the place of professional care. These and other lay programs, including other 12-step programs, may be helpful as adjunctive supports but they should be entered with clinician knowledge and approval, and with the knowledge that their superficial treatment (and sometimes outright denial) of medical, nutritional, and psychodynamic issues may be harmful.

307.50 EATING DISORDER NOS

Clinically significant eating disorders that do not meet specific DSM-IV criteria may respond to one or more of the treatment principles outlined above.

CHAPTER 24

SLEEP DISORDERS

Although many complex sleep disorders are listed in the DSM-IV for nomenclature completeness, most psychiatrists and other mental health professionals will deal primarily with only a few (e.g., insomnia, nightmare disorder, somnambulism). Such disorders as narcolepsy and sleep apnea (the latter often presenting with complaints of snoring or hypersomnia) usually should be referred to a sleep specialist. Their treatment is briefly summarized in this chapter. Child psychiatrists often see more patients with parasomnias than do clinicians who treat only adults, and should be generally familiar with their diagnosis and treatment.

DYSSOMNIAS

307.42 PRIMARY INSOMNIA

One should be conservative when considering treatment for insomnia. Patients' perceptions of difficulty attaining or maintaining sleep are often inaccurate, and there are many variations of normal sleep. It is often useful to have patients carefully keep a "sleep diary," which can aid diagnosis and at the same time show some patients that they are sleeping more than they realize.

In the absence of stimulating syndromes such as hypomania, truly decreased sleep causes daytime fatigue or sleepiness, which, if chronic or recurring, may be a gauge for starting treatment. On the other hand, mere complaints of sleeplessness deserve the clinician's attention, especially in the elderly. In normal individuals, average total sleep time decreases gradually but continuously after age 35; stage III and IV sleep time in geriatric patients often total less than an hour (Tomasovic, 1989).

TABLE III.24-1

Sleep Hygiene

1. Establish and maintain a regular sleep and wakefulness schedule. Do not sleep late the morning after you were unable to get to sleep, and do not nap during the day.
2. Establish the bed (and bedroom, if possible) as a place for sleep (or sexual activity). Some authors suggest not watching television or reading in bed; we would disagree for many patients.
3. Create a routine in which things related to sleep (e.g., being in bed, wearing sleep attire) are not associated with wakeful activities.
4. Keep the bedroom slightly cool.
5. Consider a light snack before retiring.
6. Avoid evening stimulants, including caffeine.
7. Mask environmental noise with "white noise" or earplugs.
8. If sleep does not come, or if it is interrupted, do not simply lie in the dark. Read, watch television, or perform some other mild activity until sleepy.

Nonpharmacologic approaches

Morin *et al.* (1994) found that over 75% of patients can improve with nonpharmacologic treatments such as stimulus control and sleep restriction. Relaxation therapies may help as well. Maintenance of improvement appears good, although onset of improvement often takes days or weeks. In some cases, hypnotic medication may be prescribed for short-term gains while pursuing stimulus control or sleep restriction.

Stimulus control, sometimes described as similar to *sleep hygiene,* can alleviate mild insomnia and other dyssomnias in some patients, although it is rarely effective for more serious disorders. The type of procedure is described in Table III.24-1.

In *sleep restriction,* the therapist tells the patient to spend only as much time in bed as he or she can sleep. Thus, if a patient reports four hours of sleep a night, he or she is only allowed to spend four hours in bed every night. The time is gradually increased over several weeks when it is clear that the patient is actually sleeping almost all of the time when in bed. The technique is described in detail by Spielman *et al.* (1987).

It is not clear whether such methods as meditation are helpful in inducing sleep. Although relaxing, many patients describe them as invigorating rather than soporific (cf., exercise before retiring).

Cognitive strategies to alter destructive thought patterns, such as those that lead the patient into a cycle of can't sleep → worry about it → try harder to sleep → no success → more worry → try harder, are often helpful. Misconceptions about causes or consequences of lack of sleep, unrealistic expectations of treatment, and the like can be addressed, for example, by telling the patient with benign insomnia that the body will naturally see that he or she gets enough sleep (Morin *et al.*, 1993).

Chronotherapy is discussed under "Circadian Rhythm Sleep Disorder," below.

Sleeping Medications

Many drugs can safely induce sleep. The main issues of clinical concern include whether or not the sleep produced is physiologically useful, duration of drug effect, development of tolerance and/or dependence, and patient reaction when the medication is discontinued. The initial dose should be small, especially in older patients. Most patients require medication for only a short time, so that tolerance and dependence are not often an issue; however, abuse potential should be considered.

Some nonmedical hospital surveyors from accrediting or certifying agencies occasionally consider sleeping medications "psychotropic drugs" for purposes of special polypharmacy or consent requirements. It will be obvious to most clinicians that although some hypnotics are benzodiazepines or tricyclics, they should not be considered psychotropics in the same sense as medications specifically prescribed for anxiolytic or antidepressant purposes.

Benzodiazepines and similarly acting drugs that bind to benzodiazepine receptors are the most often-recommended hypnotics. In general, they have an anxiolytic effect that may be difficult to separate from their hypnotic effect, are susceptible to tolerance, can be abused, and can potentially aggravate sleep apnea (although the effects are minimal in mild to moderate cases at routine doses). Long-acting preparations, such as flurazepam, quazepam, and nitrazepam, produce daytime drowsiness (and sometimes ataxia) which is often unacceptable, particularly in the elderly. Short- and medium-acting drugs (e.g., estazolam, temazepam, triazolam, zolpidem, zopiclone) are usually a better choice, but may cause rebound insomnia after several days of use. Vogel and Morris (1992) reported good results with estazolam in elderly patients.

The clinical importance of withdrawal insomnia is probably exaggerated in the literature. Patient surveys suggest that withdrawal insomnia is uncommon (Balter & Uhlenhuth, 1992), and both intermittent use and tapering of the dose are effective preventive measures. Zolpidem and zopiclone have fewer rebound effects than do the true benzodiazepines (Nishino *et al.*, 1995).

All benzodiazepines may occasionally cause transient anterograde amnesia and may very rarely be associated with "paradoxical" dyscontrol reactions. Problems with dependence and withdrawal among benzodiazepine recipients have probably been overstated, particularly in patients taking them as hypnotics (Shader & Greenblatt, 1993). Time spent in stage II sleep is increased; stages III and IV are decreased (cf., their effectiveness in treating nightmares, sleep terrors, and sleepwalking); and REM time is minimally decreased. Minor REM decreases are generally offset by increases in overall sleep time (Nishino *et al.*, 1995).

Barbiturates are excellent sedatives, safe in therapeutic doses and free of most common side effects. Nevertheless, they suppress REM and stage III and IV sleep, and are associated with tolerance and significant withdrawal after chronic use (sometimes even at therapeutic doses). These drawbacks, coupled with their relatively dangerous overdose potential, make them a poor choice as a hypnotic for most patients.

Barbiturate- and Alcohol-like Drugs. Chloral hydrate, ethchlorvynol, and similar drugs, sometimes described by their alcohol-like properties, have a short half-life and preserve REM sleep. They are associated with tolerance with chronic use and potentially severe respiratory depression in overdose. For most patients, there is little reason to choose them over the benzodiazepine-receptor drugs. Glutethimide, methyprylon, and similar sedatives were once popular, but their propensity for tolerance, considerable danger in overdose, and frequent hepatic effects make them poor choices for the modern clinician.

Most over-the-counter soporifics are antihistamines (e.g., diphenhydramine). They may be useful for helping patients get to sleep, but do not increase sleep time (Reite *et al.*, 1990). If patients are kept awake by itching or allergic reactions, they may be useful.

Two naturally-occurring substances have been used to induce sleep. L-tryptophan, a serotonin precursor, is an effective soporific with very few side effects at 1 to 2 grams per night (Schneider-Helmert & Spinweber, 1986). In spite of the fears of a few years ago, brought on by impurities in one company's product, it is a safe and inexpensive substitute for prescribed drugs when decreased sleep latency is the clinical goal. Melatonin has recently received considerable lay attention, and controlled studies are underway. Preliminary indications suggest that it is safe and effective for inducing sleep; its effect on sleep architecture is less well understood (James *et al.*, 1990).

A few *antidepressants* have hypnotic qualities that appear separate from their other effects. Trimipramine (unlike other tricyclics) and trazodone exert their effects with little REM suppression (Nierenberg *et al.*, 1994; Buysse *et al.*, 1995).

Other Somatic Treatments

A double-blind study of low-energy emission therapy (LEET), in which very small (imperceptible) currents induce electromagnetic fields through a conducting mouthpiece, found significant decreases in sleep latency with no side effects or additional treatment (Reite *et al.*, 1994). Acupuncture is occasionally suggested, but the allopathic medical literature contains few case reports or studies (Xie & Dong, 1994).

307.42 INSOMNIA RELATED TO AN AXIS I OR AXIS II DISORDER

Successful treatment of the primary mental disorder should address the sleep disorder as well. The specific insomnia treatments described above may be necessary in the interim, or when the initial disorder does not respond (Nofzinger *et al.*, 1993).

307.44 PRIMARY HYPERSOMNIA

There are several forms of hypersomnia. Most patients' symptoms can be traced to some form of sleep deprivation or interruption; other, "primary," syndromes occur in the presence of normal or excessive nighttime sleep. Polysomnography, a multiple sleep latency test (MSLT) (Richardson *et al.*, 1978), a family history, and other diagnostic procedures should be undertaken to determine the cause and suggest a direction for treatment. Several of the structural (e.g., noncentral sleep apnea), neurological (e.g., narcolepsy, restless-leg syndrome, central sleep apnea), and depression-related dyssomnias present with severe daytime sleepiness. The treatments discussed immediately below address idiopathic hypersomnia.

Most patients already know the dangers of severe daytime sleepiness (e.g., unsafe driving); they should be cautioned not to decrease their safeguards (e.g., by operating a car or machinery) until the treatment has been shown consistently effective. When danger to others is an issue, it is appropriate (sometimes mandatory) to notify motor vehicles agencies, employers, and the like. The patient should be consulted before such notification, but it may be required even when he or she refuses to give permission.

Nonpharmacologic Approaches

Regularly scheduled brief naps, similar to those recommended in narcolepsy, may be helpful for some patients. On the other hand, this is often inconsistent with routine nighttime sleep hygiene, which is more effective for sleep-deprived hypersomniacs. Specific approaches to breathing-related sleep disorders (e.g., sleep apnea) are discussed in that section of this chapter.

Medications

Once one has ruled out sleep deprivation as a cause of the hypersomnia, stimulants may be considered. Alertness can be encouraged with methylphenidate (usually 10 to 30 mg), pemoline (one to three 37.5-mg doses), or dextroamphetamine (10 mg b.i.d. or t.i.d.). One should start with lower, morning doses, warn the patient of side effects and potential medication problems, and avoid evening stimulation. Bastuji and Jouvet (1988) reported success with modafinil, but we are not aware of any follow-up studies.

307.44 HYPERSOMNIA RELATED TO AN AXIS I OR AXIS II DISORDER

Successful treatment of the primary mental disorder should address the sleep disorder as well. The specific hypersomnia treatments described above may be necessary in the interim, or when the initial disorder does not respond (Nofzinger *et al.*, 1993). Daytime sedation is a possible side effect of many psychiatric medications.

347 NARCOLEPSY

Narcolepsy, frequently accompanied by cataplexy or hypnagogic phenomena, has physical, social, and vocational effects on the patient. Management should include attention to the dangers of falling asleep in settings requiring alertness (e.g., while operating machinery or carrying breakable items). Reporting the patient's condition to the state driver's license bureau, other appropriate agencies (e.g., Department of Transportation for commercial drivers, Federal Aviation Administration for pilots), or the employer is often necessary, and legally mandated in most or all states when the physician has reason to be concerned about the safety of others.

Stimulant medication is the foundation of treatment. Methylphenidate, pemoline, and dextroamphetamine in divided doses, avoiding times that interfere with nighttime sleep, have long been the drugs of choice. Mazindol may also be tried (Iijima *et al.*, 1986), but there is little reason to use it as the first-line treatment. Parasomnic symptoms, such as cataplexy or hypnagogic hallucinations, often respond to low doses of tricyclic antidepressants or monoamine oxidase inhibitors. Selective serotonin reuptake inhibitors may be effective, but have not yet been established for this indication.

Controversy often arises about providing stimulants to people who may abuse them (or who may malinger the diagnosis in the first place). Nevertheless, after a reliable sleep workup has established the diagnosis, medication should be prescribed unless strongly clinically contraindicated.

Highly regulated nighttime sleep schedules and one or more naps scheduled throughout the day may decrease unpredictable sleep attacks. The effect of brief naps usually lasts less than an hour; however, they may decrease the need for stimulant medication (Aldrich, 1990). Some authors suggest one long afternoon nap rather than several short ones (Garma & Marchand, 1994; Mullington & Broughton, 1993).

780.59 BREATHING-RELATED SLEEP DISORDERS (SLEEP APNEA)

There are many breathing-related sleep syndromes. The cause may lie in the central nervous system, in the peripheral neuroanatomy, or, most commonly, in the airway and neck structure (often related to obesity). Most treatments are beyond the scope of both this book and general psychiatric practice; some issues are addressed in **Part I.** One should ask about signs of the disorder before prescribing drugs with significant sedative effects, and should discourage evening alcohol use by susceptible patients.

Conservative approaches, effective in some cases of mild or structural abnormality (e.g., those that merely cause snoring), include weight loss and training or devices for sleep positioning (e.g., avoiding sleeping on one's back). Over-the-counter appliances, such as nasal splints, may or may not be helpful, but should not overshadow the need for medical evaluation to rule out more serious dysfunction and/or poor oxygen saturation.

More complex treatments include maintaining positive pressure in the airway through either continuous positive airway pressure appliances (CPAP) or, less often, bilevel appliances (BiPAP). A mask is tightly fitted to the face and a compressor keeps a gentle pressure that permits normal breathing but does not allow the upper respiratory system to collapse passively. Most patients learn to tolerate the encumbrance, especially when they begin to reap the benefits of uninterrupted sleep with full blood oxygenation. For those who do not respond to, or tolerate, CPAP or BiPAP, surgical alteration or removal of specifically targeted soft oropharyngeal structures may be helpful, but is not always associated with long-term relief. Tracheostomy is effective in difficult cases (McCall, 1995). There are no broadly effective drug treatments.

307.45 CIRCADIAN RHYTHM SLEEP DISORDER (SLEEP-WAKE SCHEDULE DISORDER)

The causes of this disorder vary from jet travel, shift work, or noncircadian environments (e.g., underwater or space laboratories) to physical damage to the suprachiasmic hypothalamic nuclei. In noncircadian environments, sleep schedules should be normalized to prevent sleep-wake schedule disorder. Working on one shift for a long time rather than frequently changing shifts is also preventive. Once the symptoms develop, treatment consists of resetting the circadian "clock" with chronotherapy, phototherapy, or temporary medication.

There are two forms of *chronotherapy*. In one, sleep and (especially) wake times are rigidly set at the desired timetable, forcing a return to normal scheduling as soon as possible. In the other, sleep and wake times are gradually shifted forward two to three hours per day toward the desired period. Other markers of circadian rhythms (or *zeitgebers*) that may be scheduled as part of treatment include work periods and mealtimes. Under controlled circumstances, gradual shifting is quite effective; however, outpatient compliance is difficult to establish.

Phototherapy (bright light therapy) involves exposure to bright (about 5,000 lux) sunlight-like (full-spectrum) light for one or two hours just after awakening or in the evening, to delay sleep onset (Bunnell *et al.,* 1992). Satlin *et al.* (1992) found that two hours of bright light before bedtime alleviated sleep-wake disorder and "sundowner syndrome" in some patients with Alzheimer's disease.

Medications may be helpful for forcing a scheduled bedtime after travel or a shift change. Taking a short-acting benzodiazepine such as triazolam or zolpidem, at the new bedtime is effective for starting sleep, but users should understand the possibility of amnesia for the period in which the drug is active (and thus probably should avoid taking it preventively, such as during a long plane trip).

307.47 DYSSOMNIA NOT OTHERWISE SPECIFIED

Restless leg syndrome and periodic leg movement disorders are common complaints of elderly patients. Treatments include late afternoon exercise, clonazepam, levodopa, carbamazepine, and, for a minority of patients, iron or vitamin B_{12} supplements (Montplaisir *et al.*, 1992; McCall, 1995). A combination preparation containing both levodopa and carbidopa is also available. Benzodiazepines are not usually effective for the movement disorder (Mitler *et al.*, 1986), but may increase sleep time. Ancoli-Israel *et al.* (1986) reported success with specialized biofeedback, but their study has not been replicated to our knowledge.

PARASOMNIAS

307.47 NIGHTMARE DISORDER (DREAM ANXIETY DISORDER)

This disorder should not be confused with sleep terror disorder, discussed below. Syndromes related to Axis I disorders, such as posttraumatic stress disorder or drug withdrawal, should be considered in the differential diagnosis and treated accordingly. Most other nightmares are transient, requiring only psychiatric support and/or a short course of medication. Some syndromes respond to either a REM-conserving hypnotic (for non-REM syndromes) or low doses of a REM-suppressing tricyclic antidepressant.

When stress, anxiety, or fear precipitates nightmares, appropriate psychotherapy (e.g., relaxation, cognitive therapy, or desensitization) is often helpful. Such therapy is reportedly at least partially successful in most cases, even after only one session (Neidhardt *et al.*, 1992; Krakow *et al.*, 1993), although controlled studies are lacking. Pellicer (1993) reported a case of a child treated with "eye movement desensitization."

307.46 SLEEP TERROR DISORDER

Sleep terrors are deep non-REM phenomena that are extremely disturbing to the patient. Their treatment or control is similar to that of somnambulism (see below). The disorder is far more common in children than in adults; parents can be reassured that the syndrome is unlikely to persist as the child matures (although it may return briefly during periods of adolescent or adult stress).

Specific hypnosis paradigms may be effective for either children or adults (Hurwitz *et al.*, 1991). Bedtime benzodiazepines, either hypnotics or anxiolytics, have been associated with relief in several reports, as have low doses of tricyclic antidepressants (Fisher *et al.*, 1973; Cooper, 1987). Balon (1994) recently reported successful treatment of a child with trazodone after failure of several other drugs. Contrary to common myth, awakening the sleeper, or trying to arouse him or her further after the terror episode, is not particularly dangerous, provided it is done gently.

307.46 SLEEPWALKING DISORDER (SOMNAMBULISM)

Like sleep terrors, sleepwalking is generally a deep non-REM phenomenon, is usually benign, and is less often associated with psychopathology than is generally believed. Far more common in children than in adults, parents can be reassured that sleepwalking is unlikely to persist beyond age eight or ten. Adult episodes are usually associated with physical or emotional stress (e.g., significant loss, military service, sleep deprivation, or fatigue), medication side effects, or drug withdrawal. The likelihood of injuring oneself or others is often exaggerated.

Hypnotic learning paradigms are often effective (Hurwitz *et al.*, 1991). The author has trained patients to end their trance when their feet touch the floor, a response that quickly generalized to prevent sleepwalking (Reid *et al.*, 1981). Anticipatory awakening, much as sometimes used for enuresis, may also be tried (Tobin, 1993)

Medication is often the treatment of choice, especially when sleepwalking occurs frequently. As with sleep terrors, low H.S. doses of benzodiazepines (e.g., diazepam, medium-duration preparations [Reid *et al.*, 1981]) are safe and effective for most patients. The drug should have a long enough half-life to remain in the system for most of the night. It can generally be discontinued after a few weeks, but tolerance is rarely a problem in those who require it for longer periods. Tricyclics may be tried as well. In the elderly, low doses of a high-potency neuroleptic may be a safer choice than a benzodiazepine because of the central nervous system depression associated with the latter.

OTHER SLEEP DISORDERS

780.XX SLEEP DISORDER DUE TO A GENERAL MEDICAL CONDITION —-.- SUBSTANCE-INDUCED SLEEP DISORDER

Treatments of these disorders are discussed in **Part I** and **Part II** of this book.

CHAPTER 25

IMPULSE CONTROL DISORDERS NOT ELSEWHERE CLASSIFIED

GENERAL TREATMENT PRINCIPLES

There have been very few studies of the treatment of these disorders. Clinical and case reports often speak of impulsive (or compulsive) behaviors without actually linking them to DSM-III-R or DSM-IV criteria. In addition, treatment studies, and treatment itself, are complicated by the secrecy or shame associated with many of the syndromes. Finally, the symptoms described are often found with other primary psychiatric disorders, with treatment for the primary disorder leading to improvement in the impulse control problem. This section will not address treatments of other diagnoses (e.g., clozapine for psychosis, carbamazepine or lithium for bipolar disorder) unless the treatment is used specifically for impulse control.

McElroy *et al.* (1992) are among those who believe that even when properly diagnosed, disorders of impulse control are often related to each other and to mood, anxiety, and substance use disorders. For example, doses of antidepressants associated with reductions in the frequency and intensity of impulses and impulsive behaviors (see below) are typically in the range associated with treatment of depressive disorders. Relationships with obsessive-compulsive disorder (Swedo *et al.*, 1989) and mixtures of disorders (Kafka & Coleman, 1991) have also been suggested. There thus has been a great deal of interest recently in drugs that affect serotonin availability.

Treatment Planning and Integration

One should not focus too narrowly on particular therapies, the *components* of treatment, at the expense of overall treatment planning and integration of biological and psychosocial factors. Eichelman (1992) and Tardiff (1992) note that aggressive syndromes, for example, are complex, and that although the biological factors in "explosive" disorders are usually important, they often do not fully explain the interaction of stresses, cues, and other conditions that contribute to many patients' episodic rage.

312.34 INTERMITTENT EXPLOSIVE DISORDER AND OTHER SYNDROMES OF IMPULSIVE VIOLENCE

Intermittent explosive violence may be seen as a lack of modulation of anger or, perhaps in a separate group of patients, as a seizurelike condition of idiosyncratic behavior that cannot easily be placed on a spectrum of "normal" to "abnormal" impulse control. A few patients have may have "paradoxical" reactions to benzodiazepines or alcohol with a concomitant rage response. These are discussed in **Part II.**

Medications

Although no single pharmacologic approach has been routinely successful in the variety of aggressive syndromes that are described as impulsive, many drugs are helpful in some cases. The initial drug choice is based on clinical presentation and whether or not the clinician believes the violence is ictal, characterologic, situational, serotonergically mediated, or related to another Axis I disorder.

Propranolol and other β-blockers have long been suggested by Elliott (1977, 1978) and others who have described episodic dyscontrol phenomena (Monroe, 1981). More recently, Jenkins and Maruta (1987) discussed eight patients with intermittent explosive disorder, five of whom experienced substantial improvement with propranolol. Several other reports describe some success with β-blockers in rage disorders and temper outbursts (Mattes 1986a, 1986b, 1990). Metoprolol, a selective β_1-adrenoreceptor blocker, may be more specific (Mattes, 1985). Both drugs are generally prescribed within their usual medical range; Silver and Yudofsky (1995) suggest that most patients will not require more than 800 mg/day of propranolol. Silver and Yudofsky summarize a number of β-blockers in the context of behavioral indications and provide a useful, if somewhat dated, table for propranolol dosing (Yudofsky *et al.*, 1987).

One need not see specific ictal activity to consider anticonvulsant therapy. Carbamazepine, considered as either an anticonvulsant or a mood stabilizer, is often the initial drug of choice (unless the patient is taking clozapine). The physician should monitor the blood level and complete blood count, especially early in treatment. Phenytoin was described as potentially useful in a review by Finkel

(1984). Mattes (1992) reported on valproate in the mentally retarded. Combinations of the more common anticonvulsants, with or without other drugs (e.g., thioridazine), have also been tried, with limited success.

Lithium is often prescribed for mood or behavioral instability. Although it has never become popular for control of social violence (as contrasted with that arising from a psychiatric disorder), a lengthy study by Tupin *et al.* (1973) found lithium effective for decreasing violence in prisoners. Sheard *et al.* (1976) found similarly positive results. Lithium's antiaggressive effect may be mediated through tryptophan availability in the serotonergic (5-HIAA) system.

Tryptophan itself has aggression-reducing qualities in both animals and humans (Garza-Trevino, 1994). Supplements of up to several grams a day have been suggested in intractable, primitive aggression, although we are not aware of any controlled studies. Other drugs that increase serotonin availability (e.g., fluoxetine and other selective serotonin reuptake inhibitors, clomipramine, trazedone, buspirone) have shown varying success (Coccaro *et al.*, 1990; Lion & Scheinberg, 1995).

Although controlled studies are not available, patients who respond to anxiolytics tend to be those whose outbursts are related to difficulty handling anxiety or affect (e.g., obsessive-compulsive patients). In spite of rare reports of paradoxical reactions with benzodiazepines, they act rapidly, have few side effects, and can be effective in as-needed PRN doses. Fairly high doses of buspirone were effective in some mentally retarded patients with impulsive violence (but who did not meet the criteria for an impulse control disorder) studied by Ratey *et al.* (1991).

Neuroleptics are often considered in violence and agitation, but their effect on impulsive violence is difficult to separate from their sedative and antipsychotic properties. The author has anecdotally observed risperidone to be helpful and well tolerated in potentially violent schizophrenic outpatients. Effective antipsychotic treatment of any kind may be as useful.

Antiandrogens such as medroxyprogesterone acetate (MPA) and cyproterone acetate (CPA) are sometimes considered, since testosterone is associated with aggression and anabolic steroids precipitate rage under some conditions. In North America, the use of MPA and CPA in men has generally been limited to paraphilias and sexual violence, for which they are sometimes quite effective.

Neurosurgical Approaches

Stereotactic surgery showed considerable promise in animal studies a few years ago. Unfortunately, research on humans has been limited.

Behavioral Treatments

Behavioral treatments have a role in many violent syndromes, although not usually a primary one. Token, decelerative, and symptom-replacement paradigms can be very effective in controlled settings such as hospitals and residential programs (Silver & Yudofsky, 1995). They should not be relied on alone without careful consideration and, at least initially, close monitoring.

Psychotherapy

Psychotherapy is rarely a primary treatment for impulsive aggression. On the other hand, disorders with behavioral symptoms are almost never completely treated using biological means. The therapist should have experience with potentially violent patients or obtain consultation from an experienced colleague.

For the patient who has difficulty recognizing or modulating affect or behavior, treatment may include biofeedback, desensitization, group therapy, and counseling that encourages behavior exploration (such as keeping a diary of explosive impulses, the events that precede them, and the behaviors that follow).

Psychotherapy often defines and deals with primary (i.e., unconscious, internal) gain. If biological treatment is successful, psychotherapy may help the patient and his or her family adapt to his or her becoming a nonviolent person (which requires different coping skills and mechanisms than were previously employed). The family is likely to have been in some sort of precarious equilibrium before treatment; any change, even for the better, requires restabilization. Therapy can also address depression related to the loss of symptoms and a particular kind of identity. Finally, the patient must deal with the wish or hope that his or her chronic disorder is "cured" (or with his or her unconscious wishes *not* to be cured), which often leads to medication noncompliance.

Safety Issues in Release and Follow-up Care

Preventing recurrence of violence is the main concern in this and many other potentially dangerous syndromes. No form of treatment short of continuous monitoring or incarceration can guarantee protection from future violence. Legal, ethical, and therapeutic considerations suggest that most patients eventually will be released from the hospital or incarceration. It is important to prepare for that day while the patient is under some form of social and medical control.

Those who decide whether or not to release a patient with a known propensity for serious violence should take their task very seriously, whether the release is to be permanent, a furlough or parole, a brief pass, or a transfer to a less secure setting. They should have access to relevant information about the patient's past behavior (often not just hospital records), and should have as much knowledge and experience as feasible for the setting involved.

This does not mean that all past records must be exhaustively reviewed in every situation, and especially not by every psychiatrist or other clinician who sees the patient or participates in a pass or release. However, accurate information about known significant danger or violence, past and present, should be available in the current record, and should be generally understood by prominent caregivers and treatment team leaders.

The extent to which past information is, or should be, known to the treating setting (e.g., hospital, residential treatment facility, court referral clinic) deserves discussion. It seems inappropriate, sometimes even foolhardy, to accept an intermittently explosive or impulsively violent patient without amassing enough information about his or her behavior to plan for the safety of staff and other patients, and to know something of the patient's behavior (and potential precipitants of dangerous behavior) in the community. While it is impossible to gather detailed information in every case, and the information that can be obtained may be biased or inaccurate, reasonable efforts should be made to do so. Clinicians should not allow themselves to be pressured into pass or release decisions with insufficient data.

In many cases, treatment decision makers have access to courts with jurisdiction over the patient, and may wish to get judicial authorization for passes, furloughs, discharges, or changes in the treatment plan that significantly alter external monitoring or control. The court should not prescribe treatment, but it may have a legitimate interest in dangers posed by the patient. Court notification or review is also a useful risk management procedure.

Both the patient and staff members should understand that confidentiality must take a back seat to the safety of the patient, family, clinic staff, or others. In order to obtain a good history, the clinician should ask relatives, friends, and relevant others to share data about the patient, even when the therapist cannot give out information in return. That is, collateral contact can be made and the outside information received in a one-way stream from source to clinician, while explaining to the source that one is constrained from supplying information about the patient (and sometimes even the fact that the person is a patient).

There should be clear communication about significant violence potential with family, physicians, other therapists, hospital staff, and, in some cases, employers and licensing agencies (e.g., related to a driver's license or pilot's certificate). Such communications often need not be detailed, and should take place with the patient's knowledge and consent whenever feasible; however, one generally should not accept and treat a patient whom one knows to be potentially dangerous without some consideration of other clinicians and foreseeable victims. One may encourage the patient and his or her family to notify such individuals or agencies themselves; however, certain reporting by the clinician may be required.

Not taking prescribed medication is a major cause of symptom return. Every effort should be made to monitor and encourage medication compliance. Depot preparations are available for violent syndromes associated with psychosis (fluphenazine decanoate, haloperidol decanoate) and sexual violence (depot medroxyprogesterone acetate or cyproterone acetate), and should be considered when appropriate. Medications that require regular visits for laboratory monitoring (e.g., clozapine, carbamazepine) provide an extra measure of control as well. Simply having the patient return to the clinic frequently can be effective, particularly when outpatient compliance is made a requirement of discharge or parole.

One should not allow a potentially dangerous patient to avoid outpatient monitoring. If appointments are missed, efforts should be made to find him or her and evaluate the situation. Similarly, the clinician should resist the temptation to reduce the frequency of visits too early, even when caseloads are high and resources are limited, since most causes of intermittent violence are not cured with time or symptomatic treatment.

Prediction of future danger is very difficult, and may be impossible. When human life or limb is at stake, decision makers should try to err on the side of caution. Potential danger is usually best assessed in a realistic setting, not in a hospital or prison. Passes and furloughs are often critical for accurate evaluation of the patient's ability to get along in the community. A hierarchy of passes, first brief and closely monitored, later longer and more independent, is recommended. When feasible, there should be some way to obtain feedback about the patient's behavior on pass, such as from a family member. Evidence of failure, whether actual violence or behavior associated with past violence (e.g., drinking, drug abuse, going to places associated with past violence), should be evaluated before a decision is made to continue.

312.32 KLEPTOMANIA

There are very few studies of persons with kleptomania, and almost none that use standard diagnostic criteria. McElroy *et al.* (1991a) blindly assessed 20 cases that met DSM-III-R criteria and found that all had met major mood disorder criteria at some time in their lives. Most had had diagnosable anxiety or eating disorders. Ten of 18 patients receiving antidepressant medication had good responses. Several other papers describe a relationship with mood disorders, sometimes postulating either a "depressive spectrum disorder" or compulsive stealing as a means of obtaining punishment and decreasing self-worth (Fishbain, 1987). This has led to case reports of treatment success with lithium, fluoxetine, fluoxetine and lithium, trazodone, tranylcypromine, perphenazine, and amitriptyline (Burstein, 1992; Fishbain, 1988; McElroy *et al.*, 1989; Rocha & Rocha, 1992). McElroy, Pope, *et al.* (1991) cite several positive reports of the use of electroconvulsive therapy (ECT), alone or in combination with antidepressants.

The traditional treatment of kleptomania is psychotherapy. In some patients, discovery of the defensive factors alone is sufficient to allow behavioral change. When the onset of the disorder is not acute or associated with some identifiable event, however, reports of therapeutic success become less common. Guilt and the need to be caught and punished are fairly accessible dynamics. Others are more subtle, including efforts to find objects that help the patient maintain control over destructive aggression (Cierpka, 1986). Behavioral treatment using covert sensitization (described in Chapter 22 on the treatment of paraphilias) was reported by Glover (1985).

312.33 PYROMANIA

Pyromania in the professional literature is almost entirely limited to fire-setting behavior that has not been scrutinized according to DSM criteria, especially that associated with antisocial syndromes or Axis I disorders. There are few reported cases with DSM-IV or DSM-III diagnoses. In practice, most fire setters other than criminals-for-profit are either juveniles or adults whose behavior is related to another psychiatric disorder; neither are true pyromaniacs.

Most of the treatment literature refers to child or adolescent fire setters. Many strategies attempt to interrupt fire-setting behavior by correlating events, feelings, and behavior, sometimes graphically (Bumpass *et al.*, 1985). These are often part of community fire department programs, which treat more fire setters than do most mental health clinics, and are frequently quite successful (Webb *et al.*, 1990). They usually stress parents' teaching children how to ignite and extinguish fires appropriately, and allowing children to assist (under adult supervision) in igniting fires for barbecues or in fireplaces (Baizerman & Emshoff, 1984). The National Firehawk Foundation offers juvenile programs that emphasize fire safety and link fire setters with volunteer firefighters (Kolko, 1988).

Issues of mastery, in which the child creates a situation the child believes he or she can control, then panics when he or she cannot do so, can often be successfully addressed by having the parent or therapist start a fire, put it out (thus controlling the situation), and help the child predict that which is controllable and that which is not (Dalton *et al.*, 1986).

Adler and colleagues (1994) found that a multicomponent program that included satiation (allowing the children to light and extinguish many fires) was no more effective than safety education alone. Wolff (1984) reported a case in which a seven-year-old was apparently successfully treated with some 100 satiation sessions. Koles and Jenson (1985) described success in a "severely behaviorally disturbed" boy treated with education, response cost, visits to a hospital burn unit, and relaxation training.

True pyromania is an obsessive, often fetishistic behavior that in the past was addressed (usually with little success) through psychotherapy (Barnett & Spitzer, 1994). The characteristics of neurotic defensive structure in pyromania appear to be similar to those of kleptomania; however, the causative psychodynamics and the age of the patient may be quite different. The driven or sexual quality of many recidivists suggests involvement of serotonergic systems and the possibility that SSRIs would be effective; however, we found no reference to SSRI treatment in a recent literature review.

Safety Issues

General safety and confidentiality issues are similar to those discussed under "Intermittent Explosive Disorder." Geller (1992) notes that a particular danger of fire setting (and part of its internal dynamic) is that the outcome is not controllable by the perpetrator. The risk of treating the patient outside a highly controlled setting is obvious. Even in hospitals, the danger of fire must be recognized and the patient appropriately monitored. After treatment, recidivism is generally fairly high, although adult follow-up studies have not been done. Recidivism probably decreases when the fire setting assumes a dysphoric character for the patient and/or impulse control can be biologically restored (e.g., through successful medication), and not before.

312.31 PATHOLOGICAL GAMBLING

Treatment programs should be multifaceted, with psychosocial, and sometimes pharmacologic, strategies available. Addiction models are common, attract therapists who view obsessive behavior in this way, and often report good results (although there are no good follow-up studies in the literature). An inpatient/ residential phase of treatment (two to four weeks of structured program) may be necessary for patients whose behavior is so intractable and destructive that they are in danger of destroying family resources and livelihood, or when comorbid disorders, such as depression, become serious. Blume (1989) describes one such hospital program with psychiatric leadership and a multifaceted approach. Taber *et al.* (1987) reported total abstinence six months after hospitalization in almost half the patients treated in their Brecksville unit. Abstinence, reduction of the urge to gamble, and restoration of social functioning were the principal objectives during a four-week program. Non-hospital addiction-model programs sometimes do not include medical participation, although those authors recommend it.

Lopez-Ibor and Carrasco (1995) describe several important factors in successful psychosocial treatment, including abstinence, reduction of environmental cues and stimuli, cognitive restructuring related to unrealistic expectations of winning or other reward, dealing with negative internal states such as dysphorias, and self-help groups and programs.

Behavioral approaches, particularly aversive conditioning, are based on the tremendous reinforcing characteristic of gambling for the patient. Although by the time treatment is sought the gambling itself is not particularly pleasurable, it has provided reinforcement on a variable-ratio, variable-intensity schedule that is very difficult to extinguish. Aversive therapies are less popular today than in the past. McElroy and her colleagues (1992), in an excellent review of impulse control disorder, noted that imaginal desensitization was more effective than aversive therapy in reducing gambling urge and behavior (McConaghy *et al.,* 1983).

Psychotherapy, especially psychodynamic or psychoanalytic treatment, appears in anecdotal reports to be more effective for pathological gambling than for other impulse control disorders. There are no controlled studies of results or follow-up.

Medication

McElroy and associates (1995) cite a few case reports from the small literature on medication for pathological gambling. Some authors, noting the obsessive quality of the disorder, report limited success with such drugs as clomipramine (Hollander *et al.*, 1992). Lithium received some support in the past, although there are no recent studies (Moskowitz, 1980). Serotonergic drugs such as fluoxetine have been suggested by a few authors (Rosenthal & Lorenz, 1992), but no controlled studies have been completed.

Comorbidity

There is an increased prevalence of affective disorders, suicidal behavior, substance abuse, and sexual dysfunction among pathological gamblers. These should be considered in any comprehensive treatment strategy. Taber and associates (1987) reported that 18% of their socially and vocationally successful patients continued to have problems with depression.

Follow-up

Follow-up is critical to relapse prevention. Taber and associates (1987) attributed much of the postresidential success of their program to Gamblers Anonymous (GA). Various GA programs, GA-related family groups, and other self-help groups are available throughout the country, and should be recommended to patients and families. No matter what the approach, treatment and follow-up should include attention to the patient's family environment, social and vocational situations, and debts.

Responsibility for One's Behavior

Actions to obtain money for gambling should be separated from the act of gambling with that money. Although behaviors that are a very direct result of craving (i.e., gambling behavior itself) may be looked on by some as outside the person's control, it is therapeutically important (and clinically accurate) to give him or her responsibility for those actions. The first step in the 12-step program, in which the person acknowledges helplessness, refers to the obsessive or addictive behavior (in this case, gambling *per se*). It should not be allowed to conflict with the steps that follow, in which the patient accepts responsibility for the damage he or she has caused. Certainly, less direct actions to support gambling (e.g., embezzling, misappropriating funds) should not be considered out of the patient's control, any more than one's need to support a drug habit exonerates him or her from burglary charges.

312.39 TRICHOTILLOMANIA

Although usually seen in children, in whom spontaneous remission is common and the main serious complication is a bezoar, trichotillomania in adults is more likely to be chronic or associated with another psychiatric disorder. Successful treatment of the primary disorder (e.g., a psychosis or anxiety disorder) often leads to remission of the trichotillomania.

Biological Treatment

Addressing trichotillomania generically, as a compulsion, may be the best approach (although it may also be seen as a habit or tic-like syndrome). Tricyclics have been recommended in the past, with most recent reports focusing on clomipramine. Swedo *et al.* (1989) found clomipramine effective in a controlled study in which 9 of 20 patients with trichotillomania also described themselves as obsessive-compulsive. Pollard *et al.* (1991) had similar success with four patients taking antidepressant doses of clomipramine. A few case reports describe use of monoamine oxidase inhibitors; Krishman *et al.* (1984) discuss treating a patient whose hair pulling may have been related to severe depression and anxiety who received 30 mg/day of isocarboxazid, after which her symptoms stopped for some four months.

Fluoxetine has been investigated in several small studies and case reports, sometimes with conflicting results. Christenson *et al.* (1991a) at first reported that a placebo-controlled, double-blind study found no measurable response to fluoxetine. Streichenwein and Thornby (1995) found similarly negative results in 23 patients taking up to 80 mg/day for over seven months. Other studies, however, have been more positive. A later study by Christenson and several other reports indicate significant decreases in symptoms using the drug (Koran *et al.*, 1992; Winchel *et al.*, 1992; Christenson *et al.*, 1994). One of Christenson's patients also received hypnosis, and another, who did not respond to fluoxetine, later responded to a combination of hypnosis, behavioral monitoring, competing response training, and positive reinforcement.

Addition of low doses of pimozide to serotonergic drugs was associated with success in several trichotillomanic patients treated by Stein and Hollander (1992). Mahr (1993) reported a case in which the serotonin-agonist anorectic fenfluramine, reportedly effective in some obsessive-compulsive disorders, completely eradicated long-standing hair-pulling urges at 20 mg three times a day. The patient previously had a partial response to fluoxetine, sertraline, and a combination of sertraline (100 mg/day) and alprazolam (1 mg/day). We are unaware of reports regarding other SSRI antidepressants. A few papers describe limited response to lithium carbonate (Christenson *et al.*, 1991b).

Psychotherapies

Several psychotherapies and behavioral approaches have been tried with varying success. Dynamic and/or family therapy was associated with remission in children and adolescents in some older reports (Sticher *et al.*, 1980).

Hypnosis is often a component of successful treatment, and may be added to biological approaches (Christenson *et al.*, 1994). Useful techniques include direct suggestion, substituting other behaviors, and in-trance scripts discussing the benefits of not pulling out one's hair. One of the benefits of hypnosis is that once the procedure is learned, the patient can continue the work between office visits.

Behavioral or cognitive therapies that address hair pulling as a bad habit are sometimes successful as well. Simple feedback, positive reinforcement (even simple praise), mild aversive conditioning (e.g., by snapping a rubber band), and response competition have all been recommended at times. We were unable to find documented results of the common practice of using mittens or other barriers for children.

Follow-up and Special Considerations

Recurrence is common, and may be precipitated by physical or emotional crises, including exacerbations of skin disorders such as acne. Skin disorders and permanent hair loss are the most common physical sequelae in adults. Treating the skin in the affected area (e.g., with dermatologic agents) may be helpful, whether the skin problems preceded or were caused by the hair pulling. Gastrointestinal blockage due to bezoars can be a serious complication, since hair is indigestible and sometimes is unaffected by normal gastric motility. Bezoars are much more common in children (especially girls who mouth or eat their hair), but occasionally seen in adults with comorbid severe mental illness.

312.30 IMPULSE CONTROL DISORDER NOS

Conditions that appear clinically similar to one or more of the foregoing disorders often respond to similar treatments. For example, several syndromes usually viewed as habit disorders or tic-like behaviors have been reported to respond to serotonergic approaches similar to those for trichotillomania (e.g., nail biting [onychophagia] and picking at oneself), whether the symptoms are independent or related to other syndromes (e.g., Prader-Willi syndrome) (Leonard *et al.*, 1991; Warnock, 1993). McElroy, Satlin, *et al.* (1991) and McElroy *et al.* (1992) describe case reports using fluoxetine for compulsive shopping. The use of SSRIs in eating disorders is discussed elsewhere in this text. Because of the variety of treatments recommended for different impulse control disorders, ranging from multifaceted milieu treatment of pathological gambling to complex biological management of some intermittent explosive disorders, the clinician should consider consultation with or referral to a colleague who often works with similar patients.

CHAPTER 26

ADJUSTMENT DISORDERS

GENERAL PRINCIPLES

By definition, adjustment disorders are maladaptive reactions to identifiable psychosocial stressors. The tasks of treatment are to deal with acute symptoms and to promote either a return to a healthy premorbid state or effective coping with a chronic stressor. Strain (1995) mentions the military BICEPS approach to acute treatment (True & Benway, 1992), which stresses brevity, immediacy, centrality, expectance, proximity, and simplicity.

Symptoms are expected to remit or disappear once the stressor is gone, or to evolve into a more permanent (effective or ineffective) coping mechanism if the stressor persists. The clinician should be alert to signs of such evolution and to the possibility that the diagnosis is in error, so that more definitive treatment can be implemented.

In a number of the disorders, support is important while the patient draws on his or her own resources for improvement and growth. Support and active psychotherapeutic involvement may also prevent regressive or disabling resolution of the adjustment disorder.

PSYCHOTHERAPY

Crisis intervention, brief psychotherapy, behavioral therapy, counseling, and education are all commonly used and generally effective. Brief environmental change may be helpful; however, simplistic advice, such as, "Take a few days of vacation," is usually insufficient for patients who meet the criteria for these diagnoses. Some specific guidelines for brief dynamic psychotherapy, particularly for patients who need more than transient support, are presented by Horowitz (1986).

Group therapy, particularly that which focuses on enhancing self-image while showing the patient how to improve in a supportive environment, may be helpful. Patients with adjustment disorders often need individual attention, however, although it need not be intensive in nature. For those whose stressors continue (e.g., persons with a chronic illness), a consistent group therapy environment in which transient problems can be effectively resolved may be very useful.

While much of treatment involves the patient alone, family members are often concerned and can benefit from reassurance, with the patient's permission, concerning the treatability and transience of the disorder. This is best done in a conjoint or family session soon after the initial evaluation.

MEDICATION

One view, generally shared by the author, holds that medication usually should not be emphasized unless the patient is unable to manage without it. When not completely necessary, anxiolytic agents and antidepressants can rob the patient of the opportunity to use—or to learn to use—emotional resources to deal with the crisis or stressor, and to feel good about it. In addition, using medications encourages the patient to see himself or herself as sicker than necessary, decreases the amount of meaningful communication between doctor and patient, promotes masking of symptoms or feelings, and exposes the patient to risks of side effects or medication abuse.

On the other hand, there are at least three reasons to consider pharmacotherapy when psychotherapy is slow or ineffective. The first is simple alleviation of discomfort. Second, more chronic syndromes and disorders may be prevented by the active alleviation of acute symptoms, either because the pathological process has been blocked or because symptom relief allows one to devote more inner resources to adaptive or psychotherapeutic work. Third, some conditions, such as depression, often respond more readily to medication that addresses the brain problem directly (e.g., serotonin blockade) than to treatments that act only indirectly (e.g., cognitive therapy).

Nonmedical psychotherapists often ask psychiatrists or primary care physicians for medications for their uncomfortable patients, and payers, such as managed care systems, often suggest drugs instead of counseling or psychotherapy, to decrease costs. When the diagnosis is adjustment disorder, however, the psychiatrist should carefully consider whether there is some temporary need for medication, whether there is no real need, or whether the diagnosis is inaccurate. If the patient appears to require chronic medication, the clinician should entertain the possibility of either an erroneous original diagnosis or an evolving of the adjustment disorder toward a chronic, pathological resolution.

SUBTYPES OF ADJUSTMENT DISORDER

309.0 ADJUSTMENT DISORDER WITH DEPRESSED MOOD

Patients with depressive symptoms are often more uncomfortable than those with other adjustment disorders, and may appear more disabled, experience more behavioral change (e.g., sleep disturbance, lack of energy), appear more regressed, and/or present with suicidal ideation. Unless the patient has other symptoms of major affective or bipolar disorder (in which case the adjustment disorder diagnosis is probably inappropriate), medication should be used only after considering the caveats discussed above. Temporary use of short-acting soporifics may be an exception.

The support and availability of the clinician, with reassurance that the current experience is transient, are important for these patients. Simple, practical recommendations—not necessarily pharmacological ones—for complaints of sleeplessness, lack of energy, and the like often produce good results.

The patient should be asked about suicidal thoughts, and any suicidal ideation or behavior should be openly discussed. In patients with an adjustment disorder, thoughts of suicide are likely to produce anxiety and to be efforts at resolving real problems within the patient's fantasy world. Nevertheless, the clinician must assure the patient that this topic can be discussed just as any other, and that if further treatment or protection becomes necessary, it is readily available.

309.24 ADJUSTMENT DISORDER WITH ANXIETY

In addition to the principles outlined in the "General Treatment Considerations" above, reassuring the patient that the symptoms are transient, and that the clinician and patient together can alleviate them, is useful. Nonintrusive support, crisis intervention techniques, relaxation, meditation, hypnosis, or biofeedback may be used by those therapists experienced in one or another of these techniques. Brief dynamic psychotherapy that explores the symbolic meaning of conflict-producing stressors and/or cognitive exploration of "errors" in thinking that produce symptoms beyond those normally expected from the stressor are effective for psychologically minded patients. Temporary antianxiety medication may be considered, with the caveats already described. Emphasis on the patient's ability to weather the stress and praise for his or her ability to strengthen coping mechanisms are helpful.

309.3 ADJUSTMENT DISORDER WITH DISTURBANCE OF CONDUCT

It is important to understand the difference between this disorder and other, more chronic, antisocial conditions (e.g., adult antisocial behavior, antisocial personality disorder). Treatment or management of antisocial behaviors at the time they present as an adjustment disorder lowers the probability that the antisocial symptoms will continue as a chronic pattern of coping or adaptation after the initial stress is removed (or as chronic stress continues).

Countertransference issues and the temptation to take a harsh approach to persons with this disorder should be carefully monitored. In spite of the inconvenience or injury that has been caused to others, acceptance and attempts to have the patient understand that his or her symptoms are characteristics of a difficulty in adjusting—not indications of some deep inner criminality or character disorder—are very important. This allows the patient to see treatment as something logical and accomplishable, whose explorations and anxieties can be tolerated.

Continuing responsibility for one's own actions should be expected. The therapist's acceptance of the patient's condition does not imply acceptance of antisocial acts that place people and property in jeopardy. For example, adjustment disorders *per se* do not generally exonerate patients from responsibility for criminal acts.

309.4 ADJUSTMENT DISORDER WITH MIXED DISTURBANCE OF EMOTIONS AND CONDUCT

This disorder should be treated using the principles already outlined, both at the beginning of this chapter and in the paragraphs on individual disorders. It should be noted that treatment for one kind of symptom (e.g., benzodiazepines for anxiety) may have either a positive or negative effect on other symptoms (e.g., recklessness or self-destructive behavior). The risks and benefits of each must be weighed. The self-destructive nature of many reckless or antisocial-appearing acts should not be overlooked.

SPECIAL CONSIDERATIONS

RESPONSES TO MEDICAL CONDITIONS

Medical illness or injury is often a precipitating stressor. Adjustment to loss, pain, or the fear of either is the usual dynamic, and can be seen in a wide variety of medical settings. There are often time constraints for treatment, such as the patient's expected hospital stay or an approaching date for surgery. Psychotherapy skills, relaxation techniques (including hypnosis), and often the ability to explain more about the illness or medical procedure involved (as might be done by a psychiatrist or nurse therapist) are all helpful. Bibliotherapy, or the use of selected reading material as an adjunct to treatment, can help, although one should not substitute a few books or pamphlets for the therapeutic relationship.

Sometimes rapid alleviation of acute situational anxiety, depression, or psychosis cannot be accomplished without psychoactive drugs. Consideration should be given to interactions with medications already being prescribed, and to the effects of the psychotropic drug on the primary illness. Most antidepressants and neuroleptics do not act quickly. Small doses of amphetamines or methylphenidate may be considered for their rapid action in depression, particularly in elderly patients.

Communication with the referring physician (and the ward staff if the patient is in a hospital) is a large part of the consultative treatment of medical patients. An outline of the psychiatrist's findings, prescribed treatment, and recommendations for other caregivers, concise and free of jargon, should be placed in the chart. Recommendations or instructions should be clear, since the psychiatrist may not be personally involved in the next steps of patient care.

UNUSUAL GRIEF REACTIONS

Although uncomplicated bereavement is discussed elsewhere, it is appropriate to consider "complicated" bereavement or "aberrant grief reaction" in a section on adjustment disorders. The principles discussed often also apply to other forms of loss, including divorce, amputation, or other disability.

If grief remains unresolved for a particularly long time, with persistent yearning, overidentification with the deceased, and/or inability to express sadness or rage, some sort of grief-resolution therapy should be offered. This may include helping the patient to make a decision to grieve, using guided imagery or guided mourning, and helping to construct a life and identity without the lost object.

OTHER SUBTYPES OF ADJUSTMENT DISORDERS

Other subtypes (Adjustment Disorder with Mixed Anxiety and Depressed Mood [309.28] and Adjustment Disorder NOS [309.9] may be treated using the principles outlined above.

CHAPTER 27

PERSONALITY DISORDERS

GENERAL PRINCIPLES

The nature of personality disorders suggests that treatment is unlikely to alter them in any significant way. Restructuring psychotherapy (generally psychoanalysis, often after extended preparatory therapy) has been successful for selected patients seen by highly specialized therapists; however, there is no evidence that biological, behavioral, or other psychotherapeutic modalities affect the core disorder. This refractoriness is in part a reflection of the ego-syntonic nature of the disorders, but probably is primarily due to their roots in very early development—personal, familial, and perhaps physiological.

This is not to say that the accompanying behaviors and affects, and to some extent their clinical presentation, cannot be modified. The sections that follow address ways in which the psychiatrist or other clinician can attempt to alter destructive and/or painful syndromes such as depression, suicidal behavior, violence, other antisocial behavior, intolerance of closeness or intimacy, and occasional psychotic symptoms. Treatment is usually designed to decrease social or emotional disability and to deal with society's need for management of, for example, the antisocial person. No treatment is universally helpful, and many require considerable time and resources.

Countertransference and related feelings in the psychiatrist or psychotherapist are major issues in the treatment of the personality disorders. The frustration of dealing with treatment-resistant and/or primitive patients, who (unless dismissed by the therapist) may be seen over many years, is obvious. Less obvious is the problem of the therapist's true countertransference, seeing in the patient frightening or distasteful aspects of his or her own angry, sexual, or dependent impulses.

Medications have a limited role in the treatment of core symptoms of most personality disorders (as contrasted with temporary overlying depression or anxiety). In some, the role of psychopharmacology is more prominent. The sections on borderline and schizotypal personality contain the most detailed discussions of prescribing. Since many other personality disorders are commonly comorbid with them, or at least contain borderline or schizotypal traits, the reader may wish to review their medications sections when treating other characterologic syndromes.

301.0 PARANOID PERSONALITY DISORDER

Persons with paranoid personality rarely come to treatment unless they are in crisis or develop an Axis I disorder. Those who do present to the psychiatrist may do so to prove to others that "there is nothing wrong with me," or may consult the clinician as a peer or colleague about some problem the patient is perceiving as external. Resolution of the crisis is usually their sole concern, although some patients seek help for acute symptoms such as depression (Quality Assurance Project, 1990).

> A physician telephoned the author for assistance in ferreting out corruption in the health care system. He eventually agreed to an interview to discuss circumstances under which a state agency was threatening to revoke his professional license. There was no history of delusions, hallucinations, or substance abuse. He perceived routine peer review as harassment and an unfair imposition on his practice, and he was considering filing a lawsuit to make his point.

While many therapists would choose not to continue what appears to be an unrewarding interaction with such a person, there may be some value in allowing a benign relationship to form within which current and future problems may be handled. The relationship should be a professional one; the temptation to befriend or humor the patient should be resisted.

Psychoanalytically oriented psychotherapy involves issues similar to those in other "self-centered" character problems, including the probability that the "curative effects of insight" are outweighed by negative effects of interpretation (Jimenez, 1993).

Pharmacotherapy is not indicated unless psychotic decompensation appears to be approaching. When the patient feels anxiety about loss of control, he or she may accept, and benefit from, low doses of neuroleptics from a physician in whom there is some trust. The patient should never be treated surreptitiously.

Although usually merely irritable and unpleasant to be around, patients whose judgment about the world around them is clouded by paranoia occasionally become troublesome, and even dangerous. Their feelings of entitlement, which have little chance of being mollified, can create—to them—a rationale for actions that others normally see as inappropriate. In forensic settings, such actions generally should not be viewed as outside the person's responsibility unless there is evidence of an acute psychotic disorder.

301.20 SCHIZOID PERSONALITY DISORDER

These patients rarely come to treatment in the absence of some form of crisis or decompensation, which may be triggered by unavoidable shifts in the external environment (e.g., serious illness or family crisis). Crisis treatment should be symptomatic.

Anecdotal experience in psychotherapy, particularly recent work in the understanding and restructuring of primitive developmental phenomena, suggests intensive psychotherapy; however, it is available to few patients. Appel (1974) suggests that therapeutic goals should include a sense of optimism that the patient's basic needs can be met without encountering overwhelming "collapse or supplication." The most useful therapeutic interaction is consistent and supportive, with clear rules, an ability for the patient to set therapeutic distance as needed, and some tolerance for acting out.

Distance in the therapeutic relationship and sensitivity to criticism are major stumbling blocks to intensive work. Those who are able to sustain a therapeutic relationship have a higher probability of benefit from psychodynamic work than do patients with a paranoid or schizotypal personality. Cognitive therapy that focuses on social skills may be useful (Quality Assurance Project, 1990). In some patients, fantasy games, hypnosis, and other innovative ways to encourage affect in a "safe" setting have met with some limited success (Blackmon, 1994; Scott, 1989).

Medications are generally not useful except as temporary aids in cases of extraordinary anxiety. Neuroleptics should be reserved for signs of psychotic decompensation. Antidepressants should not be prescribed in the absence of clinical signs of a mood disorder.

301.22 SCHIZOTYPAL PERSONALITY DISORDER

There has been considerable psychotherapeutic experience with schizotypal patients, particularly in day treatment programs that specialize in character disorders (Karterud *et al.*, 1992). They are often seen in long-term treatment programs, usually accompanied by other (e.g., Axis I) disorders. Reports frequently discuss treatment of schizotypal and borderline patients together, one author (Stone, 1985a) noting that the two are similar, and that schizotypal personality was derived from the "borderline schizophrenia" concept.

Medications

Schizotypal patients often present with symptoms for which medication is indicated, and frequently are treated in inpatient settings. As with borderline patients, low doses of high-potency neuroleptics such as thiothixene or haloperidol may be effective, even in the absence of frank psychosis. One should expect only modest gains, however. At times, the dose may approach that used in chronic psychosis. In severe cases, newer, nontraditional neuroleptics such as clozapine and risperidone may be tried, although controlled studies in this patient population are lacking.

At least one open study of fluoxetine has shown encouraging results at fairly high doses (80 mg/day). Patients treated were both "pure" schizotypal and, as is common in clinical practice, of mixed schizotypal and borderline personality disorders (Markovitz *et al.*, 1991). Other new or recently introduced antidepressants may be prescribed, but have not been studied for the core symptoms of this population. Tricyclics, such as amitriptyline, have shown little effect, except for occasional provoking of paranoia and hostility (Gitlin, 1993).

Medication compliance tends to be relatively poor, at least for traditional drugs. Patients often appear highly sensitive to side effects (Hymowitz *et al.*, 1986).

The treatment of superficial symptoms, such as acute psychosis or depression, is often successful. On the other hand, Axis I disorders accompanied by schizotypal personality (and other personality disorders) tend to be harder to treat than those presenting alone. The response of the schizotypal personality to tricyclic antidepressants and alprazolam is usually disappointing. There are anecdotal reports of success with monoamine oxidase inhibitors (MAOIs).

Treatment outcome is better than that for schizophrenia, but worse than that for mood disorders or other personality disorders (including borderline personality in some studies). Even with continuing treatment, the course is usually one of instability, hospitalization, and poor social function (McGlashan, 1986; Mehlum *et al.*, 1991; Plakun *et al.*, 1985). Outcome may be enhanced when the patient is able to remain in lengthy, restorative psychotherapy, provided he or she meets the usual criteria for analytically oriented work (Stone, 1985b). Supportive and educational aspects of therapy must often be allowed to intervene in the psychodynamic work.

In spite of an absence of reported studies, it is tempting to recommend community support approaches, such as assertive community treatment, that enhance social functioning and decrease the need for hospitalization in many chronically mentally ill patients. Because of patients' difficulty with social skills and comfort, group therapy and behavior modification are often symptomatically helpful. The principles discussed in the section on borderline personality, below, often apply.

301.7 ANTISOCIAL PERSONALITY DISORDER

General Principles

Very few outcome studies on treatment of antisocial personality disorder (APD) have been carried out. Many, perhaps most, available papers use unreliable diagnostic criteria, often confusing APD with other antisocial behaviors and syndromes. Treatment candidates are more often delinquent, violent, or criminal than carefully diagnosed and representative of the entire APD population.

Since there is widespread agreement that true APD does not respond consistently to any specific treatment, the importance of differentiating antisocial personality from other psychiatric diagnoses and nonillness conditions (e.g., adult or adolescent antisocial behavior, V71.01, V71.02) cannot be overstated. Clinicians should not treat antisocial *symptoms and behaviors* as if they represent the personality disorder itself. Adult continuation of childhood attention-deficit/hyperactivity disorder (ADHD) is especially important to differentiate; its symptoms mimic APD but are often quite treatable.

When confronting APD itself, one may wish to recall three principles enumerated by the Australia-New Zealand Quality Assurance Project (Quality Assurance Project, 1991): seek out and clarify the real reason that help is being sought, treat intercurrent conditions, and expect remission during middle or late life (at which time the patient must live with the consequences of a "misspent youth"). This author disagrees in part with the premise that APD always remits late in life, and would suggest that the changes seen are more often related simply to the manner in which it manifests itself. Other general guidelines include assessing the likelihood of legal involvement and, in some cases, assuring the safety of clinical personnel.

Prediction of treatability may be enhanced by gaining an understanding of the patient's underlying psychodynamics and personality structure (Meloy, 1995; Gacono & Meloy, 1991). Patients who barely meet the DSM-IV criteria for APD but who do not have characteristics of the deeper psychopathy syndrome described by Meloy (1994), Hare (1991), or Reid (1978) may have a better prognosis in both psychotherapy and residential programs. Those with Axis I symptoms, such as anxiety or depression, have a marginally better prognosis.

Psychotherapy

Most characterologically antisocial persons do not actively seek therapy; however, they may come to treatment in a variety of ways, most commonly in a forensic setting. Without the internal motivation necessary for the work of therapy, it is difficult (but not always impossible) for the patient to find reasons to continue treatment. In a few circumstances, usually late in life, the patient may begin to experience some form of chronic dysphoria.

Insight-oriented treatment of sufficient intensity and duration to penetrate the psychopathic defensive structure requires extraordinary dedication on the part of both patient and therapist. The former is generally unwilling to take on the psychotherapeutic task; the latter may not wish to spend his or her time treating such a potentially unrewarding patient. Powerful countertransference feelings (e.g., of seduction and revulsion) are so compelling that consultation or supervision is highly recommended for even the experienced clinician.

For those patients who do become engaged in long-term psychotherapeutic treatment, the most reliable sign of progress is eventual development of true affect. The first affect seen is often depression, which is both surprising and uncomfortable for a patient not accustomed to such feelings. To prevent flight from treatment, the therapist must become supportive and empathic (while monitoring countertransference), helping the patient to understand that the discomfort is a sign of progress, that it is bearable, and that the patient and therapist will work together to understand it.

Hospital Treatment

Most APD patients in the United States are not treated in hospitals. Nevertheless, there is evidence that APD can respond to highly specialized residential treatment. The absence of long-term inpatient programs in North America today may reflect decisions about funding and freedom of patients to refuse treatment more than outcome itself.

Successful inpatient programs involve long-term, strictly structured hierarchical settings in which every aspect of the patient's life affects, and is affected by, his or her progress. Successful programs control the patient's administrative status (e.g., whether and when he may be discharged), as well as other parts of his life from the day he enters the hospital. The staff must be experienced in the treatment of characterologically disordered patients. Care should be taken to be certain staff members are well trained, experienced, well supervised, and caring (as contrasted with punitive). All must understand the lengths to which the patient will go to manipulate and sabotage treatment, and all must be able to tolerate those efforts by the patient without showing any deterioration in their professional demeanors. The environment must be limited to severe antisocial syndromes. Hospital units that mix antisocial and nonantisocial patients do little to help either, and can be dangerous for the latter.

In addition to rigorous structure, there should be time for reflection. Particularly during early stages of treatment, the patient needs a place to become emotional without exposing himself completely to others. Later in the program, sharing one's feelings is a necessary part of treatment (Reid, 1985). Consistent support, short of coddling, is extremely important; the very basic fragility of the patient's self-image must be recognized in spite of his or her tough exteriors.

Communication among staff members for mutual support and a consistent treatment approach is critical. Many institutions use the same staff for both inpatient and outpatient treatment; the period of transition between the hospital and community should be monitored especially carefully. Control over discharge, such as through close relationships between treating staff and the paroling authority, is important.

Carney (1978) notes particular deficits in the truly psychopathic patient that must be addressed during such intensive residential treatment: the inability to trust, to fantasize, to feel affect, and to learn from experience. As the patient slowly moves through a hierarchy of levels and privileges, he acquires more and more self-esteem, awareness of his emotional life, and social and interpersonal competence, leading to a lessened need for the antisocial character style.

The reader may wish to consult the work of Georg Stürup for more detailed program descriptions (Stürup, 1968; Stürup & Reid, 1981).

Medications

Medications have not proved helpful in APD, although they are sometimes prescribed for specific situational symptoms (e.g., anxiety, depression) that are often better treated with brief counseling. One exception to this general premise is the treatment of severe depression in older patients and those whose treatment has allowed restructuring of the antisocial personality. These patients are sometimes suicidal, and may benefit from antidepressant medication.

Several medications have been studied to address aggressive behavior in antisocial personality and other diagnoses. Lithium carbonate has decreased fighting in some nonbipolar prison populations. Methylphenidate or antidepressants may be useful in patients whose antisocial behavior is linked to childhood ADHD. Eichelman and Hartwig (1993) provide a concise discussion of the pharmacotherapy of aggression.

Other Treatment Approaches

Community Programs. Some specialized community programs, particularly those patterned after the Probationed Offenders Rehabilitation and Treatment (PORT) program designed in Rochester, Minnesota, by Francis Tyce, provide a successful alternative for many offenders who are not mentally ill. Although not specifically designed for antisocial personality, they share some characteristics with the longer, more intensive residential approaches just described (e.g., hierarchical structures). The offender is expected to become employed or enroll in full-time school, to be responsible for his own behavior *and that of his peers in the program*, to arrange restitution to victims, and to engage completely in a program that lasts about six months (Reid & Solomon, 1981).

These programs should not be confused with halfway houses. Although the doors are not locked, many antisocial individuals find the pressures of responsibility, affect, and noncriminal lifestyles highly stressful; up to 50% drop out.

Wilderness and Physical Challenge Programs. Another treatment modality, helpful for antisocial people but not specifically designed for antisocial personality, is the specialized wilderness program, with challenging physical and social settings designed specifically for adolescent and adult offenders. Such programs usually consist of three phases, which take about three weeks to complete: orientation and learning about the survival and interpersonal skills that will be required, a wilderness trip with several offenders and a few counselors working together to achieve a complex physical goal in a natural setting, and a solo phase during which the individual experiences himself or herself and the wilderness alone (Reid & Matthews, 1980).

Some such programs include only the wilderness component, with little or no follow-up. Others provide as much as a year of residential activity designed to increase personal and social competence and to prepare the patient for reentering the community. A few similar programs use urban settings instead of wilderness. Recidivism rates are considerably better than those for incarceration or for easy or nonspecialized wilderness trips (e.g., ordinary camping).

Longer residential experiential programs, some lasting up to one year, have been successful for adolescents with chronic social inadequacy and antisocial behavior. It should be noted that the patients/clients in such programs are too young to have adult antisocial personality, although it seems likely that, without the treatment program, many would qualify for the diagnosis later in life.

Prison Programs. Treatment programs in correctional settings are usually not aimed at changing personality disorders, although they may be valuable for treating schizophrenic, affective, and substance abuse disorders. Substance abuse treatment programs often address antisocial behavior, but are not comprehensive programs for antisocial personality.

Community follow-up of released felons should not be confused with treatment of characterologic psychopathology. It is clear, however, that smooth transfer to the community mental health center, case management, and vigorous monitoring help decrease decompensation and recidivism related to Axis I disorders.

APD and Substance Abuse

Abuse of alcohol or other substances is a common concomitant of, and a complicating factor in, APD. Several studies suggest that substance abusers with APD have a worse prognosis in alcohol and substance abuse programs (Poldrugo & Forti, 1988; Shuckit, 1985). On the other hand, although specific treatments for substance-related symptoms, such as desipramine in cocaine abuse, are less successful in patients with APD (Arndt *et al.*, 1994), other reports indicate that APD may not always predict worse outcome (Cacciola *et al.*, 1995; Longabaugh *et al.*, 1994).

The Patient's Family

The family often deserves counseling. Psychopathic offspring or spouses who cause repeated social and family problems routinely engender (particularly in parents) confusion, guilt, inappropriate temptation to make restitution, and the frustration of loving someone who refuses treatment (or to whom treatment is not offered). Encouraging family members to eschew guilt and go on with their own lives is very important. The author has found it helpful to suggest that they read Hervey Cleckley's *The Mask of Sanity* (1976/1988).

Outcome

Black *et al.* (1995) note that outcome for most persons with APD not only is dismal, but is in some ways worse than that for depression or schizophrenia. This is not merely a disorder of social adaptation (cf., the term "sociopathy"), but one of chronic impairment on many levels.

301.83 BORDERLINE PERSONALITY DISORDER (BPD)

Note: Borderline personality disorder (BPD) will be addressed in more detail than the other personality disorders, in part because it is so common and in part because of the vast number of clinical symptoms and presentations it may entail. Many general principles of personality disorder treatment are reflected in borderline personality.

General Principles

The patient with BPD may appear quite healthy. Nevertheless, he or she has severe internal deficits often associated with extraordinary social dysfunction, certain kinds of vulnerability, and emotional instability. Treatment must be considered a chronic process, even when care must be limited to crisis visits.

The patient's often exquisite sensitivity to loss and his or her dysfunctional ways of coping with intrapsychic issues portend problems and crises that are often unpredictable. It is tempting for the inexperienced therapist either to assume that the patient is incapable of self-control and responsibility (and thus assume a role of rescuer or "parent"), or to view the patient's behavior as merely a series of immature whims and demands (and thus assume a rigid or punitive role). Neither is appropriate. The complexity and nuances of treatment demand that the clinician (and others involved in care) have a sophisticated understanding of, and sensitivity to, both the disorder and the person being treated.

Past sexual abuse and the concept of BPD as posttraumatic stress disorder (PTSD) are widely discussed in the current literature. Thinking of BPD as PTSD may seem to consolidate a complex and confusing clinical picture, but this view is at best an oversimplification and at worst a therapeutic disservice highly vulnerable to lack of valid or corroborating history. As important as severe childhood abuse or neglect may be, it should not form the single platform on which the treatment plan is constructed. *Adult* functioning, self-image, and expectations are important to positive outcome.

Comorbidity. Patients with BPD almost always have characteristics of other personality disorders (especially those from the same "cluster"), and often meet criteria for other Axis I and Axis II diagnoses. Stone (1994) describes Axis II subtypes of BPD that can suggest therapeutic direction and prognosis. The poorest prognosis is associated with antisocial traits. Obsessive-compulsive traits are associated with better outcome. The presence of BPD in an Axis I disorder almost always predicts poorer treatment outcome than for the Axis I disorder alone.

Therapist Response and Countertransference. In addition to knowing how to treat the patient, therapists working with BPD must contend with strong personal feelings and impulses of their own. Most arise from a combination of the patient's pathology or manipulations and the clinician's own vulnerabilities. Supervision is recommended, particularly when treatment is provided by a single therapist rather than by a team whose members regularly discuss their experiences.

Suicide and Suicidal Behavior

Self-destructive impulses and behavior in BPD are often extremely difficult to assess and manage. Consciously or not, these patients frequently use "suicidal" conversation, superficial self-harm, and even suicide attempts for nonsuicidal purposes (e.g., to decrease anxiety, soothe themselves, or manipulate others and their environment). One cannot ignore even the most "superficial" suicidal behavior. The knowledge that as many as 9% of BPD patients eventually die by their own hand (Stone, 1993) makes the prospect of helping/allowing the patient to deal with strong affects and impulses independently—a primary goal in treatment—daunting indeed.

The work of Linehan *et al.* (1994) with specialized ("dialectical") cognitive-behavioral treatment (DBT) suggests success with suicidal impulses and behaviors. Sabo *et al.* (1995) reported that suicidal behavior in treated patients decreased over several years, but there was no decrease in suicidal *ideation*. A trend toward a decrease in self-harm (as contrasted with suicidal behavior) was not significant. Maltsberger (1994) discusses aspects of treatment of "intractably suicidal" patients, including "calculated risks" and legal liability.

Psychotherapy

Cognitive therapies are widely applied in BPD. Linehan describes the goals of her DBT in both group (primarily coping skills) and individual interventions (suicidal behavior, behavior that interferes with therapy, behavior that interferes with one's quality of life, acquisition of social/emotional skills, PTSD-related feelings and behaviors, feelings and behaviors related to self-respect). She focuses on modifying specific behaviors. Staff training in DBT is quite specialized, requiring considerable commitment (Linehan, 1993).

Perris (1994) uses cognitive-behavioral techniques to, in his words, "restructure dysfunctional working models of self and environment." Arntz (1994) offers a treatment protocol that illustrates the depth and duration necessary to address core symptoms adequately. Five stages are described (development of the working relationship, gaining control of symptoms, correction of errors of thinking, emotional processing and cognitive reevaluation of childhood trauma, and termination).

A review by Goldstein (1993) provides a concise introduction to other well-known psychotherapeutic treatment methods, including those used by Adler, Meissner, Chessick, Giovacchini, Kernberg, and Stone.

Medications

Studies of biological treatments have reported only short- and medium-term results. The fluctuating nature of borderline symptoms suggests caution in interpreting either improvement or worsening after only a few weeks or months.

With the possible exception of the MAOIs, atypical neuroleptics (such as clozapine), and newer antidepressants (such as the selective serotonin reuptake inhibitors (SSRIs), the effectiveness of pharmacological treatment is generally limited to (but sometimes quite helpful for) acute symptoms and psychosis. Doses of traditional neuroleptics should be fairly low (often in the range of 50 to 200 mg/day chlorpromazine equivalent). Trial clozapine, olanzapine, and risperidone doses are not yet established for this indication. The psychiatrist may attempt to target specific areas of dysfunction, such as affective instability, depression, cognition, or impulse control (Soloff *et al.* 1993). Patients with BPD are often overly sensitive to side effects. Controlled studies are often small or lacking.

Fluoxetine has shown broadly positive effects and good patient tolerance in several open studies (Gitlin, 1993). Tranylcypromine and other MAOIs are sometimes useful for atypical depressive and suicidal symptoms and impulse control problems (Cowdry & Gardner, 1988). The author knows of no recent studies of lithium in BPD, although carbamazapine has been found to curb behavioral outbursts in many patients (Cowdry & Gardner, 1988). Alprazolam, once widely prescribed for BPD patients, appears to have fallen into disrepute; recent studies indicate little reason to consider it an early choice.

Table III.27-1 summarizes some general medication considerations for short-term, targeted prescribing.

TABLE III.27-1

Target Symptom Effectiveness in Reported Studies

(Adapted from Phillips & Gunderson, 1994)

	Cognition	*Affect*	*Impulsivity* (Including Affective Instability)	*Anxiety*
Neuroleptics*	Modest	Modest	Good	Modest
TCAs[+]	Variable	Modest	Variable	Variable
MAOIs[+]	Unknown	Modest	Variable	Modest
SSRIs[+]	Good	Good	Good	Modest
Carbamazepine	Modest	Variable	Good	Unknown
Benzodiazepines	Unknown	Variable	?Worsen	Modest

*Except for clozapine, the dose is usually below that for Axis I psychotic disorders.
[+]TCA = tricyclic antidepressant; MAOI = monoamine oxidase inhibitor; SSRI = selective serotonin reuptake inhibitor.

A few recent studies deserve individual mention. Frankenburg and Zanarini (1993) treated 15 borderline patients with clozapine. Blind ratings two to nine months later showed significant improvement of both positive and negative symptoms on BPRS and the Global Assessment Scale. This author's anecdotal experience supports those findings, although further study is needed. A short, open study of low doses (3 mg/day) of flupenthixol, not currently available in the United States, in carefully diagnosed borderline adolescents indicated significant improvement over eight weeks (Kutcher *et al.*, 1995). Cornelius *et al.* (1993) studied the effectiveness of 16 weeks of low-dose (up to 6 mg/day) haloperidol versus phenelzine (up to 90 mg/day) in BPD patients whose crisis symptoms had abated. Neither group did very well; the haloperidol patients had comparatively fewer positive responses, more side effects, and a higher dropout rate.

Hospital Treatment

Acute-Care Hospitalization. This is often reserved for management of crises that present a serious danger to a patient. In addition, the inpatient setting can be useful for efficient and comprehensive multidisciplinary assessment. Hospital containment and protection may also be needed to begin complex treatment programs that would be difficult (or dangerous) to initiate on an outpatient basis.

The clinician must be cautious when deciding whether the apparent need for hospitalization is related to acute suicidal danger, chronic suicidality, or the patient's primarily seeking an anxiety-reducing environment. While hospitalization is often countertherapeutic, the consequences of refusing admission or continued stay can range from suicide to other ways of acting out feelings of anger or abandonment (with concomitant complicating of the treatment relationship). Denying or limiting inpatient care may be consistent with lowering treatment costs; however, such decisions should be based primarily on the best interests of the patient.

Long-Term Active Hospital Treatment. Hospital treatment aimed at personal growth and long-term character restructuring must be differentiated from that for specific behaviors and symptoms. Prolonged hospitalization for definitive, intensive psychotherapy—not merely extended care or social support—should not be considered simply an expansion of the concept of acute care. The goal is quite different, and its unique efficacy in truly changing selected patients should not be underemphasized. Nevertheless, today's dearth of such programs for severe and primitive personality disorders is a fact of life for most patients. The author is left to recommend that such care be sought, knowing it may not be found.

Intermediate Care

There is, of course, a place for intermediate care—between outpatient and inpatient settings. Supportive living environments (including day- or night-"hospital") with staff members who can contain regression and promote social and affective stability can be a crucial adjunct to outpatient therapy and the success of psychosocial programs. Staff members should be more sophisticated than those commonly employed for case management, since they will have to recognize and deal with a variety of strong (and sometimes confusing) affects and behaviors.

Outcome

Chronic parasuicidal *behavior* is significantly reduced in patients who complete a one-year program of Linehan's dialectical behavior therapy, as compared with those who receive little or no focused treatment (Linehan *et al.*, 1991). There is no difference in depressive or suicidal *ideation*. Treatment dropout rates are comparatively low (Shearin & Linehan, 1994).

Pessimism about long-term outcome in BPD is rebutted in part by Stone (1993), who reports that up to half of borderline patients are clinically recovered at 10- to 25-year follow-up, but that 3 to 9% have committed suicide. He describes factors that suggest a higher probability of recovery (e.g., particular talents or skills), and others that predict failure (e.g., parental cruelty). Stevenson and Meares (1992) describe continued significant treatment gains one year after 12 months of "well-defined," supervised psychotherapy by psychotherapist trainees. Individual sessions took place twice a week using a self-psychology model. Other authors are much less optimistic about long-term findings. Rosowsky and Gurian (1992) note that core symptoms may manifest themselves differently late in life than when one is young or middle-aged.

There are no recent controlled studies of psychoanalytic psychotherapy in BPD, but case reports suggest that many patients do fairly well. Those who are less inclined to extreme destructiveness and acting out tend to be more successful. Patients who, for whatever reason, are not able to complete most or all of treatment tend to do poorly, no matter what the treatment type.

301.50 HISTRIONIC PERSONALITY DISORDER

For those persons with histrionic personality who wish to change the disorder itself, psychoanalytic psychotherapy is the preferred treatment. Horowitz (1991, 1995) suggests a long-term psychotherapeutic approach that pursues symptoms and attempts character restructuring in several phases: clarifying symptoms and establishing the therapeutic alliance, managing "shifts in state of mind," dealing with defensive systems, and helping the patient to change irrational beliefs and self-images. Psychoanalysis is helpful for patients whose underlying narcissism and view of self allow tolerance of the analytic process. Briefer therapies can be symptomatically useful for patients who are already functioning well, or for those in crisis.

Superficial symptoms, some of which may interfere significantly with one's quality of life and/or relationships, often respond to briefer treatments. Winston *et al.* (1994) note good results with brief, "adaptive" psychotherapy.

301.81 NARCISSISTIC PERSONALITY DISORDER

There is no single recommended treatment for narcissistic personality, and controlled studies have not been reported. Treatment for symptoms associated with its various presentations—such as antisocial behavior or control of inner rage, relationship problems, maladaptive style of work or management, distress at difficulty feeling strong affect, or reaction to overwhelming narcissistic injury—has been variously described and is best used in patients who are functioning well in spite of their personality disorder. The resilience of youth often wears thin with age, prompting dysphoria and the seeking of (or referral for) treatment.

Psychodynamically oriented therapy may have some limited success, given reasonable expectations by the therapist. Some patients may tolerate psychoanalytic work; however, in those with more primitive presentations (e.g., prominent borderline or antisocial features), therapies that promote limit setting and support expressive experience are preferred.

An understanding of modern theory concerning narcissism and careful attention to countertransference are important for successful treatment of narcissistic traits wherever they appear (e.g., in marital or family problems, work-related conflict, bulimia, or paranoia). Characterologically narcissistic patients are very difficult for the unsupervised new or inexperienced psychotherapist.

Medications have not proved helpful for narcissistic symptoms or personality *per se*, although, as in other personality disorders, they may be useful for Axis-I-like symptoms.

301.82 AVOIDANT PERSONALITY DISORDER

Psychotherapy is the only well-accepted approach for the treatment of core avoidant characteristics. Some newer medications show promise, but have not been studied extensively for this indication.

Psychotherapy and Social Skills Training

Patients with avoidant features are often seen, erroneously, as being too fragile for active exploration. If the therapist is too cautious, the patient may sense that he or she is being protected, adding to his view that the world is a risky place (or, more accurately, that the patient is in danger of unleashing dangerous impulses). Conversely, pressing too vigorously for change will drive the patient away. Group therapy, with its obvious combination of social experience and safety, is often the treatment of choice. As in other disorders, patients who make some progress in controlling their fears and trying new environments may continue to improve after therapy has ceased.

Features common to both avoidant personality and social phobia (and, in some ways, agoraphobia) may be treated symptomatically (e.g., with cognitive or behavioral approaches, desensitization, or exposure techniques), as suggested in Chapter 18 on Axis I anxiety disorders. While often successful for target symptoms, one should not expect wholly positive results, since the psychopathologic issues in avoidant personality are far more ingrained and complex than those of an ordinary phobia.

Stravynski *et al.* (1994) found that an intensive social skills training program enhanced social function and comfort, but lasting effects were difficult to document. Combining *in vitro* sessions with real-life training did not enhance treatment response.

Medication

Medication for target symptoms, such as panic, may be helpful. There is as yet little evidence that high-potency benzodiazepines (e.g., alprazolam, clonazepam) or MAOIs, useful for social phobia and superficial symptoms, change the personality disorder. The SSRIs (e.g., fluoxetine, paroxetine, sertraline) and buspirone are often effective for target phobic symptoms, and may also affect core manifestations (Deltito & Stam, 1989), but further study is needed before recommending them broadly.

301.6 DEPENDENT PERSONALITY DISORDER

Psychotherapy

Patients with dependent personality disorder may seek treatment after an actual or threatened loss that has precipitated anxiety or depression. Many tolerate exploratory therapy well, although the therapist must be aware that their anxiety about loss or independence creates special transference problems. As in the case of avoidant personality, overattention to outwardly fragile aspects of the patient generates inappropriate dependence. Even simply being directive often suggests to the patient that he or she may rely on the clinician's strength and comfortably bond to the treatment environment, without working toward improvement and autonomy. On the other hand, the therapist should also be alert to evidence of a depriving—even punitive—countertransference.

More superficial approaches, such as group therapy and targeted behavioral therapy, are often helpful. The gains attained may increase with practice even after treatment has come to an end.

Sometimes a dependent lifestyle has its rewards. Friends or family may consciously or unconsciously reward the dependent symptoms. Although attention to primary and secondary gain is important, and family intervention may help some symptoms, the core disorder is ultimately one that exists within the patient, not the environment.

Medications

Although not useful for core symptoms, medications may be helpful in adjustment-related anxiety or depressive disorders.

301.4 OBSESSIVE-COMPULSIVE PERSONALITY DISORDER

Although the two may coexist, obsessive-compulsive personality is qualitatively different from the generally ego-dystonic Axis I obsessive-compulsive disorder (OCD). One thus should consider their treatments separately.

Psychotherapy

Psychotherapy has long been considered the mainstay of treatment for characterologic obsessive-compulsive syndrome. Brief (16 sessions) therapy can have significant results, according to Primac (1993), but there are few other recent studies that address the core symptoms. An older review suggests short-term psychotherapy or a cognitive-behavioral approach (Quality Assurance Project, 1985). Simple exposure and response prevention, useful in Axis I OCD, is not particularly helpful. Group therapy that dilutes control issues and power struggles among participants may allow the patient to experience different cognitive styles, explore true affect, and modulate his or her punitive superego.

Intensive or psychoanalytic psychotherapy is helpful for many patients. The resilience of obsessive-compulsive defenses (e.g., intellectualization) makes treatment lengthy and arduous, with countertransference pitfalls in the obsessive-compulsive character traits found in many therapists and analysts.

Medications

The SSRIs, often helpful for obsessions and compulsions themselves, have not been well studied in the treatment of the core symptoms of obsessive-compulsive personality. Stein and Hollander (1993) suggest that they may be of use. Otherwise, drugs are, at this point, merely aids in accompanying symptoms such as depression.

301.9 PERSONALITY DISORDER NOS

Disorders of personality functioning that do not meet criteria for any other DSM-IV pesonality disorder, including mixed syndromes, may be treated using the principles outlined above.

CHAPTER 28

OTHER CONDITIONS THAT MAY BE A FOCUS OF CLINICAL ATTENTION

PSYCHOLOGICAL FACTORS AFFECTING MEDICAL CONDITION

316 SPECIFIC PSYCHOLOGICAL FACTORS AFFECTING GENERAL MEDICAL CONDITION

These syndromes and conditions take several forms (mental disorder, psychological factor, personality trait, coping style, maladaptive health behavior, or stress response affecting medical condition), all sharing a detrimental impact on a medical condition. The enormous array of medical conditions and possible psychological factors cannot be addressed in this general text. Many related topics are discussed in other chapters and sections (e.g., "Somatoform Disorders," "Substance-Related Disorders").

There are several general principles of treatment or management.

(1) The treating physician or other health care provider must recognize that a psychological factor or behavior is affecting the overall treatment situation.

(2) Psychiatric referral (or psychological care by the primary care physician) must be available and accepted by the patient (and often family).

(3) The psychological condition and/or relationship of the psychological condition to the general medical illness must be accurately diagnosed.

(4) The psychiatric/psychological intervention chosen must be both effective and compatible with the general medical condition and its treatment.

Mental health clinicians, especially psychiatrists, should not only be alert for specific psychological effects. They also should be prepared to assist patients in health-promoting behaviors (such as smoking cessation and weight loss), stress reduction, acceptance of or adaptation to medical illness, recognition of psychological impediments to treatment success, and creation of emotional states that encourage treatment compliance and healing, enhance quality of life, or extend survival.

MEDICATION-INDUCED MOVEMENT DISORDERS

332.1 NEUROLEPTIC-INDUCED PARKINSONISM
333.92 NEUROLEPTIC MALIGNANT SYNDROME
333.7 NEUROLEPTIC-INDUCED ACUTE DYSTONIA
333.99 NEUROLEPTIC-INDUCED ACUTE AKATHISIA
333.82 NEUROLEPTIC-INDUCED TARDIVE DYSKINESIA

Each of the neuroleptic-related disorders is addressed in Chapter 16, Schizophrenia and Other Psychotic Disorders.

333.1 MEDICATION-INDUCED POSTURAL TREMOR

Several nonneuroleptic psychotropic medications can cause tremor. Most, like lithium-induced tremor, are dose related and decrease with reductions in medication. Unlike neuroleptic-related tremor, significant postural tremor with other drugs (e.g., lithium) usually suggests a toxicity for which medication decrease or discontinuation should be considered.

333.90 MEDICATION-INDUCED MOVEMENT DISORDER NOS
995.2 ADVERSE EFFECTS OF MEDICATION NOS

Other medication-induced disorders, including movement disorders, may respond to the principles discussed above and elsewhere in the text; however, the large number of possible physiologic effects and medication interactions suggest careful individual assessment. The reader is referred to more specialized texts for guidance.

RELATIONAL PROBLEMS

**V61.9 RELATIONAL PROBLEM RELATED TO A MENTAL DISORDER OR
   GENERAL MEDICAL CONDITION
V61.20 PARENT-CHILD RELATIONAL PROBLEM
V61.1 PARTNER RELATIONAL PROBLEM
V61.8 SIBLING RELATIONAL PROBLEM
V62.81 RELATIONAL PROBLEM NOS**

Relational problems are usually best dealt with by involving the relationship participants in the treatment process. With some exceptions, family or couples therapy cannot be adequately accomplished when important members are missing. On the other hand, family members who do not live at home, and sometimes late adolescents who are in the process of healthy separation from their parents, may reasonably be excluded when they are peripheral to the primary relational issues (e.g., some family matters involving younger children that are comparatively extraneous to late adolescents).

In the absence of other mental disorder, including adjustment disorder, the goals of the therapist are generally to provide information and counseling, to be an objective observer, to recognize problems in communication and facilitate their resolution, and to avoid overdiagnosis (see below). The therapist may wish to become a negotiator to some extent; however, most authors recommend against placing oneself in the position of "referee."

Therapists or counselors are often in a position to influence important family or couple decisions (e.g., whether or not to separate, divorce, or obtain an abortion). It is strongly recommended that one not use one's personal views in this way, since it immediately shifts the therapist's role and purpose away from objective contribution. If the counselor has strong disagreement with, for example, a couple's wish to avoid abortion, they should be referred to a more impartial person. This does not mean, however, that counselors should not attempt to influence clients whom they believe are engaging in potentially harmful or countertherapeutic practices, or when their behavior is clearly immoral or illegal.

In the author's opinion, a therapist who is working with a couple or family on relational issues should usually avoid seeing the members separately after the initial assessment. Although it is tempting to seek individual viewpoints or to accede to requests from one party for some "special" time, this almost always interferes with the therapist's proper role in the relational issue. In addition, if members of the family or couple are seeing individual therapists, it is usually best to keep the relational counseling separate and free of collaboration among caregivers, even in the name of "communication" or preventing "splitting."[1]

---

[1] This caveat does not apply to clinical supervision or to communications about serious dangers or health issues. Inpatient treatment of severe mental illness, in which family therapy is a part of an overall team approach, may be another exception.

When family or partner difficulty is related to a severe or chronic mental illness, therapists sometimes misunderstand the illness's effect on treatment. Although one should be wary of removing a participant's *responsibility* for his or her part in a relationship (e.g., for violence), it is often unreasonable to expect subtly psychotic or severely depressed individuals to respond to counseling processes that require unattainable cognition, attention, insight, or persistence.

Divorce and Child Custody

Counseling for relational problems is often related to divorce or child custody. In such cases, the therapist must decide who the patient is, and be alert to external distractions from treatment goals. For example, if a child is referred for help adjusting to his or her parents' divorce, it should be clear from the outset that the counselor is not there to carry out a parent's divorce-related "agenda," but to assist the child. Therapists should also be very cautious about making supporting statements—in letters or court testimony, for example—that are more appropriately referred to a qualified forensic psychiatrist or psychologist with access to broader information.

Overdiagnosis is a common problem in the treatment of relational problems. One may be tempted to label one or another person as the problem's source or sustaining factor, especially when third-party payers require a DSM-IV diagnosis for compensation. The therapist should remember that intentional overdiagnosis is unethical and, in a reimbursement context, illegal. Purposeful or not, it can also be quite harmful to patients. Since this kind of treatment is often done by counselors who lack doctoral or postdoctoral training in diagnosis, experienced clinical supervision is recommended before diagnosis in all but the most straightforward cases.

Boundary Violations

Patients or clients in relational counseling are usually outwardly healthy. At various times, they may appear attractive, titillating, or as candidates for "rescue." They often seek, consciously or not, substitute relationships of various kinds. The counseling setting is thus fertile ground for displacement and transference.

The presence of displacement and transference *per se* is not the boundary issue. Rather, problems may arise related to the therapist's inappropriate use of the patient's material and feelings, the therapist's inability to recognize signs of inappropriate use (by patient or counselor), and sometimes the imprudent encouraging of strong or intimate feelings in a relatively superficial "counseling" environment (compared, for example, with psychoanalytic psychotherapy by a qualified analyst).

Even therapists who have no intention of exploiting patients or otherwise acting improperly may become inappropriately involved with them. While legal and professional reactions to a therapist's peccadillos may sometimes seem out of proportion to the intent or damage incurred, the patient must be the first consideration, not the therapist's needs. Serious patient exploitation is a worst-case scenario that is sometimes preventable (e.g., through clinician training, supervision, or psychotherapy), but sometimes extremely subtle or even purposeful (e.g, in situations involving dishonest or predatory therapists).

PROBLEMS RELATED TO ABUSE OR NEGLECT

V61.21 PHYSICAL ABUSE OF CHILD
V61.21 SEXUAL ABUSE OF CHILD
V61.21 NEGLECT OF CHILD
V61.1 PHYSICAL ABUSE OF ADULT
V61.1 SEXUAL ABUSE OF ADULT

Abuse or neglect in this section will refer to that which occurs within families, against family members. Professional or institutional abuse or neglect, or other forms that may occur outside the home, are not addressed here.

A finding of abuse or neglect is a very serious matter. Clinicians want desperately to prevent tragedy, but we must protect the rights of all concerned. Government agencies (e.g., those charged with child protective services) are usually quite experienced, but specific procedures or caseworkers may be unsuitable for such individualized work. Agency staffs often have insufficient resources to evaluate or follow cases properly, causing extremely important decisions about children, other victims, and families to be made with inadequate information. Unfortunately, some investigators or decision makers may also have personal agendas or intentions that overestimate family problems in the otherwise commendable name of victim protection. This section is designed to address situations in which serious abuse or neglect is not merely suspected but has actually occurred.

Confidentiality and patient privilege are often confused in presentations of abuse and neglect. It may be helpful to note that, with regard to release of information, *privilege* is the *p*atient's *r*ight to control the use of his or her information and *c*onfidentiality is the *c*linician's *o*bligation to protect that privilege.[2] All U.S. states have laws that allow and require mental health professionals to report suspected child abuse or neglect to an appropriate agency. Most (perhaps all) also require reporting of abuse or neglect of the elderly, disabled, and other vulnerable persons. This means that the uncovering of suspected abuse or neglect in psychotherapy is not protected by therapist-patient or doctor-patient privilege. If a child or other vulnerable person is reasonably suspected of being in danger, the professional must report it. Readers should consult the laws of their own jurisdictions for details.

---

[2]Thanks to Thomas Gutheil, M.D., for this pneumonic.

V61.21, V61.1 PERPETRATOR TREATMENT/MANAGEMENT

There is an extensive literature on the individual and family treatment of abusive individuals. Some authors focus primarily on treatment efforts that may keep the family together; others believe that the integrity of the family is usually less important than protecting current and potential victims and/or punishing the perpetrator(s). *Separation from the victim is recommended when there is reasonable probability of serious injury, and in any case in which child abuse or neglect is probable.*

Emphasis on social stresses in the causation and amelioration of abusive behavior is, in our opinion, misplaced. There is little objective evidence that poverty, unemployment, inadequate housing, and the like cause otherwise reasonable people to abuse those who are unable to defend themselves. Conversely, there is much to suggest that character pathology and Axis I mental disorders play an enormous role. In addition, studies of the intergenerational transmission of abusive behavior, purporting that abused children become abusive adults, are often flawed by both nonrandom subject selection and partisan reporting (Oliver, 1993). Studies reviewed by Oliver often concluded that perhaps one third of severely abused children grow up to be "inept, neglectful, or abusive" parents; however, the reasons are complex, and not limited to the factors commonly cited by many social advocates.

The author agrees with Oliver (1993) who found no justification for the popular view of causation that "apportion(s) responsibility between the 'sins of the parents' and the failings of society." Familial abusive situations are far more complex than "like father, like son." The retrospective finding that many, perhaps most, abusers of children and others were abused as children is interesting, but has less predictive value than commonly assumed. Although a lack of family models for parenting is correlated with later poor parenting skills, and although the early family is the single most important source of adult conscience and values, there is no evidence that most children who are abused or neglected will later place their own offspring in physical danger.

The expectation that the perpetrator is responsible for his or her actions should be underscored. Even many (but not all) people with mental illness can conform their behavior to societal norms most or all of the time, if expected to do so. There is a significant likelihood that the abuse is related to treatment-resistant perpetrator characteristics. Whether the behavior results from serious Axis I mental illness (e.g., schizophrenia or paraphilia) or simply an antisocial or sadistic character, psychiatric treatment may well not affect it in the long run.

Even when the perpetrator has a disorder that responds to treatment, the long-term reliability of improvement is the important issue. Depression (especially postpartum) is one of the few severe Axis I disorders associated with abuse or neglect for which effective treatment usually confers reasonable reliability that the harmful behavior will not recur without advance warning. If relapse is likely, for any reason, caution should be the first priority.

Perpetrators of child sexual abuse should usually be considered pedophiles for purposes of treatment. They (and some observers) do not consider their actions violent, and may employ a great deal of denial that their actions constitute abuse (e.g., in nonpenetrating sexual activity or actions with the "consent" of an older child). Treatment is discussed with the paraphilias, Chapter 22.

995.5, 995.81 VICTIM PROTECTION AND TREATMENT

Five aspects of victim issues are briefly discussed in the following. Readers who plan to treat victims of abuse or neglect should consult more specialized texts to acquire a better understanding of these complex issues. One should recall that in almost all instances abuse or neglect must be promptly communicated to the appropriate government agency. When feasible, reporting should be done in a context of discussion with the patient. While there is no question about reporting abuse of young children, some adult or late-adolescent victims may ask the therapist not to divulge their abuse. Therapists should be familiar with the law in this regard.

The reporting requirement sometimes interferes with psychotherapy. A review by Roback and Shelton (1995) indicates that for persons at risk of serious sociolegal consequences, mandatory reporting serves as a barrier to therapeutic disclosure or entry into treatment. For example, a victim or perpetrator may be reluctant to discuss certain topics for fear of setting uncomfortable social or legal processes into motion. Similarly, a warning by the therapist that certain topics are reportable or not confidential may cast a pall over trust in treatment.

Prevention

Prevention is the most sought-after form of treatment. There are a number of statistically significant correlates of abuse and neglect. Until the behavior actually occurs, however, reliable individual predictions are not possible in populations without serious mental illness. Once abuse or neglect occurs in a family setting, no matter what the form, and with or without treatment of the perpetrator, recurrence is likely. It is very difficult to prevent further injury so long as the perpetrator is allowed extended, unsupervised contact with the vulnerable abuse victim. Parents or relatives who neglect children or disabled persons are similarly unlikely to change their behavior unless the neglect was due to lack of knowledge or skills, or to some remediable form of negligence (e.g., depression or substance abuse).

Although we disagree with some authorities that environmental stressors cause substantial abuse, they often make abusive behavior more likely in predisposed perpetrators. Attention to such stressors may be indicated, but should not be considered sufficient *per se*.

Recognition

Early recognition by teachers, doctors, emergency room staff, neighbors, and other family members is a key to preventing further injury. Some signs are well known, such as characteristic fractures or burn patterns in children. Others are difficult to find. Awareness of the possibility of abuse or neglect in students or emergency room patients is very important, in spite of some fraudulent allegations and overly zealous reporting.

Recognition by family members is at least as important as that by doctors and teachers. A mother, for example, may deny or ignore child or elder abuse by her husband, perhaps in a misguided attempt to preserve the marriage or family. This makes the problem far more serious, increasing the person's exposure to danger and adding to the number of important adults who have betrayed his or her trust.

Protection

Protection from harm is not as straightforward as it may appear. Once a vulnerable person is known to be in danger, many factors can stand in the way of adequate physical safety.

In cases of possible child abuse or neglect, it is very difficult to remove the child from the abuser's environment (or vice versa), and be prepared to make the separation permanent. The level of proof required to remove the child or perpetrator is high enough that a large number of children are forced to remain in harmful, sometimes lethal, situations. Similarly, children, spouses, and the elderly often choose to remain in abusive or neglectful settings, for reasons too complex to address here. Nevertheless, we believe that when serious physical or emotional damage to a vulnerable person is reasonably likely, the immediate priority must rest with protecting the potential victim.

Fraudulent reporting and agency misunderstandings can cause severe hardship (sometimes devastation) for entire families. We know of no good answers to the double binds of protection versus rights of the accused perpetrator, protection versus fraudulent accusations by angry spouses or children, or protection versus overzealousness and poor investigation by overburdened social service agencies.

Treatment

Victim treatment is a very broad topic, which cannot be adequately addressed in this section. Physical injuries usually heal better and faster than emotional ones. The effects of betrayal and damage by a person who is ordinarily trusted and loved are significant, and become worse as the abuse or neglect becomes more chronic or repetitious.

Crisis intervention is not enough. Victims, especially abused children, deserve complete psychiatric assessment and individual (and usually family) therapy. If safe for the victim, the family should be supported and strengthened.

Many forms of individual, group, and family therapy have been used for victims of abuse and neglect. Whatever the primary modalities, treatment should begin promptly, with the understanding that the absence of currently apparent symptoms does not mean an absence of significant and lasting damage. Major treatment issues include trust and betrayal of trust, amelioration of inappropriate guilt, and creation of a feeling of success to replace failure and shame. If the patient is old enough and has obvious symptoms, associations may be drawn between the symptoms and feelings and memories about the abuse or neglect. Memories should be seen as material for therapeutic purposes, and not as exact validation of specific events (see below).

Some clinicians use therapy as a way further to diagnose or clarify the physical events of the abuse (e.g., in children or in adults with child abuse histories). We believe this should be approached with great caution, and that treatment should focus on symptoms, psychopathology, and rehabilitation, not truth seeking. The psychotherapy setting encourages many thoughts, feelings, and impressions that assist the treatment effort, but the material elicited is necessarily colored by the effects of emotion, point of view, transference, and the patient's perception of the therapist's expectations. The products of therapy sessions should not be considered absolutely factual, often change over time, and are sometimes quite at odds with documented facts. The more intensive the therapy, the more this is true.

Outcome

There is no question that abuse by a family member is a terrible experience, usually with lasting emotional effects. Chronic abuse or neglect is even worse. The effects may be destructive, but often they are largely overcome by the many other important influences in one's life and development. Studies of adult "survivors" of chronic child physical and sexual abuse appear to indicate severe disability in a large proportion (Green, 1994), as well as a correlation with (but not a one-to-one prediction of) future abusive behavior. These reports are often skewed by nonrandom selection (and sometimes by reporter bias), however. It is likely that many victims became successful in life, and are indistinguishable from the general population.

Finally, "victim" or "survivor" status can become an inappropriate focus of the abused individual's identity. Therapists and families should help the person concentrate on improving and normalizing his or her life, leaving behind the abused or flawed self-image. Most victims, with or without formal treatment, function and enjoy life on an equal footing with other men and women.

ADDITIONAL CONDITIONS THAT MAY BE A FOCUS OF CLINICAL ATTENTION

V15.81 NONCOMPLIANCE WITH TREATMENT

Noncompliance in the absence of any of the mental disorders already described may be approached with education about one's illness or treatment or with counseling. Since the patient generally has a right not to comply, counseling with family members or frustrated medical staff who are having difficulty accepting the patient's decision may be indirectly helpful. For example, a clinician may ease tensions between nursing staff and the patient that might adversely affect other aspects of the patient's care.

V65.2 MALINGERING

Since, by definition, there is no primary illness to treat once malingering has been established, only a couple of management issues remain. The most obvious is to offer understanding and counsel to the person who feels he or she must use this dishonest course of action. Education about help for financial problems from social agencies, the possible consequences of dishonesty, or even the fact that faking an illness really *is* dishonest and a misuse of expensive resources may be useful.

The temptation to publicize the malingering broadly should be resisted. We disagree with some authors that one of the clinician's goals should be to publicize the malingering "diagnosis" to health, social, and legal agencies. The psychiatrist or therapist who does this runs some risk of breach of ethics, and could be answerable for slander or libel. It seems more prudent, if less personally gratifying, simply to note in the record that one is unable to find any medical or psychological basis for the individual's complaints, and that malingering is strongly suspected.

V71.01 ADULT ANTISOCIAL BEHAVIOR

Few treatment approaches are effective for repeated antisocial behavior that is not due to one of the mental disorders already discussed in the text (including an adjustment disorder). Psychotherapies, hospitalization, biological therapies, and ordinary incarceration offer little chance of change.

Specialized long-term residential forensic programs may be successful for some individuals; however, the majority of those arrested with adult antisocial behavior cannot be sentenced to years of maximum security treatment. The best option for many is a community or wilderness experiential program (Reid & Matthews, 1980; Reid & Solomon, 1981), but these are rarely available. Consistency of consequence is one of the best preventive measures (Reid, in press).

V71.02 CHILDHOOD OR ADOLESCENT ANTISOCIAL BEHAVIOR

The treatment of many of these behaviors is discussed elsewhere in the text. Persons of this age should not be given a diagnosis of antisocial personality, nor should their behavior be assumed to be a precursor to antisocial personality disorder. Some specialized forms of residential treatment (not acute-care hospitalization) may be helpful for some patients; however, the most effective "treatment" continues to be psychiatrically designed experiential approaches, such as wilderness programs (Reid & Matthews, 1980; Reid & Solomon, 1981). Psychotherapy and brief hospitalization rarely change ordinary delinquency.

Establishing very reliable consequences for antisocial behavior is crucial for any program, whether therapeutic or simply correctional. Court diversion, probation, special treatment, and very brief juvenile sentences for serious crimes (e.g., sentences that are terminated when an adolescent becomes an adult) seem humane on the surface, but actually increase antisocial behavior in both the index person and his or her peers. Investment in strict and significant punishment for crime, with little or no ability to manipulate the legal or correctional system, seems to be the best approach (Reid, in press).

Until a few years ago, it was common for children with simple antisocial behavior to be placed in psychiatric hospitals. In some cases, this was done because well-meaning judges, probation officers, or parents felt that hospitalization was preferable to juvenile detention or jail. In others, hospitalization was associated with marketing efforts of the hospitals themselves. In either case, adding an indelible record of psychiatric hospitalization and fostering a "sick" identity is rarely helpful in the long run.

V62.89 BORDERLINE INTELLECTUAL FUNCTIONING

This category, which is made up of the majority of people society calls "mentally retarded," does not represent true mental retardation (Strider & Menolascino, 1981). For the most part, these individuals get along well in the community; however, they may be prone to difficulty in areas in which one's cognitive ability or fund of knowledge is important for coping with personal or environmental problems. Supportive treatment and relevant education when such problems or crises develop are almost always helpful. One may wish to counsel the family as well, and to be sure that the person knows of available aid from social agencies (e.g., employment counseling for one who has lost a job).

Much of the frustration associated with borderline intellectual functioning is related to how such people are treated by an uninformed or prejudiced public. Discussions with community, school, or work officials may be useful. When problems are more troublesome (as in a person with an accompanying conduct disorder), practical, flexible therapeutic measures should be employed in *lieu* of traditional individual or group therapies (although some group approaches are highly effective). Institutionalization or other infantilizing procedures *per se* have no role in this condition.

780.9 AGE-RELATED COGNITIVE DECLINE

In addition to referral for a complete medical evaluation, the psychiatrist or psychotherapist may offer considerable support to both the patient and family. Some of the principles of treatment include those of "Phase-of-Life Problem" below such as education and being alert for countertransference and related issues (e.g., those of a young therapist treating an older patient). Assuming that the cognitive decline is biological in spite of the absence of a neurological diagnosis, such medications as tacrine, donepezil, ergoloid, or central nervous system stimulants may be tried.

V62.82 BEREAVEMENT

Family physicians, and sometimes psychiatrists and psychotherapists, may be consulted about some of the more striking symptoms of *normal* grief. One pitfall of treatment is overdiagnosis. The person should not be treated as if an aberrant grief reaction or serious depression is present unless he or she does not qualify for this V-code condition. Support and guidance may be given, however, with reassurance that the feelings are normal and should not be avoided. The therapist should show approval of the many feelings experienced by the grieving person, including anger at the lost object.

Counseling for the individual or for well-meaning family or friends should include a *caveat* against overprotection. Such activities as attending funeral and memorial services, returning to the home where the deceased lived, and putting away his or her possessions (and with them, memories) should be encouraged for grieving persons of all ages. The clinician should make it clear that he or she is available, but need not be intrusive.

Treatment for unresolved or aberrant grief, with persistent yearning, overidentification with the deceased, and/or inability to express sadness or rage, is briefly addressed in Chapter 26, Adjustment Disorders.

V62.3 ACADEMIC PROBLEM

Treatment of this condition in the absence of any other diagnosable mental disorder should be based on simple counseling, with exploration of possible family and environmental stresses, personal expectations, and academic skills. As with many of the other V codes, one should be aware of the dangers of overdiagnosis and mislabeling of conditions not attributable to a mental disorder.

V62.2 OCCUPATIONAL PROBLEM

The same basic treatment principles apply as were mentioned above under "Academic Problem." One may also wish to consider some of the issues discussed in Chapter 26, Adjustment Disorders.

313.82 IDENTITY PROBLEM

Identity issues that are not part of a mental disorder may be addressed with reality-based therapy. The counselor should be experienced, and avoid over-diagnosis. There should be a distinction between therapy and guidance, with each having its place in the process.

V62.89 RELIGIOUS OR SPIRITUAL PROBLEM

Counseling for religious or spiritual problems should follow many of the recommendations for "Identity Problem," above. If the person's concern is within a specific faith, an experienced pastoral counselor may be the best choice. We would advise against counselors who insist on following a rigid religious doctrine, unless the problem is defined as within that doctrine.

V62.4 ACCULTURATION PROBLEM

Adapting to a new culture is a difficult task, and one that can, albeit uncommonly, lead to serious emotional or social problems. Education and support are usually quite helpful. Many national and cultural groups have established, supportive communities in the United States and other countries, particularly in large cities. For some, such as Chinese immigrants, there are formal business and cultural networks specifically designed to assist with acculturation and social success (but not usually with associated emotional problems).

By the same token, persons from other countries usually succeed much more readily if they do not limit their contacts to people from their homeland. While older immigrants may do best when surrounded by traditional ways, it is important that young adults and children become established in the English language and American way of life. There is richness in diversity, but isolation from things that are associated with educational and occupational success is unwise.

V62.89 PHASE OF LIFE PROBLEM

The tremendous variety of problems that might fall into this category is too broad to address completely. The education and counseling principles discussed elsewhere in the text should suffice for most cases. The therapist should be alert for countertransference and related issues (e.g., those of a young therapist treating an older patient with concerns about retirement, or a therapist with particular opinions or values who attempts to give objective counseling to a patient with opposing views).

References for Part III

Abel, G. G., Becker, J. V., Cunningham-Rathner, J., *et al.* (1984): *The Treatment of Child Molesters.* Atlanta, GA: Behavioral Medicine Institute.

Abel, G. G., & Osborn, C. A. (1995): Pedophilia. In G. O. Gabbard (Ed.), *Treatments of Psychiatric Disorders* (2nd ed.). Washington, DC: American Psychiatric Press.

Abel, G. G., Osborn, C., Anthony, D., *et al.* (1993): Current treatment of the paraphilias. In J. Bancroft, C. M. Davis, & H. J. Ruppel (Eds.), *Annual Review of Sex Research.* Mount Vernon, IA: Society for the Scientific Study of Sexuality.

Adler, R., Nunn, R., Northam, E., *et al.* (1994): Secondary prevention of childhood firesetting. *Journal of the American Academy of Child and Adolescent Psychiatry,* 33(8):1194–1202.

Agency for Health Care Policy and Research, Acute Pain Management Guideline Panel: *Acute Pain Management: Operative or Medical Procedures and Trauma.* Clinical Practice Guideline (AHCPR Publ No 92–0032), Rockville, MD: U.S. Department of Health and Human Services, 1992.

Agras, S. (1994): *Journal of Psychotherapy Practice and Research.*

Agras, W. S. (1991): *Cognitive Behavior Therapy Treatment Manual for Bulimia Nervosa.* Department of Psychiatry and Behavioral Sciences, Stanford University School of Medicine.

Agras, W. S., Dorian, B., Kirkley, B. G., *et al.* (1987): Imipramine in the treatment of bulimia: A double-blind controlled study. *International Journal of Eating Disorders,* 6:29–38.

Agras, W. S., Schneider, J. A., Arnow, B., *et al.* (1989): Cognitive-behavioral and response-prevention treatments for bulimia nervosa. *Journal of Consulting and Clinical Psychology,* 57:215–221.

Agras, W. S., Rossiter, E. M., Arnow, B., *et al.* (1994): One-year follow-up of psychosocial and pharmacologic treatments for bulimia nervosa. *Journal of Clinical Psychiatry,* 55(5):179–183.

Akiskal, H. S., Djenderedjian, A. H., Rosenthal, R. H., & Khani, M. R. (1977): Cyclothymic disorder: Validating criteria for inclusion in the bipolar affective group. *American Journal of Psychiatry,* 134:1227–1233.

Aldrich, M. S. (1990): Narcolepsy. *New England Journal of Medicine,* 323:389–394.

Allen, S. N., Bloom, S. L. (1994): Group and family treatment of post-traumatic stress disorder. *Psychiatric Clinics of North America,* 17(2):425–437.

Altshuler, L. L., Post, R. M., Leverich, G. S., *et al.* (1995): Antidepressant-induced mania and cycle acceleration: A controversy revisited. *Psychiatry,* 152(8):1130–1138.

American Psychiatric Association Task Force on Electroconvulsive Therapy (1990): *The Practice of Electroconvulsive Therapy: Recommendations for Treatment, Training, and Privileging.* Washington, DC: American Psychiatric Press.

American Psychiatric Association Work Group on Eating Disorders (J. Yager, Chair) (1993): *Practice Guideline for Eating Disorders.* Washington, DC: American Psychiatric Press.

Ancoli-Israel, S., Seifert, A. R., & Lemon, M. (1986): Thermal biofeedback and periodic movements in sleep: Patients' subjective reports and a case study. *Biofeedback Self-Regulation,* 11:177–188.

Andrews, E., Bellard, J., & Walter-Ryan, W. G. (1986): Monosymptomatic hypochondriacal psychosis manifesting as delusions of infestation: Case studies of treatment with haloperidol. *Journal of Clinical Psychiatry,* 47(4):188–190.

Angst, J., & Preisig, M. (1995): Outcome of a clinical cohort of unipolar, bipolar and schizoaffective patients: Results of a prospective study from 1959 to 1985. *Schweiz Arch Neurol Psychiatr,* 146(1):17–23.

Appel, G. (1974): An approach to the treatment of schizoid phenomena. *Psychoanalytic Review,* 61:99–113.

Armstrong, K., Gorden, R., & Santorella, G. (1995): Occupational exposure of health care workers (HCWs) to human immunodeficiency virus (HIV): Stress reactions and counseling interventions. *Social Work and Health Care,* 21(3):61–80.

Armstrong, K., O'Callahan, W., & Marmar, C. R. (1991): Debriefing Red Cross disaster personnel: The multiple stressor debriefing model. *Journal of Traumatic Stress,* 4:481–491.

Arndt, I. O., McLellan, A. T., Dorozynsky, L., *et al.* (1994): Desipramine treatment for cocaine dependence. Role of antisocial personality disorder. *Journal of Nervous and Mental Diseases,* 182(3):151–156.

Arntz, A. (1994): Treatment of borderline personality disorder: A challenge for cognitive-behavioural therapy. *Behavioral Research and Therapy,* 32(4):419–430.

Assendelft, W. J., Bouter, L. M., & Kessels, A. G. (1991): Effectiveness of chiropractic and physiotherapy in the treatment of low back pain: A critical discussion of the British Randomized Clinical Trial. *Journal of Manipulative Physiological Therapy,* 14(5):281–286.

Ayuso-Gutierrez, J. L., Palazon, M., & Ayuso-Mateos, J. L. (1994): Open trial of fluvoxamine in the treatment of bulimia nervosa. *International Journal of Eating Disorders,* 15(3):245–249.

Baer, L., Rauch, S. L., Ballantine, H. T. Jr., *et al.* (1995): Cingulotomy for intractable obsessive-compulsive disorder. Prospective long-term follow-up of 18 patients. *Archives of General Psychiatry,* 52(5):384–392.

Baizerman, M., & Emshoff, B. (1984): Juvenile firesetting: Building a community-based prevention program. *Children Today,* 13(3):7–12.

Baldwin, D., & Rudge, S. (1995): The role of serotonin in depression and anxiety. *International Clinical Psychopharmacolgy,* 9(suppl 4):41–45.

Ballenger, J. C., Burrows, G., DuPont, R., *et al.* (1988): Alprazolam in panic disorder and agoraphobia: Results from a multicenter trial, I: Efficacy in short term treatment. *Archives of General Psychiatry,* 45:413–422.

Ballenger, J. C., Lydiard, R. B., & Turner, S. M. (1995): Panic disorder and agoraphobia. In G. O. Gabbard (Ed.), *Treatments of Psychiatric Disorders* (2nd ed.). Washington, DC: American Psychiatric Press.

Balon, R. (1994): Sleep terror disorder and insomnia treated with trazodone: A case report. *Annals of Clinical Psychiatry,* 6(3):161–163.

Balter, M. B., & Uhlenhuth, E. H. (1992): New epidemiological findings about insomnia and its treatment. *Journal of Clinical Psychiatry,* 53(suppl 12):34–39.

Barak, Y., Ring, A., Levy, D., *et al.* (1995): Disabling compulsions in 11 mentally retarded adults: An open trial of clomipramine SR. *Journal of Clinical Psychiatry,* 56(10):459–461.

Barlow, D. H., & Craske, M. G. (1989): *Mastery of Your Anxiety and Panic.* Albany, NY: Graywind.

Barlow, D. H., Craske, M. G., Cerny, J. A., & Klosko, J. S. (1989): Behavioral treatment of panic disorder. *Behavior Therapy,* 20:261–282.

Barnett, W., & Spitzer, M. (1994): Pathological fire-setting 1951–1991: A review. *Medical Science and Law* (England), 34(1):4–20.

Barsky, A. J. (1996): Hypochondriasis. *Psychosomatics,* 37(1):48–56.

Basoglu, M., Marks, I. M., Kilic, C., *et al.* (1994): Alprazolam and exposure for panic disorder with agoraphobia. Attribution of improvement to medication predicts subsequent relapse. *British Journal of Psychiatry* 164(5):652–659.

Bastani, J. B., & Kentsmith, D. K. (1980): Psychotherapy with wives of sexual deviants. *American Journal of Psychotherapy,* 34(1):20–25.

Bastuji, H., & Jouvet, M. (1988): Successful treatment of idiopathic hypersomnia and narcolepsy with modafinil. *Progress in Neuropsychopharmacology and Biological Psychiatry,* 12:695–700.

Bauer, M. S., & Whybrow, P. C. (1990): Rapid cycling bipolar affective disorder. Treatment of refractory rapid cycling with high-dose levothyroxine: A preliminary study. *Archives of General Psychiatry,* 47:435–440.

Beck, A. T. (1976): *Cognitive Therapy and the Emotional Disorders.* New York: International Universities Press.

Beck, A. T., Rush, A. J., Shaw, B. F., *et al.* (1979): *Cognitive Therapy of Depression: A Treatment Manual.* New York: Guilford.

Beck, A. T., Sokol, L., Clark, D. A., *et al.* (1992): A crossover study of focused cognitive therapy for panic disorder. *American Journal of Psychiatry,* 149:778–783.

Beck, J. G., Stanley, M. A., Baldwin, L. E., *et al.* (1994): Comparison of cognitive therapy and relaxation training for panic disorder. *Journal of Consulting Clinical Psychology,* 62(4):818–826.

Becker, J. V., & Kavoussi, R. J. (1994): Sexual and gender identity disorders. In R. E. Hales, S. C. Yudofsky, J. A. Talbott (Eds.), *Textbook of Psychiatry* (2nd ed.). Washington, DC: American Psychiatric Press.

Belfer, P. L., Munoz, L. S., Schachter, J., & Levendusky, P. G. (1995): Cognitive-behavioral group psychotherapy for agoraphobia and panic disorder. *International Journal of Group Psychotherapy,* 45(2):185–206.

Benjamin, J., Levine, J., Fux, M., *et al.* (1995): A double-blind, placebo-controlled, crossover trial of inositol treatment for panic disorder. *American Journal of Psychiatry,* 152(7):1084–1086.

Benton, M. K., & Schroeder, H. E. (1990): Social skills training with schizophrenics: A meta-analytic evaluation. *Journal of Consulting Clinical Psychology*, 58:741–747.

Berlin, F. S., Malin, H. M., & Thomas, K. (1995): Nonpedophiliac and nontransvestic paraphilias. In G. O. Gabbard (Ed.), *Treatments of Psychiatric Disorders* (2nd ed.). Washington, DC: American Psychiatric Press.

Black, D. W., Baumgard, C. H., & Bell, S. E. (1995): The long-term outcome of antisocial personality disorder compared with depression, schizophrenia, and surgical conditions. *Bulletin of the American Academy of Psychiatry and the Law*, 23(1):43–52.

Black, D. W., Wesner, R., Bowers, W., & Gabel J. (1993): A comparison of fluvoxamine, cognitive therapy and placebo in the treatment of panic disorder. *Archives of General Psychiatry*, 50:44–50.

Black, D. W., & Wojcieszek, J. (1991): Depersonalization syndrome induced by fluoxetine. *Psychosomatics*, 32:468–469.

Blackmon, W. D. (1994): Dungeons and dragons: The use of a fantasy game in the psychotherapeutic treatment of a young adult. *American Journal of Psychotherapy*, 48(4):624–632.

Blouin, J. H., Carter, J., Blouin, A. G., *et al.* (1994): Prognostic indicators in bulimia nervosa treated with cognitive-behavioral group therapy. *International Journal of Eating Disorders*, 15(2):113–123.

Blume, S. B. (1989): Treatment for the addictions in a psychiatric setting. *British Journal of the Addictions*, 84(7):727–729.

Bolton, D., Luckie, M., & Steinberg, D. (1995): Long-term course of obsessive-compulsive disorder treated in adolescence. *Journal of the American Academy of Child and Adolescent Psychiatry*, 34(11):1441–1450.

Borkovec, T. D., Abel, J. L., & Newman, H. (1995): Effects of psychotherapy on comorbid conditions in generalized anxiety disorder. *Journal of Consulting Clinical Psychology*, 63(3):479–483.

Borkovec, T. D., & Costello, E. (1993): Efficacy of applied relaxation and cognitive-behavioral therapy in the treatment of generalized anxiety disorder. *Journal of Consulting Clinical Psychology*, 61(4):611–619.

Boskind-Lodahl, M., & White, W. (1978): The definition and treatment of bulimarexia in college women: A pilot study. *Journal of American College Health*, 27:84–97.

Boudewyns, P. A. (1996): Posttraumatic stress disorder: Conceptualization and treatment. *Progress in Behavior Modification*, 30:165–189.

Bourin, M., & Malinge, M. (1995): Controlled comparison of the effects and abrupt discontinuation of buspirone and lorazepam. *Progress in Neuropsychopharmacology and Biological Psychiatry*, 19(4):567–575.

Bowden, C. L. (1995): Predictors of response to divalproex and lithium. *Journal of Clinical Psychiatry*, 56(suppl 3):25–30.

Bowden, C. L., Brugger, A. M., Swann, A. C., *et al.* (Depakote Mania Study Group) (1994): Efficacy of divalproex vs. lithium and placebo in the treatment of mania. *Journal of the American Medical Association*, 271:918–924.

Bowden, C. L., Janicak, P. G., Orsulak, P., *et al.* (1996): Relation of serum valproate concentration to response in mania. *American Journal of Psychiatry*, 153(6):765–770.

Bradford, J. M. W. (1985): Organic treatments for the male sexual offender. *Behavior Science and Law*, 3:355–375.

Bradford, J. M. W. (1994): Can pedophilia be treated? *Harvard Mental Health Letter*, 10:8.

Bradford, J. M. W., & Greenberg, D. M. (1996): Pharmacological treatment of deviant sexual behaviour. In R. C. Rosen, C. M. Davis, & H. J. Ruppel, Jr. (Eds.), *Annual Review of Sex Research,* Vol. 7. Mount Vernon, IA: Society for the Scientific Study of Sexuality.

Bradford, J. M. W., Martindale, J. J., Goldberg, M., *et al.* (1995): Sertraline in the treatment of pedophilia: An open label study. *New Research Abstracts,* NR 441, American Psychiatric Association Annual Meeting.

Bradford, J. M. W., & Pawlak, A. (1987): Sadistic homosexual pedophilia: Treatment with cyproterone acetate: A single case study. *Canadian Journal of Psychiatry,* 32:22–31.

Bradford, J. M. W., & Pawlak, A. (1993): A double-blind placebo crossover study of CPA in treatment of paraphilias. *Archives of Sexual Behavior,* 22:383–402.

Brady, K. T., Sonne, S., & Lydiard, R. B. (1993): Valproate treatment of comorbid panic and affective disorders in two alcoholic patients. *Journal of Clinical Psychopharmacology,* 13:292–295.

Brady, K. T., Sonne, S. C., & Roberts, J. M. (1995): Sertraline treatment of comorbid posttraumatic stress disorder and alcohol dependence. *Journal of Clinical Psychiatry,* 56(11):502–505.

Briere, J. N. (1992): *Child Abuse Trauma: Theory and Treatment of the Lasting Effects.* Newbury Park, CA: Sage.

Brodaty, H. (1993): Think of depression—atypical presentations in the elderly. *Australian Family Physician,* 22(7):1195–1203.

Brown, G. R. (1995): Transvestism. In G. O. Gabbard (Ed.), *Treatments of Psychiatric Disorders* (2nd ed.): Washington, DC: American Psychiatric Press.

Brown, T. A., & Barlow, D. H. (1995): Long-term outcome in cognitive-behavioral treatment of panic disorder: Clinical predictors and alternative strategies for assessment. *Journal of Consulting Clinical Psychology,* 63(5):754–765.

Brown, T. A., Barlow, D. H., & Liebowitz, M. R. (1994): The empirical basis of generalized anxiety disorder. *American Journal of Psychiatry,* 151(9):1272–1280.

Buchele, B. J. (1993): Group psychotherapy for persons with multiple personality and dissociative disorders. *Bulletin of the Menninger Clinic,* 57(3):362–370.

Buffum, J. (1992): Prescription drugs and sexual function. *Psychiatric Medicine,* 10(2):181–198.

Bumpass, E. R., Brix, R. J., & Preston, B. (1985): A community-based program for juvenile firesetters. *Hospital and Community Psychiatry,* 36(5):529–533.

Bunnell, D. E., Treiber, S. P., Phillips, N. H., *et al.* (1992): Effects of evening bright light exposure on melatonin, body temperature and sleep. *Journal of Sleep Research,* 1:17–23.

Burstein, A. (1992): Fluoxetine-lithium treatment for kleptomania. *Journal of Clinical Psychiatry,* 53:28–29.

Butler, G., Fennell, M., Robson, P., *et al.* (1991): Comparison of behavior therapy and cognitive behavior therapy in the treatment of generalized anxiety disorder. *Journal of Consulting Clinical Psychology,* 59:167–175.

Buysse, D. J., Morin, C. M., & Reynolds, C. F. (1995): Sleep disorders. In G. O. Gabbard (Ed.), *Treatments of Psychiatric Disorders* (2nd ed.). Washington, DC: American Psychiatric Press.

Byrne, A., & Yatham, L. N. (1989): Pimozide in pathological jealousy. *British Journal of Psychiatry,* 155:249–251.

Cacciola, J. S., Alterman, A. I., Rutherford, M. J., & Snider, E. C. (1995): Treatment response of antisocial substance abusers. *Journal of Nervous and Mental Diseases,* 183(3):166–171.

Calabrese, J. R., Kimmel, S. E., Woyshville, M. J., *et al.* (1996): Clozapine for treatment-refractory mania. *American Journal Psychiatry,* 153(6):759–764.

Calabrese, J. R., & Woyshville, M. J. (1995): A medication algorithm for treatment of bipolar rapid cycling? *Journal of Clinical Psychiatry* 56(suppl 3):11–18.

Carney, F. (1978): Inpatient treatment programs. In W. H. Reid (Ed.), *The Psychopath: A Comprehensive Study of Antisocial Disorders and Behaviors.* New York: Brunner/Mazel.

Carpenter, W. T., Jr., Conley, R. R., Buchanan, R. W., *et al.* (1995): Patient response and resource management: Another view of clozapine treatment of schizophrenia. *American Journal of Psychiatry,* 152(6):827–832.

Centorrino, F., Baldessarini, R. J., Frankenburg, F. R., *et al.* (1996). Serum levels of clozapine and norclozapine in patients treated with selective serotonin reuptake inhibitors. *American Journal of Psychiatry,* 153(6):820–822.

Chambless, D. L., & Gillis, M. M. (1993): Cognitive therapy of anxiety disorders. *Journal of Consulting Clinical Psychology,* 61:248–260.

Chow, E. W., Collins, E. J., Nuttall, S. E., & Bassett, A. S. (1995): Clinical use of clozapine in a major urban setting: One year experience. *Journal of Psychiatry and Neuroscience,* 20(2):133–140.

Christenson, G. A., MacKenzie, T. B., & Mitchell, J. E. (1994): Adult men and women with trichotillomania. *Psychosomatics,* 35(2):142–149.

Christenson, G. A., Mackenzie, T. B., Mitchell, J. E., & Callies, A.L. (1991a): A placebo-controlled, double-blind crossover study of fluoxetine in trichotillomania. *American Journal of Psychiatry,* 148(11):1566–1571.

Christenson, G. A., Popkin, M. K., Mackenzie, T. B., *et al.* (1991b): Lithium treatment of chronic hair pulling. *Journal of Clinical Psychiatry,* 52:116–120.

Christison, G. W., Kirch, D. G., & Wyatt, R. J. (1991): When symptoms persist: Choosing among alternative somatic treatments for schizophrenia. *Schizophrenia Bulletin,* 17:217–245.

Cierpka, M. (1986): Zur psychodynamik der neurotisch bedingten kleptomanie. *Psychiatric Prax,* 13(3):94–103.

Cleckley, H. M. (1976): *The Mask of Sanity.* St. Louis: Mosby (privately reprinted, Emily Cleckley, 1988).

Coccaro, E. F., Astil, J. L., Herbert, J., *et al.* (1990): Fluoxetine treatment of impulsive aggression in DSM-III-R personality disorder patients. *Journal of Clinical Psychopharmacology,* 10:373–375.

Cohen, L. S., Sichel, D. A., Robertson, L. M., *et al.* (1995): Postpartum prophylaxis for women with bipolar disorder. *American Journal of Psychiatry,* 152(11):1641–1645.

Cole, J. O., & Yonkers, K. A. (1995): Nonbenzodiazepine anxiolytics. In A. F. Schatzberg & C. B. Nemeroff (Eds.), *American Psychiatric Press Textbook of Psychopharmacology.* Washington, DC: American Psychiatric Press.

Coons, P. M. (1986): Treatment progress in twenty patients with multiple personality disorder. *Journal of Nervous and Mental Diseases,* 174(12):715–721.

Cooper, A. J. (1987): Treatment of coexistent night-terrors and somnambulism in adults with imipramine and diazepam. *Journal of Clinical Psychiatry,* 48:209–210.

Cooper, A. J., Sandhu, S., Losztyn, S., *et al.* (1992): A double-blind placebo controlled trial of medroxyprogesterone acetate and cyproterone acetate with seven pedophiles. *Canadian Journal of Psychiatry,* 37:687–693.

Cooper, P. J., Coker, S., & Fleming, C. (1994): Self-help for bulimia nervosa: A preliminary report. *International Journal of Eating Disorders,* 16(4):401–404.

Cooper, T. B., Bergner, P. E., & Simpson, G. M. (1973): The 24-hour serum lithium level as a prognosticator of dosage requirements. *American Journal of Psychiatry,* 130:601–603.

Cornelius, J. R., Soloff, P. H., Perel, J. M., & Ulrich, R. F. (1993): Continuation pharmacotherapy of borderline personality disorder with haloperidol and phenelzine. *American Journal of Psychiatry,* 150(12):1843–1848.

Cottraux, J., Note, I. D., Cungi, C., *et al.* (1995): A controlled study of cognitive behaviour therapy with buspirone or placebo in panic disorder with agoraphobia. *British Journal of Psychiatry,* 167(5):635–641.

Cowdry, R. W., & Gardner, D. L. (1988): Pharmacotherapy of borderline personality disorder: Alprazolam, carbamazepine, trifluoperazine and tranylcypromine. *Archives of General Psychiatry,* 45:111–119.

Craske, M. G., Mohlman, J., Yi, J., *et al.* (1995): Treatment of claustrophobias and snake/spider phobias: Fear of arousal and fear of context. *Behavior Research and Therapy,* 33(2):197–203.

Cross-National Collaborative Panic Study Second Phase Investigators (1992): Drug treatment of panic disorder: Comparative efficacy of alprazolam, imipramine, and placebo. *British Journal of Psychiatry* 160:191–202 (see also corrections in *British Journal of Psychiatry,* 161:724).

Croughan, J. L., Saghir, M., Cohen, R., *et al.* (1981): A comparison of treated and untreated male cross-dressers. *Archives of Sexual Behavior,* 10(6):515–528.

Cullington, C. J. (1976): Psychosurgery: National commission issues surprisingly favorable report. *Science,* 194:229–301.

Cumming, S., Hay, P., Lee, T., & Sachdev, P. (1995): Neuropsychological outcome from psychosurgery for obsessive-compulsive disorder. *Australia and New Zealand Journal of Psychiatry* 29(2):293–298.

Curran, H. V., Bond, A., O'Sullivan, G., *et al.* (1994): Memory functions, alprazolam and exposure therapy: A controlled longitudinal study of agoraphobia with panic disorder. *Psychological Medicine,* 24(4):969–976.

Curtis, J. M. (1995): Elements of critical incident debriefing. *Psychological Reports,* 77(1):91–96.

Dalton, R., Haslett, N., & Baul, G. (1986): Alternative therapy with a recalcitrant firesetter. *Journal of the American Academy of Child Psychiatry,* 25(5):715–717.

Dantzler, A., & Salzman, C. (1995): Treatment of bipolar depression. *Psychiatric Services,* 46(3):229–238.

Davidson, J. R., Beitman, B., Greist, J. H., *et al.* (1994): Adinazolam sustained-release treatment of panic disorder: A double-blind study. *Journal of Clinical Psychopharmacology,* 14(4):255–263.

Davidson, J. R., Petts, N., Richichi, E., *et al.* (1993): Treatment of social phobia with clonazepam and placebo. *Journal of Clinical Psychopharmacology,* 13:423–428.

de Beurs, E., van Balkom, A. J., Lange, A., *et al.* (1995): Treatment of panic disorder with agoraphobia: Comparison of fluvoxamine, placebo, and psychological panic management combined with exposure and of exposure *in vivo* alone. *American Journal of Psychiatry,* 152(5):683–691.

Delini-Stula, A., Mikkelsen, H., & Angst, J. (1995): Therapeutic efficacy of antidepressants in agitated anxious depression: A meta-analysis of moclobemide studies. *Journal of Affective Disorders,* 9;35(1–2):21–30.

Delle Chiaie, R., Pancheri, P., Casacchia, M., *et al.* (1995): Assessment of the efficacy of buspirone in patients affected by generalized anxiety disorder, shifting to buspirone from prior treatment with lorazepam: A placebo-controlled, double-blind study. *Journal of Clinical Psychopharmacology,* 15(1):12–19.

Deltito, J. A., & Stam, M. (1989): Pharmacological treatment of avoidant personality disorder. *Comprehensive Psychiatry,* 30:498–504.

den Boer, J. A., Westenberg, H. G., De Leeuw, A. S., & van Vliet, I. M. (1995): Biological dissection of anxiety disorders: The clinical role of selective serotonin reuptake inhibitors with particular reference to fluvoxamine. *International Clinical Psychopharmacology,* 9(suppl 4):47–52.

den Boer, J. A., van Vliet, I. M., & Westenberg, H. G. (1995): Recent developments in the psychopharmacology of social phobia. *European Archives of Psychiatry and Clinical Neuroscience,* 244(6):309–316.

Dencker, S. J., & Dencker, K. (1994): Does community care reduce the need for psychiatric beds for schizophrenic patients? *Acta Psychiatrica Scandinavica,* 382(suppl):74–79.

de Vito, R. A. (1993): The use of amytal interviews in the treatment of an exceptionally complex case of multiple personality disorder. In R.P. Kluft & C. G. Fine (Eds.), *Clinical Perspectives on Multiple Personality Disorder.* R.P. Washington, DC: American Psychiatric Press.

Dewulf, L., Hendrickx, B., & Lesaffre E. (1995): Epidemiological data of patients treated with fluvoxamine: Results from a 12 week non-comparative multicentre study. *International Clinical Psychopharmacology,* 9(suppl 4):67–72.

Dilsaver, S. C., Swann, A. C., Shoaib, A. M., *et al.* (1993): Depressive mania associated with nonresponse to antimanic agents. *American Journal of Psychiatry,* 150:1548–1551.

Dobson, D. J., McDougall, G., Busheikin, J., & Aldous, J. (1995): Effects of social skills training and social milieu treatment on symptoms of schizophrenia. *Psychiatric Services,* 46(4):376–380.

Dominguez, R. A., & Mestre, S. M. (1994): Management of treatment-refractory obsessive-compulsive disorder patients. *Journal of Clinical Psychiatry,* 55(suppl):86–92.

Drug Administration Office (Sweden) and State Drug Control (Norway) (1995): Recommendations for drug therapy in anxiety. Serotoninergic agents to replace benzodiazepines. *Lakartidningen* 92(12):1256–1261.

Dubowsky S. L. (1995): Calcium channel antagonists as novel agents for manic-depressive disorder. In A. F. Schazberg & C. B. Nemeroff (Eds.), *American Psychiatric Press Textbook of Psychopharmacology.* Washington, DC: American Psychiatric Press.

Dubovsky, S. L. & Thomas, M. (1992): Psychotic depression: Advances in conceptualization and treatment. *Hospital and Community Psychiatry,* 43(12):733–745.

Earle, J. R., Jr., & Folks, D. G. (1986): Factitious disorder and coexisting depression: A report of successful psychiatric consultation and case management. *General Hospital Psychiatry,* 8(6):448–450.

Eckman, T. A., Wirshing, W. C., Marder, S. R., *et al.* (1992): Technique for training schizophrenic patients in illness self-management: A controlled trial. *American Journal of Psychiatry,* 149(11):1549–1555.

Ehlers, A. (1995): A 1-year prospective study of panic attacks: Clinical course and factors associated with maintenance. *Journal of Abnormal Psychology,* 104(1):164–172.

Eichelman, B. (1992): Aggressive behavior: From laboratory to clinic. Quo vadit? *Archives of General Psychiatry,* 49:488–492.

Eichelman, B., & Hartwig, A. (1993): The clinical psychopharmacology of violence. *Psychopharmacology Bulletin,* 29:57–63.

Eisendrath, S. J. (1989): Factitious physical disorders: Treatment without confrontation. *Psychosomatics,* 30:383–387.

Elkin, I., Shea, M. T., Watkins, J. T., *et al.* (1989): General effectiveness of treatments. Part I of the Treatment of Depression Collaborative Research Program, National Institute of Mental Health. *Archives General Psychiatry,* 46:971–982.

Elliott, F. A. (1977): Propranolol for the control of belligerent behavior following acute brain damage. *Annals of Neurology,* 1:489–491.

Elliott, F. A. (1978): Neurological aspects of antisocial behavior, In W.H. Reid (Ed.), *The Psychopath: A Comprehensive Study of Antisocial Disorders and Behaviors* New York: Brunner/Mazel.

Elliott, F. A. (1990): Neurology of aggression and episodic dyscontrol. *Seminars in Neurology,* 10:303–311.

Emmanuel, N. P., Lydiard, R. B., & Ballenger, J. C. (1991): Fluoxetine treatment of voyeurism. *American Journal of Psychiatry,* 148:950.

Essa, M. (1986): Grief as a crisis: Psychotherapeutic interventions with elderly bereaved. *American Journal of Psychotherapy,* 40(2):243–251.

Fahy, T. A., & Eisler, I., & Russell, G. F. (1993): A placebo-controlled trial of d-fenfluramine in bulimia nervosa. *British Journal of Psychiatry,* 162:597–603.

Fahy, T. A., & Russell, G. F. (1993): Outcome and prognostic variables in bulimia nervosa. *International Journal of Eating Disorders,* 14(2):135–145.

Fairburn, C. G., Jones, R., Peveler, R. C., *et al.* (1991): Three psychological treatments for bulimia nervosa: A comparative trial. *Archives of General Psychiatry,* 48:463–469.

Fallon, B. A., Campeas, R., Schneier, F. R., *et al.* (1992): Open trial of intravenous clomipramine in 5 treatment-refractory patients with obsessive-compulsive disorder. *Journal of Neuropsychiatry and Clinical Neuroscience,* 4:70–75.

Fallon, B. A., Liebowitz, M. R., Salman, E., *et al.* (1994): Fluoxetine for hypochondriacal patients without major depression. *Journal of Clinical Psychopharmacology,* 13:438–441.

Faravelli, C., Paterniti, S., & Scarpato, A. (1995): 5-year prospective, naturalistic follow-up study of panic disorder. *Comprehensive Psychiatry,* 36(4):271–277.

Fava, G. A., Grandi, S., Zielezny, M., *et al.* (1994): Cognitive behavioral treatment of residual symptoms in primary major depressive disorder. *American Journal of Psychiatry,* 151(9):1295–1299.

Fava, G. A., Zielezny, M., Savron, G., & Grandi S. (1995): Long-term effects of behavioural treatment for panic disorder with agoraphobia. *British Journal of Psychiatry*, 166(1):87–92.

Fava, M., Rosenbaum, J. F., Pava, J. A., *et al.* (1993): Anger attacks in unipolar depression, Part 1: Clinical correlates and response to fluoxetine treatment. *American Journal of Psychiatry*, 150(8):1158–1163.

Fedoroff, J. P. (1988): Buspirone hydrochloride in the treatment of transvestic fetishism. *Journal of Clinical Psychiatry*, 49:408–409.

Fedoroff, J. P. (1992): Buspirone hydrochloride in the treatment of an atypical paraphilia. *Archives of Sexual Behavior*, 21:401–406.

Fedoroff, J. P. (1993): Serotonergic drug treatment of deviant sexual interests. *Annals of Sex Research*, 6:105–121.

Fenton, W. S., & Cole, S. A. (1995): Psychosocial therapies of schizophrenia: Individual, group, and family. In G. O. Gabbard (Ed.), *Treatments of Psychiatric Disorders*, (2nd ed.), Washington, DC: American Psychiatric Press.

Finkel, M. J. (1984): Phenytoin revisited. *Clinical Therapeutics*, 6(5):577–591.

Fishbain, D. A. (1987): Kleptomania as risk-taking behavior in response to depression. *American Journal of Psychotherapy*, 41:598–603.

Fishbain, D. A. (1988): Kleptomanic behavior response to perphenazine-amitriptyline combination. *Canadian Journal of Psychiatry*, 33(3):241–242.

Fisher, C., Kahn, E., Edwards, A., *et al.* (1973): A psychophysiological study of nightmares and night terrors: The suppression of stage 4 night terrors with diazepam. *Archives of General Psychiatry*, 28:252–259.

Flor, H., Fydrich, T., & Turk, D. C. (1992): Efficacy of multidisciplinary pain treatment centers: A meta-analytic review. *Pain*, 49:221–230.

Fluoxetine Bulimia Nervosa Collaborative Study Group (1992): Fluoxetine in the treatment of bulimia nervosa: A multicenter, placebo-controlled, double blind trial. *Archives of General Psychiatry*, 49:139–147.

Foa, E. B., Davidson, J., & Rothbaum, B. O. (1995): Posttraumatic stress disorder, In G.O. Gabbard (Ed.), *Treatments of Psychiatric Disorders*, (2nd ed.), Washington, DC: American Psychiatric Press.

Foa, E. B., Hearst-Ikeda, D., & Perry, K. J. (1995): Evaluation of a brief cognitive-behavioral program for the prevention of chronic PTSD in recent assault victims. *Journal of Consulting Clinical Psychology*, 63(6):948–955.

Foa, E. B., & Riggs, D. S. (1993): Post-traumatic stress disorder in rape victims, In J. Oldham, M. B. Riba, & A. Tasman (Eds.), *American Psychiatric Press Review of Psychiatry*, vol 12. Washington DC: American Psychiatric Press.

Folks, D. G., & Freeman, A. M., III (1985): Munchausen syndrome and other factitious illness. *Psychiatric Clinics of North America*, 8(2):263–278.

Ford, C. V. (1995): Conversion disorder and somatoform disorder NOS. In G.O. Gabbard (Ed.), *Treatments of Psychiatric Disorders* (2nd ed.), Washington, DC: American Psychiatric Press.

Frances, A., & Wise, T. N. (1987): Treating a man who wears women's clothes. *Hospital and Community Psychiatry*, 38(3):233–234.

Frank, E., Kupfer, D. J., Perel, J. M., *et al.* (1990): Three year outcomes for maintenance therapies in recurrent depression. *Archives of General Psychiatry*, 48:1093–1099.

Frankel, F. H. (1993): Adult reconstruction of childhood events in the multiple personality literature. *American Journal of Psychiatry,* 150:954–958.

Frankenburg, F. R., & Zanarini, M. C. (1993): Clozapine treatment of borderline patients: A preliminary study. *Comprehensive Psychiatry,* 34(6):402–405.

Freeman, C. P., Trimble, M. R., Deakin, J. F., et al. (1994): Fluvoxamine versus clomipramine in the treatment of obsessive compulsive disorder: A multicenter, randomized, double-blind, parallel group comparison. *Journal of Clinical Psychiatry,* 55(7):301–305.

Freund, K. (1980): Therapeutic sex drive reduction. *Acta Psychiatrica Scandinavica,* 287:5–38.

Friedman, R. A., Mitchell, J., & Kocsis, J. H. (1995): Retreatment for relapse following desipramine discontinuation in dysthymia. *American Journal of Psychiatry,* 152(6):926–928.

Frommer, M. S., Ames, J. R., Gibson, J. W. et al. (1987): Patterns of symptom change in the short-term group treatment of bulimia. *International Journal of Eating Disorders,* 6:469–476.

Frye, M. A., Altshuler, L. L., Szuba, M. P., et al. (1996): The relationship between antimanic agent for treatment of classic or dysphoric mania and length of hospital stay. *Journal of Clinical Psychiatry,* 57(1):17–21.

Gabbard, G. O. (1994): Mind and brain in psychiatric treatment. *Bulletin of the Menninger Clinic,* 58(4):427–446.

Gacono, C., & Meloy, J. R. (1991): A Rorschach investigation of attachment and anxiety in antisoocial personality disorder. *Journal of Nervous and Mental Diseases,* 179:546–552.

Gaffan, E. A., Tsaousis I., & Kemp-Wheeler, S. M. (1995): Researcher allegiance and meta-analysis: The case of cognitive therapy for depression. *Journal of Consulting and Clinical Psychology,* 63(6):966–980.

Gamino, L. A., Elkins, G. R., & Hackney, K. V. (1989): Emergency management of mass psychogenic illness. *Psychosomatics,* 30:446–449.

Garfinkel, P. E., & Goldbloom, D. S. (1993): Bulimia nervosa. *Journal of Psychotherapy Practice and Research,* 2(1):38–50.

Garma, L., Marchand, F. (1994): Non-pharmacological approaches to the treatment of narcolepsy. *Sleep* 17(suppl 8):S97–S102.

Garner, D. M., Fairburn, C. G., & Davis, R. (1987): Cognitive-behavioral treatment of bulimia nervosa. *Behavior Modification,* 11:398–431.

Garza-Trevino, E. S. (1994): Neurobiological factors in aggressive behavior. *Hospital and Community Psychiatry,* 45(7):690–699.

Gelernter, C. S., Uhde, T. W., Cimbolic, P., et al. (1991): Cognitive-behavioral and pharmacological treatments of social phobia: A controlled study. *Archives of General Psychiatry,* 48:938–945.

Geller, J. L. (1992): Arson in review. From profit to pathology. *Psychiatric Clinics of North America,* 15(3):623–645.

George, W. H., Marlatt, G. A. (1990): *Relapse Prevention With Sexual Offenders: A Treatment Manual.* Tampa, FL: Florida Mental Health Institute.

George, M. S., Wassermann, E. M., Williams, W. A., et al. (1995): Daily repetitive transcranial magnetic stimulation (rTMS) improves mood in depression. *Neuroreport,* 2;6(14):1853–1856.

Geracioti, T. D. Jr. (1995): Venlafaxine treatment of panic disorder: A case series. *Journal of Clinical Psychiatry*, 56(9):408–410.

Gitlin, M. J. (1993): Pharmacology of personality disorders: Conceptual framework and clinical strategies. *Journal of Clinical Psychopharmacology* 13(5):343–353.

Gitlin, M. J., Swendsen J., Heller T. L., & Hammen, C. (1995): Relapse and impairment in bipolar disorder. *American Journal of Psychiatry*, 152(11):1635–1640.

Glazer, W. M. & Kane, J. M. (1992): Depot neuroleptic therapy: An underutilized treatment option. *Journal of Clinical Psychiatry*, 53(12):426–433.

Glazer, W. M., Morgenstern, H., Schooler, N., *et al.* (1990): Predictors of improvement in tardive dyskinesia following discontinuation of neuroleptic medication. *British Journal of Psychiatry*, 157:585–592.

Glover, J. H. (1985): A case of kleptomania treated by covert sensitization. *British Journal of Clinical Psychology*, 24:213–214.

Goisman, R. M., Warshaw, M. G., Steketee, G. S., *et al.* (1995): DSM-IV and the disappearance of agoraphobia without a history of panic disorder: New data on a controversial diagnosis. *American Journal of Psychiatry*, 152:1438–1443.

Goldberg, J. F., Harrow, M., & Grossman, L. S. (1995a): Recurrent affective syndromes in bipolar and unipolar mood disorders at follow-up. *British Journal of Psychiatry*, 166(3):382–385.

Goldberg, J. F., Harrow, M., & Grossman, L. S. (1995b): Course and outcome in bipolar affective disorder: A longitudinal follow-up study. *American Journal of Psychiatry*, 152(3):379–384.

Goldbloom, D. S., & Olmsted, M. P. (1993): Pharmacotherapy of bulimia nervosa with fluoxetine: Assessment of clinically significant attitudinal change. *American Journal of Psychiatry*, 150:770–774.

Goldman, H. W., Cooper, I. S., Simpson, G. M., *et al.* (1985): Reversal of severe tardive dyskinesia and dystonia following bilateral CT-guided stereotactic thalatomy (abstract). Fourth World Congress of Biological Psychiatry, Philadephia.

Goldstein, W. N. (1993): Psychotherapy with the borderline patient: An introduction. *American Journal of Psychotherapy*, 47(2):172–183.

Goodnick, P. J. (1993): Verapamil prophylaxis in pregnant women with bipolar disorder (letter). *American Journal of Psychiatry*, 150(10):156.

Grame, C. J. (1993): Internal containment in the treatment of patients with dissociative disorders. *Bulletin of the Menninger Clinic*, 57(3):355–361.

Green, A. H. (1994): Victims of child abuse. In *American Psychiatric Press Review of Psychiatry* vol. 13. Washington, DC: American Psychiatric Press.

Gregoire, A. J., Kumar, R, Everitt, B., *et al.* (1996): Transdermal oestrogen for treatment of severe postnatal depression. *Lancet*, 347(9006):930–933.

Greist, J. H. (1994): Behavior therapy for obsessive compulsive disorder. *Journal of Clinical Psychiatry*, 55 (suppl):60–68.

Greist, J. H., Jefferson, J. W., Kobak, K. A., *et al.* (1995): Efficacy and tolerability of serotonin transport inhibitors in obsessive-compulsive disorder: A meta-analysis. *Archives of General Psychiatry*, 52(1):53–60.

Hage, J. J., Karim, R. B., Bloem, J. J., *et al.* (1994): Sculpturing the neoclitoris in vaginoplasty for male-to-female transsexuals. *Plastic and Reconstructive Surgery*, 93(2):358–364.

Haldeman, D. C. (1994): The practice and ethics of sexual orientation conversion therapy. *Journal of Consulting Clinical Psychology,* 62(2):221–227.

Haldeman, S., & Rubinstein, S. M. (1993): The precipitation or aggravation of musculoskeletal pain in patients receiving spinal manipulative therapy. *Journal of Manipulative Physiological Therapy,* 16(1):47–50.

Halmi, K. A. (1994): Eating disorders: Anorexia nervosa, bulimia nervosa, and obesity. In R. E. Hales, S. C. Yudofsky, & J. A. Talbott (Eds.), *American Psychiatric Association Textbook of Psychiatry,* (2nd ed.) Washington, DC: American Psychiatric Press.

Hardy, G. E., Barkham, M., Shapiro, D. A., *et al.* (1995): Impact of cluster C personality disorders on outcomes of contrasting brief psychotherapies for depression. *Journal of Consulting Clinical Psychology,* 63(6):997–1004.

Hare, R. D. (1991): *The Hare Psychopathy Checklist, Revised* (manual). Toronto: Multi-Health Systems.

Hedges, B. E., Dimsdale, J. E. & Hoyt, D. B. (1995): Munchausen syndrome presenting as recurrent multiple trauma. *Psychosomatics,* 36(1):60–63

Heim, N., & Hursch, C. J. (1979): Castration for sexual offenders: Treatment or punishment? A review and critique of recent European literature. *Archives of Sexual Behavior,* 8:281–304.

Heimberg, R. G., Salzman, D. G., Holt, C. S., *et al.* (1993): Cognitive behavioral group treatment for social phobia: Effectiveness at five-year follow-up. *Cognitive Therapy Research,* 17:325–339.

Hellerstein, D. J., Yanowitch, P., Rosenthal, J., *et al.* (1993): Randomized double-blind study of fluoxetine versus placebo in the treatment of dysthymia. *American Journal of Psychiatry,* 150(8):1169–1175.

Hemmeter, U., Seifritz, E., Hatzinger, M., *et al.* (1995): Serial partial sleep deprivation as adjuvant treatment of depressive insomnia. *Progress in Neuropsychopharmacology and Biological Psychiatry* 19(4):593–602.

Herman, J. L. (1992): *Trauma and Recovery.* New York: Basic Books.

Hirschfeld, R. M. A., Clayton, P., Cohen, I., *et al.* (1995): *American Psychiatric Association Practice Guideline for Treatment of Patients with Bipolar Disorder.* Washington, DC: American Psychiatric Press.

Hiss, H., Foa, E. B., & Kozak, M. J. (1994): Relapse prevention program for treatment of obsessive-compulsive disorder. *Journal of Consulting and Clinical Psychology,* 62(4):801–808.

Hodgkiss, A. D., Malizia, A. L., Bartlett, J. R., & Bridges, P. K. (1995): Outcome after the psychosurgical operation of stereotactic subcaudate tractotomy, 1979–1991. *Journal of Neuropsychiatry and Clinical Neuroscience,* 7(2):230–234.

Hoehn-Saric, R., Borkovec, T. D., & Nemiah, J. C. (1995): Generalized anxiety disorder. In G. O. Gabbard (Ed.), *Treatments of Psychiatric Disorders (2nd ed.).* Washington, DC: American Psychiatric Press.

Hoehn-Saric, R., Lipsey, J. R., & McLeod, D. R. (1990): Apathy and indifference in patients on fluvoxamine and fluoxetine. *Journal of Clinical Psychopharmacology,* 10:343–345.

Hoffart, A. (1993): Cognitive treatments of agoraphobia: A critical evaluation of theoretical basis and outcome evidence. *Journal of Anxiety Disorders* 7:75–91.

Hoffart, A. (1995): A comparison of cognitive and guided mastery therapy of agoraphobia. *Behavior in Research and Therapy,* 33(4):423–434.

Hollander, E., & Cohen, L. J. (1994): The assessment and treatment of refractory anxiety. *Journal of Clinical Psychiatry,* 55(suppl):27–31.

Hollander, E., Frenkel, M., DeCaria, C., *et al.* (1992): Treatment of pathological gambling with clomipramine. *American Journal of Psychiatry,* 149:710–711.

Hollander, E., Liebowitz, M. R., DeCaria, C., *et al.* (1990): Treatment of depersonalization with serotonin reuptake blockers. *Journal of Clinical Psychopharmacology,* 10:200–203.

Hollon, S. D., DeRubeis, R. J., Evans, M. D., *et al.* (1992): Cognitive therapy and pharmacotherapy for depression: Singly and in combination. *Archives of General Psychiatry,* 49:774–781.

Honigfeld, G. (1995): Sandoz Clozaril Database. Information available from Sandoz (now Novartis) Pharmaceuticals Corp., East Hanover, NJ.

Hope, D. A., Heimberg, R. G., & Bruch, M. A. (1995): Dismantling cognitive-behavioral group therapy for social phobia. *Behavior Research and Therapy* 33(6):637–650.

Hopkins, H. S., & Gelenberg, A. J. (1994): Treatment of bipolar disorder: How far have we come? *Psychopharmacology Bulletin,* 30(1):27–38.

Horowitz, M. J. (1986): Stress-response syndromes: A review of posttraumatic and adjustment disorders. *Hospital and Community Psychiatry,* 37(3):241–249.

Horowitz, M. J. (1991): *Hysterical Personality Style and the Histrionic Personality Disorder.* Northvale, NJ: Jason Aronson.

Horowitz, M. J. (1995): Histrionic personality disorder. In G. O. Gabbard (Ed.), *Treatments of Psychiatric Disorders,* (2nd ed.). Washington, DC: American Psychiatric Press.

Hucker, S. J., Langevin, J., & Bain, J. (1989): A double-blind trial of sex drive reducing medication in pedophiles. *Annals of Sexual Research,* 1:227–242.

Hughes, P. L., Wells, L. A., Cunningham, C. J., & Ilstrup, D. M. (1986): Treating bulimia with desipramine: A double-blind placebo-controlled study. *Archives of General Psychiatry,* 43:182–186.

Hurlbert, D. F. (1993): A comparative study using orgasm consistency training in the treatment of women reporting hypoactive sexual desire. *Journal of Sex and Marital Therapy,* 19(1):41–55.

Hurwitz, T. D., Mahowald, M. W., Schnenck, C. H., *et al.* (1991): A retrospective outcome study and review of hypnosis as treatment of adults with sleepwalking and sleep terror. *Journal of Nervous and Mental Disease,* 179:228–233.

Hyler, S. B., Sussman, N. (1981): Chronic factitious disorder with physical symptoms (the Munchausen syndrome). *Psychiatric Clinics of North America,* 4(2):365–377.

Hymowitz, P., Frances, A., Jacobsberg, L. B. *et al.* (1986): Neuroleptic treatment of schizotypal personality disorder. *Comprehensive Psychiatry,* 27(4):267–271.

Iijima, S., Sugita, Y., Teshima, Y., & Hishikawa, Y. (1986): Therapeutic effects of mazindol on narcolepsy. *Sleep,* 9(1):265–268.

Ito, L. M., Marks, I. M., de Araujo, L. A., & Hemsley, D. (1995): Does imagined exposure to the consequences of not ritualising enhance live exposure for OCD? A controlled study. II. Effect on behavioural *v.* subjective concordance of improvement. *British Journal of Psychiatry* 167(1):71–75.

Jacobsen, F. M. (1993): Low-dose valproate: A new treatment for cyclothymia, mild rapid-cycling disorders, and premenstrual syndrome. *Journal of Clinical Psychiatry* 54(6):229–234.

Jacobsen, F. M. (1995): Risperidone in the treatment of affective illness and obsessive-compulsive disorder. *Journal of Clinical Psychiatry* 56(9):423–429.

Jacobson, N. S., Wilson, L., & Tupper, C. (1988): The clinical significance of treatment gains resulting from exposure-based interventions for agoraphobia: A reanalysis of outcome data. *Behavior Therapy,* 19:539–554.

James, I. A., & Blackburn, I. M. (1995): Cognitive therapy with obsessive-compulsive disorder. *British Journal of Psychiatry,* 166(4):444–450.

James, S. P., Sack, D. A., Rosenthal, N. E., & Mendelson, W. B. (1990): Melatonin administration in insomnia. *Neuropsychopharmacology* 3:19–23.

Jefferson, J. W. (1995): Social phobia: A pharmacologic treatment overview. *Journal of Clinical Psychiatry,* 56(suppl)(5):18–24.

Jefferson, J. W., & Greist, J.H. (1994): Mood disorders. In R. E. Hales, S. C. Yudofsky, & J. A. Talbott, (Eds.), *American Psychiatric Press Textbook of Psychiatry* (2nd ed.). Washington, DC: American Psychiatric Press.

Jefferson, J. W., Griest, J. H., Ackerman, D. L., *et al.* (1987): *Lithium Encyclopedia for Clinical Practice* (2nd ed.). Washington, DC: American Psychiatric Press.

Jenkins, S. C., & Maruta, T. (1987): Therapeutic use of propranolol for intermittent explosive disorder. *Mayo Clinic Proceedings,* 62(3):204–214.

Jiggetts, S. M., & Hall, D. P., Jr. (1995): Helping the helper: 528th Combat Stress Center in Somalia. *Military Medicine,* 160(6):275–277.

Jimenez, J. P. (1993): A fundamental dilemma of psychoanalytic technique: Reflections on the analysis of a perverse paranoid patient. *International Journal of Psychoanalysis,* 74 (3):487–504.

Joffe, R. T., & Swinson, R. P. (1990): Tranylcypromine in primary obsessive-compulsive disorder. *Journal of Anxiety Disorders* 4:365–367.

Johnson, C., Shenoy, R. S., & Langer, S. (1981): Relaxation therapy for somatoform disorders. *Hospital and Community Psychiatry,* 32(6):423–424.

Johnson, D. R., Feldman, S. C., Lubin, H., & Southwick, S. M. (1995): The therapeutic use of ritual and ceremony in the treatment of post-traumatic stress disorder. *Journal of Traumatic Stress* 8(2):283–298.

Jorgensen, P. (1994): Course and outcome in delusional beliefs. *Psychopathology,* 27(1–2):89–99.

Kafka, M. P. (1991): Successful treatment of paraphiliac coercive disorder (a rapist) with fluoxetine hydrochloride. *British Journal of Psychiatry,* 158:844–847.

Kafka, M. P. (1994): Sertraline pharmacotherapy for paraphilias and paraphilia-related disorders: An open trial. *Annals of Clinical Psychiatry* 6(3):189–195.

Kafka, M. P., & Coleman, E. (1991): Serotonin and paraphilias: The convergence of mood, impulse, and compulsive disorders. *Journal of Clinical Psychopharmacology,* 11:223–224.

Kafka, M. P., & Prentky, R. (1992): Fluoxetine treatment of nonparaphiliac sexual addictions and paraphilias in men. *Journal of Clinical Psychiatry,* 53:351–358.

Kaplan, H. S. (1986): *Sexual Aversions, Sexual Phobias, and Panic Disorders.* New York: Brunner/Mazel.

Kaplan, H. S. (1993): Post-ejaculatory pain disorder. *Journal of Sex and Marital Therapy,* 19:91–103.

Kaplan, H. S. (1995): *The Disorders of Sexual Desire: Dysfunctional Control of Sexual Motivation.* New York: Brunner/Mazel.

Kaplan, K. H., Goldenberg, D. L., & Galvin-Nadeau, M. (1993): The impact of a meditation-based stress reduction program on fibromyalgia. *General Hospital Psychiatry*, 15(5):284–289.

Karasu, T. B., Docherty, J. P., Gelenberg, A., *et al.* (1993): *American Psychiatric Association Practice Guideline for Major Depressive Disorder in Adults.* Washington, DC: American Psychiatric Press.

Karterud, S., Vaglum, S., Friis, S., *et al.* (1992): Day hospital therapeutic community treatment for patients with personality disorders. An empirical evaluation of the containment function. *Journal of Nervous and Mental Disease,* 180(4):238–243.

Kashner, T. M., Rost, K., Cohen, B., *et al.* (1995): Enhancing the health of somatization disorder patients. *Psychosomatics,* 36(5):462–470.

Keck, P. E., McElroy, S. L., Strakowski, S. M., *et al.* (1996): Factors associated with maintenance antipsychotic treatment of patients with bipolar disorder. *Journal of Clinical Psychiatry,* 57(4):147–151.

Keck, P. E., Taylor, V., Tugrul, K. C., *et al.* (1993): Valproate treatment of panic disorder and lactate-induced panic attacks. *Biological Psychiatry,* 33:542–546.

Keijsers, G. P., Hoogduin, C. A., & Schaap, C. P. (1994): Predictors of treatment outcome in the behavioural treatment of obsessive-compulsive disorder. *British Journal of Psychiatry,* 165(6):781–786.

Kellner, R. (1992): Diagnosis and treatments of hypochondriacal syndromes. *Psychosomatics,* 33(3):278–289.

Kellner, R., Abbott, P., Winslow, W. W., *et al.* (1989): Anxiety, depression, and somatization in DSM-III hypochondriasis. *Psychosomatics,* 30:57–64.

Kennedy, S. H., Piran, N., Warsh, J. J., *et al.* (1988): A trial of isocarboxazid in the treatment of bulimia nervosa. *Journal of Clinical Psychopharmacology,* 8:391–396.

Kent, D. A., Tomasson, K., & Coryell, W. (1995): Course and outcome of conversion and somatization disorders. A four-year follow-up. *Psychosomatics,* 36(2):138–144.

King, S. A., & Stoudemire, A. (1995): Pain disorders. In G. O. Gabbard (Ed.), *Treatments of Psychiatric Disorders,* (2nd ed.). Washington, DC: American Psychiatric Press.

Kinon, B. J., Kane, J. M., Johns, C., *et al.* (1993): Treatment of neuroleptic-resistant schizophrenic relapse. *Psychopharmacology Bulletin,* 29:309–314.

Klein, D. F., Zitran, C. M., & Woerner, M. G. (1983): Treatment of phobias, II: Behavior therapy and supportive psychotherapy: Are there any specific ingredients? *Archives of General Psychiatry,* 40:139–145.

Klonoff, E. A., Youngner, S. J., Moore, E. J., *et al.* (1983): Chronic factitious illness: A behavioral approach. *International Journal of Psychiatry and Medicine,* 13(3):173–183.

Klosko, J. S., Barlow, D. H., Tassinari, R., & Cerny, J. A. (1990): A comparison of alprazolam and behavior therapy in treatment of panic disorder. *Journal of Consulting Clinical Psychology,* 58:77–84.

Kluft, R. P. (1991): Multiple personality disorder. In A. Tasman & S.M. Goldfinger, (Eds.), *Annual Review of Psychiatry,* Washington, DC: American Psychiatric Press.

Kluft, R. P. (1993): The treatment of dissociative disorder patients: An overview of discoveries, successes and failures. *Dissociation,* 6:87–101.

Kluft, R. P. (1995): Dissociative identity disorder. In G. O. Gabbard (Ed.), *Treatments of Psychiatric Disorders,* (2nd ed.), Washington, DC: American Psychiatric Press.

Koehler, K., & Sauer, H. (1983): First rank symptoms as predictors of ECT response in schizophrenia. *British Journal of Psychiatry,* 142:280.

Koles, M. R., & Jenson, W. R. (1985): Comprehensive treatment of chronic fire setting in a severely disordered boy. *Journal of Behavioral Therapy and Experimental Psychiatry,* 16(1):81–85.

Kolko, D. J. (1988): Community interventions for juvenile firesetters: A survey of two national programs. *Hospital and Community Psychiatry,* 39(9):973–979.

Koopmans, G. T., Meeuwesen, L., Huyse, F. J., *et al.* (1995): Effects of psychiatric consultation on medical consumption in medical outpatients with abdominal pain. *Psychosomatics,* 36(4):387–399.

Koran, L. M., Ringold, A., & Hewlett, W. (1992): Fluoxetine for trichotillomania: An open clinical trial. *Psychopharmacology Bulletin,* 28(2):145–149.

Krakow, B., Kellner, R., Neidhardt, J., *et al.* (1993): Imagery rehearsal treatment of chronic nightmares with a thirty month follow-up. *Journal of Behavioral Therapy and Experimental Psychiatry,* 24(4):325–330.

Krishman, R. R., Davidson, J., & Miller, R. (1984): MAO inhibitor therapy in trichotillomania associated with depression: Case report. *Journal of Clinical Psychiatry,* 45(6):267–268.

Kronig, M. H., Munne, R. A., Szymanski, S., *et al.* (1995): Plasma clozapine levels and clinical response for treatment-refractory schizophrenic patients. *American Journal of Psychiatry,* 152(2):179–182.

Kruesi, M. J. P., Fine, S., & Valladarcs, L. (1992): Paraphilias: A double-blind crossover comparison of clomipramine and desipramine. *Archives of Sexual Behavior,* 21:587–593.

Kutcher, S., Papatheodorou, G., Reiter, S., & Gardner, D. (1995): The successful pharmacological treatment of adolescents and young adults with borderline personality disorder: A preliminary open trial of flupenthixol. *Journal of Psychiatry and Neuroscience,* 20(2):113–118.

Lam, R. W., Goldner, E. M., Solyom, L., & Remick, R. A. (1994): A controlled study of light therapy for bulimia nervosa. *American Journal of Psychiatry,* 151(5):744–750.

Lam, R. W., Gorman, C. P., Michalon, M., *et al.* (1995): Multicenter, placebo-controlled study of fluoxetine in seasonal affective disorder. *American Journal of Psychiatry,* 152:1765–1770.

Lamontagne, Y., Lesage, A. (1986): Private exposure and covert sensitization in the treatment of exhibitionists. *Journal of Behavioral Therapy and Experimental Psychiatry,* 17(3):197–201.

Lang, A. E. (1995): Psychogenic dystonia: A review of 18 cases. *Canadian Journal of Neurological Science* 22(2):136–143.

Laws, D. R. (Ed.) (1989): *Relapse Prevention With Sex Offenders.* New York: Guilford.

Lecrubier, Y., Puech, A. J., Azcona, A., *et al.* (1993): A randomized double-blind placebo-controlled study of tropisetron in the treatment of outpatients with generalized anxiety disorder. *Psychopharmacology* (Berlin), 112(1):129–133.

Leibenluft, E., & Wehr, T. A. (1992): Is sleep deprivation useful in the treatment of depression? *American Journal of Psychiatry,* 149(2):159–168.

Leiblum, S. R., & Rosen, R. C. (1992): Couples therapy for erectile disorders: Observations, obstacles and outcomes. In R. C. Rosen, S. R. Leiblum (Eds.), *Erectile Disorders: Assessment and Treatment,* New York: Guilford.

Leitenberg, H., Rosen, J. C., Gross, J. *et al.* (1988): Exposure plus response-prevention treatment of bulimia nervosa. *Journal of Consulting Clinical Psychology,* 56:535–541.

Leitenberg, H., Rosen, J. C., Wolf, J., *et al.* (1994): Comparison of cognitive-behavior therapy and desipramine in the treatment of bulimia nervosa. *Behavior Research and Therapy,* 32(1):37–45.

Lenzi, A., Marazziti, D., Raffaelli, S., & Cassano, G. B. (1995): Effectiveness of the combination verapamil and chlorpromazine in the treatment of severe manic or mixed patients. *Progress in Neuropsychopharmacology and Biological Psychiatry,* 19(3):519–528.

Leonard, H. L., Lenane, M. D., Swedo, S. E., *et al.* (1991): A double-blind comparison of clomipramine and desipramine treatment of severe onychophagia (nail biting). *Archives of General Psychiatry,* 46:821–827.

Levinson, D. L., & Simpson, G. N. (1987): Antipsychotic drug side effects. In R. E. Hales & A. J. Francis (Eds.), *Psychiatry Update, Annual Review,* vol 6. Washington, DC: American Psychiatric Press.

Levinson, D. F., Simpson, G. M., Singh, H. *et al.* (1990): Fluphenazine dose, clinical response, and extrapyramidal symptoms during acute treatment. *Archives of General Psychiatry,* 47:761–768.

Liberman, R. P. (1992): Future prospects for psychiatric rehabilitation. In R. P. Liberman (Ed.), *Handbook of Psychiatric Rehabilitation.* New York: Macmillan.

Liberman, R. P. (1994): Psychosocial treatments for schizophrenia. *Psychiatry,* 57(2):104–114.

Lichstein, P. R. (1986): Caring for the patient with multiple somatic complaints. *Southern Medical Journal,* 79:310–314.

Licht, R. W., Gouliaev, G., Vestergaard, P., *et al.* (1994): Treatment of manic episodes in Scandinavia: The use of neuroleptic drugs in a clinical routine setting. *Journal of Affective Disorders,* 32(3):179–185.

Lichtenberg, P. A., Kimbarow, M. L., MacKinnon, D., *et al.* (1995): An interdisciplinary behavioral treatment program for depressed geriatric rehabilitation inpatients. *Gerontologist,* 35(5):688–690.

Lieberman, J. A., Safferman, A. Z., Pollack, S., *et al.* (1994): Clinical effects of clozapine in chronic schizophrenia: Response to treatment and predictors of outcome. *American Journal of Psychiatry,* 151(12):1744–1752.

Liebowitz, M. R., Quitkin, F. M., Stewart, J. W., *et al.* (1988): Antidepressant specificity in atypical depression. *Archives of General Psychiatry,* 45:129–137.

Liebowitz, M. R., Schneier, F., Campeas, R., *et al.* (1992): Phenelzine vs atenolol in social phobia: A placebo-controlled comparison. *Archives of General Psychiatry,* 49:290–300.

Lief, H. I., & Hubschman, L. (1993): Orgasm in the postoperative transsexual. *Archives of Sexual Behavior,* 22(2):145–155.

Lindskov, R., & Baadsgaard, O. (1985): Delusions of infestation treated with pimozide: A follow-up study. *Acta Derm Venereol* (Stockholm), 65(3):267–270.

Linehan, M. M. (1993): *Skills Training Manual for Treating Borderline Personality Disorder.* New York: Guilford.

Linehan, M. M., Armstrong, H. E., Suarez, A. *et al.* (1991): Cognitive-behavioral treatment of chronically parasuicidal borderline patients. *Archives of General Psychiatry,* 48(12):1060–1064.

Linehan, M. M., Tutek, D. A., Heard, H. L., & Armstrong, H. E. (1994): Interpersonal outcome of cognitive behavioral treatment for chronically suicidal borderline patients. *American Journal of Psychiatry,* 151(12):1771–1776.

Lion, J. R., & Scheinberg, A. W. (1995): Disorders of impulse control. In G. O. Gabbard (Ed.), *Treatments of Psychiatric Disorders.* Washington, DC: American Psychiatric Press.

Lipke, H. J., & Botkin, A. L. (1993): Case studies of eye movement desensitization and reprocessing (EMD/R) with chronic post-traumatic stress disorder. *Psychotherapy,* 29:591–595.

Lipsitt, D. R. (1995): Hypochondriasis and body dysmorphic disorder. In G. O. Gabbard (Ed.), *Treatments of Psychiatric Disorders* (2nd ed.). Washington, DC: American Psychiatric Press.

Longabaugh, R., Rubin, A., Malloy, P., *et al.* (1994): Drinking outcomes of alcohol abusers diagnosed as antisocial personality disorder. *Alcohol Clinics and Experimental Research,* 18(4):778–785.

Lopez-Ibor, J. J., & Carrasco, J. L. (1995): Pathological gambling. In E. Hollander & D. Stein (Eds.), *Impulsivity and Aggression.* New York: Wiley.

LoPiccolo, J. (1992): Postmodern sex therapy for erectile failure. In R. C. Rosen, & S. R. Leiblum (Eds.). *Erectile Disorders: Assessment and Treatment.* New York: Guilford.

LoPiccolo, J. (1994): Sexual dysfunction. In C. W. Craighead, W. E. Craighead, & A. E. Kazdin (Eds.), *Cognitive Behavioral Interventions.* New York: Pergamon.

LoPiccolo, J., & Daiss, S. (1988): Psychological issues in the evaluation of erectile failure. In E. Tanagho, T. F. Lue, & R. J. McClure, (Eds.). *Contemporary Management of Impotence and Infertility.* Baltimore: Williams & Wilkins.

Lorefice, L. S. (1991): Fluoxetine treatment of a fetish. *Journal of Clinical Psychiatry,* 52:41.

Lowenstein, R. J. (1995): Dissociative amnesia and dissociative fugue. In G. O. Gabbard (Ed.), *Treatments of Psychiatric Disorders.* Washington, DC: American Psychiatric Press.

Ludatscher, J. I. (1989): Stable remission of tardive dyskinesia by L-Dopa. *Journal of Clinical Psychopharmacology,* 9:39–41.

Lydiard, R. B., Ballenger, J. C. (1987): Antidepressants in panic disorder and agoraphobia. *Journal of the Affective Disorders,* 13:153–168.

Lydiard, R. B., Lesser, I. M., Ballenger, J. C., *et al.* (1992): A fixed-dose study of alprazolam 2 mg, alprazolam 6 mg, and placebo in panic disorder. *Journal of Clinical Psychopharmacology* 12:96–103.

Lydiard, R. B., Roy-Byrne, P. P., & Ballenger, J. C. (1988): Recent advances in the psychopharmacological treatment of anxiety disorders. *Hospital and Community Psychiatry,* 39:1157–1165.

Lykouras, L, Avgoustides, D., Papakostas, Y., & Stefanis C. (1995): Medication response to ECT-resistant melancholic patients. *Acta Psychiatrical Belgium* 95(3):113–121.

Lynch, P. J. (1993): Delusions of parasitosis. *Seminars in Dermatology,* 12(1):39–45.

Madhusoodanan, S., Brenner, R., Araujo, L., & Abaza, A. (1995): Efficacy of risperidone treatment for psychoses associated with schizophrenia, schizoaffective disorder, bipolar disorder, or senile dementia in 11 geriatric patients: A case series. *Journal of Clinical Psychiatry,* 56(11):514–518.

Magni, G. (1991): The use of antidepressants in the treatment of chronic pain: A review of the current evidence. *Drugs* 42:730–748.

Mahr, G. (1993): Fenfluramine and trichotillomania. *Psychosomatics,* 34(3):284.

Maj, M., Pirozzi, R., & Magliano, L. (1995): Nonresponse to reinstituted lithium prophylaxis in previously responsive bipolar patients: Prevalence and predictors. *American Journal of Psychiatry,* 152(12):1810–1711.

Maltsberger, J. T. (1994): Calculated risks in the treatment of intractably suicidal patients. *Psychiatry,* 57(3):199–212.

Marin, D. B., Kocsis, J. H., Frances, A. J., & Parides, M. (1994): Desipramine for the treatment of pure dysthymia versus double depression. *American Journal of Psychiatry,*151(7):1079–1080.

Markovitz, P. J., Calabrese, J. R., Schulz, S. C., & Meltzer, H. Y. (1991): Fluoxetine in the treatment of borderline and schizotypal personality disorders. *American Journal of Psychiatry,* 148:1064–1067.

Markowitz, J. C. (1994): Psychotherapy of dysthymia. *American Journal of Psychiatry,* 151(8):1114–1121.

Marks, I. M. (1995): Advances in behavioral-cognitive therapy of social phobia. *Journal of Clinical Psychiatry,* 56(suppl 5):25–31.

Marmar, C. R., Foy, D., Kagan, B., & Pynoos, R. S. (1993): An integrated approach for treating post-traumatic stress. In J. Oldham, M. B. Riba, & A. Tasman (Eds.), *American Psychiatric Press Review of Psychiatry,* Vol.12. Washington, DC: American Psychiatric Press.

Marshall, J. R. (1995): Integrated treatment of social phobia. *Bulletin of the Menninger Clinic,* 59(2)(suppl):A27–A37.

Marshall, W. L., Jones, R., Ward, T. *et al.* (1991): Treatment outcome with sex offenders. *Clinical Psychology Review,* 11:465–485.

Masters, W. H., & Johnson, V. E. (1970): *Human Sexual Inadequacy.* Boston: Little, Brown.

Mattes, J. A. (1985): Metoprolol for intermittent explosive disorder. *American Journal of Psychiatry,* 142:1108–1109.

Mattes, J. A. (1986a): Propranolol for adults with temper outbursts and residual attention deficit disorder. *Journal of Clinical Psychopharmacology* 6(5):299–302.

Mattes, J. A. (1986b): Psychopharmacology of temper outbursts. A review. *Journal of Nervous and Mental Disease,* 174(8):464–470.

Mattes, J. A. (1990): Comparative effectiveness of carbamazepine and propranolol for rage outbursts. *Journal of Neuropsychiatry and Clinical Neuroscience,* 2:159–164.

Mattes, J. A. (1992): Valproic acid for non-affective aggression in the mentally retarded. *Journal of Nervous and Mental Disease,* 180(9):601–602.

Mattick, R. P., Andrews, G., Hadzi-Pavlovic, D., & Christensen, H. (1990): Treatment of panic and agoraphobia: An integrative review. *Journal of Nervous and Mental Disease,* 178:567–576.

Mattick, R. P., & Peters, L. (1988): Treatment of severe social phobia: Effects of guided exposure with and without cognitive restructuring. *Journal of Consulting Clinical Psychology,* 56:251–260.

Mattick, R. P., Peters, L., & Clarke, J. C. (1989): Exposure and cognitive restructuring for social phobia: A controlled study. *Behavior Therapy,* 20:3–23.

Mavissakalian, M. (1993): Combined behavioral therapy and pharmacotherapy of agoraphobia. *Journal of Psychiatric Research,* 27 (suppl 1):179–191.

Mavissakalian, M. R., & Perel, J. M. (1995): Imipramine treatment of panic disorder with agoraphobia: Dose ranging and plasma level-response relationships. *American Journal of Psychiatry,* 152:673–682.

Max, M. B., Lynch, S. A., Muir, J., *et al.* (1992): Effects of desipramine, amitriptyline, and fluoxetine on pain in diabetic neuropathy. *New England Journal of Medicine,* 326:1250–1256.

Maxmen, J. S., & Ward, N. G. (1995): *Psychotropic Drugs Fast Facts* (2nd ed.). New York: Norton.

McCahill, M. E. (1995): Somatoform and related disorders: Delivery of diagnosis as first step. *American Family Physician,* 52(1):193–204.

McCall, W. V. (1995): Management of primary sleep disorders among elderly persons. *Psychiatric Services,* 46(1):49–55.

McCarthy, B. W. (1993): Relapse prevention strategies and techniques in sex therapy. *Journal of Sex and Marital Therapy,* 19(2):142–146.

McCarthy, B. W. (1994): Sexually compulsive men and inhibited sexual desire. *Journal of Sex and Marital Therapy,* 20(3):200–209.

McConaghy, N., Armstrong, M. S., Blaszczynski, A., *et al.* (1983): A controlled comparison of aversive therapy and imaginal desensitization in compulsive gambling. *British Journal of Psychiatry,* 142:366–372.

McCubbin, M. A., & McCubbin, H. I. (1989): Theoretical orientations to family stress and coping. In C. R. Figley (Ed.), *Treating Stress in Families.* New York: Brunner/Mazel.

McDougle, C. J., Barr, L. C., Goodman, W. K., *et al.* (1995): Lack of efficacy of clozapine monotherapy in refractory obsessive-compulsive disorder. *American Journal of Psychiatry,* 152(12):1812–1814.

McDougle, C. J., Fleischmann, R. L., Epperson, C. N., *et al.* (1995): Risperidone addition in fluvoxamine-refractory obsessive-compulsive disorder: Three cases. *Journal of Clinical Psychiatry,* 56(11):526–528.

McElroy, S. L., Hudson, J. I., Pope, H. G., Jr., *et al.* (1992): The DSM-III-R impulse control disorders not elsewhere classified: Clinical characteristics and relationship to other psychiatric disorders. *American Journal of Psychiatry,* 149:318–327.

McElroy, S. L., Keck, P. E., Jr., Pope, H. G., Jr., & Hudson, J. I. (1989): Pharmacological treatment of kleptomania and bulimia nervosa. *Journal of Clinical Psychopharmacology,* 9:358–360.

McElroy, S. L., Keck, P. E., Stanton, S. P., *et al.* (1996): A randomized comparison of divalproex oral loading versus haloperidol in the initial treatment of acute psychotic mania. *Journal of Clinical Psychiatry,* 57(4):142–146.

McElroy, S., Pope, H. G. Jr., Keck, P. E., & Hudson, J. I. (1995): Disorders of impulse control. In E. Hollander & D. J. Stein (Eds.), *Impulsivity and Aggression.* New York: Wiley.

McElroy, S. L., Pope, H. G., Jr., Hudson, J. I., *et al.* (1991a): Kleptomania: A report of 20 cases. *American Journal of Psychiatry,* 148(5):652–657.

McElroy, S. L., Satlin, A., Pope, H. G., Jr, *et al.* (1991b): Treatment of compulsive shopping with antidepressants: A report of three cases. *Annals of Clinical Psychiatry,* 3:199–204.

McFarlane, A. C. (1994): Individual psychotherapy for post-traumatic stress disorder. *Psychiatric Clinics of North America,* 17(2):393–408.

McFarlane, W. R. (1994): Multiple-family groups and psychoeducation in the treatment of schizophrenia. *New Directions in Mental Health Services,* Summer (62):13–22.

McGlashan, T. H. (1986): Schizotypal personality disorder. Chestnut Lodge follow-up study: VI. Long-term follow-up perspectives. *Archives of General Psychiatry,* 43(4):329–334.

McGlashan, T. H. (1994): What has become of the psychotherapy of schizophrenia? *Acta Psychiatrica Scandinavica,* 384(suppl):147–152.

McIvor, R. J., & Turner, S. W. (1995): Assessment and treatment approaches for survivors of torture. *British Journal of Psychiatry,* 166(6):705–711.

McNight, D. L., Nelson-Gray, R. O., & Barnhill, J. (1992): Dexmethasone suppression test and response to cognitive therapy and antidepressant medication. *Behavior Therapy* 23:99–111.

Meade, T. W., Dyer, S., Browne, W., et al. (1990): Low back pain of mechanical origin: Randomised comparison of chiropractic and hospital outpatient treatment. *British Medical Journal,* 300(6737):1431–1437.

Meade, T. W., Dyer, S., Browne, W., & Frank, A. O. (1995): Randomised comparison of chiropractic and hospital outpatient management for low back pain: Results from extended follow up. *British Medical Journal,* 311(7001):349–351.

Meadow, R. (1984): Fictitious epilepsy. *Lancet,* 2(8393):25–28.

Meeuwesen, L., Huyse, F. J., Meiland, F. J., et al. (1994): Psychiatric consultations in medical outpatients with abdominal pain: Patient and physician effects. *International Journal of Psychiatry and Medicine,* 24(4):339–356.

Mehlum, L., Friis, S., Irion, T., et al. (1991): Personality disorders 2-5 years after treatment: A prospective follow-up study. *Acta Psychiatrica Scandinavica,* 84(1):72–77.

Mellman, L. A., Gorman, J. M. (1984): Successful treatment of obsessive-compulsive disorder with ECT. *American Journal of Psychiatry,* 141:596–597.

Meloy, J. R. (1988): *The Psychopathic Mind: Origins, Dynamics and Treatment.* Northvale, NJ: Jason Aronson.

Meloy, J. R. (1995): Antisocial personality. In G. O. Gabbard (Ed.), *Treatments of Psychiatric Disorders,* (2nd ed.). Washington, DC: American Psychiatric Press.

Meltzer, H. Y., Cola, P., Way, L., et al. (1993): Cost effectiveness of clozapine in neuroleptic-resistant schizophrenia. *American Journal of Psychiatry,* 150(11):1630–1638.

Meltzer, H. Y., & Okayli, G. (1995): Reduction of suicidality during clozapine treatment of neuroleptic-resistant schizophrenia: Impact on risk-benefit assessment. *American Journal of Psychiatry,* 152(2):183–190.

Mendelberg, H. E. (1995): Inpatient treatment of mood disorders. *Psychological Reports,* 76(3,Pt 1):819–824.

Mersch, P. P. (1995): The treatment of social phobia: The differential effectiveness of exposure in vivo and an integration of exposure in vivo, rational emotive therapy and social skills training. *Behavior Research Therapy,* 33(3):259–269.

Metz, M. E., & Dwyer, S. M. (1993): Relationship conflict management patterns among sex dysfunction, sex offender, and satisfied couples. *Journal of Sex and Marital Therapy,* 19(2):104–122.

Meyer, W. J., Cole, C., & Emory, E. (1992): DepoProvera treatment for sex offending behavior: An evaluation of outcome. *Bulletin of American Academy of Psychiatry and Law,* 20(3):249–259.

Meyer, W. J., Webb, A., Stuart, C. A., et al. (1986): Physical and hormonal evaluation of transsexual patients: A longitudinal study. *Archives of Sexual Behavior,* 15:121–138.

Meyers, B. S. (1995): Late-life delusional depression: Acute and long-term treatment. *International Psychogeriatrics* 7(suppl):113–124.

Milrod, B. (1995): The continued usefulness of psychoanalysis in the treatment armamentarium for panic disorder. *Journal of the American Psychoanalytical Association,* 43(1):151–162.

Milstein, V., Small, J. G., Klapper, M. H., *et al.* (1987): Unilateral vs. bilateral ECT in the treatment of mania. *Convulsive Therapy,* 3:1–9.

Mindus, P., Rasmussen, S. A., & Lindquist, C. (1994): Neurosurgical treatment for refractory obsessive-compulsive disorder: Implications for understanding frontal lobe function. *Journal of Neuropsychiatry and Clinical Neuroscience,* 6(4):467–477.

Mitchell, J. E., Pyle, R. L., Eckert, E. D., *et al.* (1990): A comparison study of antidepressants and structured intensive group psychotherapy in the treatment of bulimia nervosa. *Archives of General Psychiatry* 47:149–157.

Mitchell, J. E. & Staff Members of the Eating Disorders Program (1991): *Bulimia Nervosa: Group Treatment Manual.* Department of Psychiatry, University of Minnesota Hospital and Clinic.

Mitler, M. M., Browman, C. P., Menn, S. J., *et al.* (1986): Nocturnal myoclonus: Treatment efficacy of clonazepam and temazepam. *Sleep,* 9:385–392.

Modigh, K., Westberg, P., & Eriksson, E. (1992): Superiority of clomipramine over imipramine in the treatment of panic disorder: A placebo-controlled trial. *Journal of Clinical Psychopharmacology,* 12:251–261.

Mok, H., & Yatham, L. N. (1994): Treatment of delusional disorders with clozapine. *American Journal of Psychiatry,* 151(9).

Monroe, R. R. (1981): The problem of impulsivity in personality disturbances. In J. R. Lion (Ed.), *Personality Disorders: Diagnosis and Management,* (2nd ed). Baltimore: Williams & Wilkins.

Montplaisir, J., Lapierre, O., Warnes, H., *et al.* (1992): The treatment of the restless leg syndrome with or without periodic leg movements of sleep. *Sleep,* 15:391–395.

Morin, C. M., Culbert, J. P., & Schwartz, S. M. (1994): Nonpharmacological interventions for insomnia: A meta-analysis of treatment efficacy. *American Journal of Psychiatry,* 151(8):1172–1180.

Morin, C. M., Stone, J., & Maghakian, C. (1993): Cognitive-behavior therapy and pharmacotherapy for late-life insomnia. *Sleep Research,* 22:240.

Mosher, L. R. (1991): Soteria: A therapeutic community for psychotic persons. *International Journal of Therapeutic Communities,* 12:53–67.

Moskowitz, J. A. (1980): Lithium and lady luck: Use of lithium carbonate in compulsive gambling. *New York State Journal of Medicine,* 80:785–788.

Mukherjee, S., Sackheim, H. A., & Lee, C. (1988): Unilateral ECT in the treatment of manic episodes. *Convulsive Therapy,* 4:74–80.

Mukherjee, S., Sackheim, H. A., & Schnur, D. B. (1994): Electroconvulsive therapy of acute manic episodes: A review of 50 years' experience. *American Journal of Psychiatry,* 151:169–176.

Mullington, J., & Broughton, R. (1993): Scheduled naps in the management of daytime sleepiness in narcolepsy-cataplexy. *Sleep,* 16(5):444–456.

Mundo, E., Bellodi, L., & Smeraldi, E. (1995): Effects of acute intravenous clomipramine on obsessive-compulsive disorder: Symptoms and response to chronic treatment. *Biological Psychiatry,* 38(8):525–531.

Munford, P. R., Hand, I., & Liberman, R. P. (1994): Psychosocial treatment for obsessive-compulsive disorder. *Psychiatry,* 57(2):142–152.

Munro, A. (1988): Monosymptomatic hypochondriacal psychosis. *British Journal of Psychiatry,* 2(suppl):37–40.

Munro, A., O'Brien, J. V., & Ross, D. (1985): Two cases of pure or primary erotomania successfully treated with pimozide. *Canadian Journal of Psychiatry,* 30(8):619–622.

Murphy, G. E., Carney, R. M., Knesevich, M. A. *et al.* (1995): Cognitive behavior therapy, relaxation training, and tricyclic antidepressant medication in the treatment of depression. *Psychological Reports,* 77(2):403–420.

Myers, W. C. (1994): Sexual homicide by adolescents. *Journal of the American Academy of Child and Adolescent Psychiatry,* 33(7):962–969.

Nagy, L. M., Krystal, J. H., Woods, S. W., & Charney, D. S. (1989): Clinical and medication outcome after short-term alprazolam and behavioral group treatment in panic disorder: A 2.5-year naturalistic follow-up study. *Archives of General Psychiatry,* 46:993–999.

Neidhardt, E. J., Krakow, B., & Kellner, R. (1992): The beneficial effects of one treatment session and recording of nightmares on chronic nightmare sufferers. *Sleep,* 15:470–473.

Neuhalfen, E. A., & Kaplan, A. (1994, March): Are you missing anything? Recent psychotropics available in Europe, but not in the United States. *Psychiatric Times,* p. 34.

Nierenberg, A. A., Adler, L. A., Peselow, E., *et al.* (1994): Trazodone for antidepressant-associated insomnia. *American Journal of Psychiatry,* 151:1069–1072.

Nishino, S., Mignot, E., & Dement, W. C. (1995): Sedative-hypnotics. In A. F. Schazberg & C. B. Nemeroff (Eds.), *American Psychiatric Press Textbook of Psychopharmacology.* Washington, DC: American Psychiatric Press.

Nitenson, N. C., & Cole, J. O. (1993): Psychotropic-induced sexual dysfunction, In D. L. Dunner (Ed.), *Current Psychiatric Therapy,* Philadelphia: Saunders.

Nofzinger, E. A., Buysse, D. J., Reynolds, C. F., & Kupfer, D. J. (1993): Sleep disorders related to another mental disorder (non-substance/primary): A DSM-IV literature review. *Journal of Clinical Psychiatry,* 54:244–255.

Nurnberg, H. G., & Levine, P. E. (1986): Schizophrenia and antipsychotic drugs. *Comprehensive Therapeutics,* 12(10):42–52.

O'Connor, K., & Robillard, S. (1995): Inference processes in obsessive-compulsive disorder: Some clinical observations. *Behavior Research and Therapy,* 33(8):887–896.

O'Sullivan, G., Noshirvani, H., Marks, I., *et al.* (1991): Six-year follow-up after exposure and clomipramine therapy for obsessive-compulsive disorder. *Journal of Clinical Psychiatry,* 52:150–155.

Oehrberg, S., Christiansen, P. E., Behnke, K., *et al.* (1995): Paroxetine in the treatment of panic disorder. A randomised, double-blind, placebo-controlled study. *British Journal of Psychiatry,* 167(3):374–379.

Oesterheld, J. R., McKenna, M. S., & Gould, N. B. (1987): Group psychotherapy of bulimia: A critical review. *International Journal of Group Psychotherapy,* 37:163–184.

Oliver, J. E. (1993): Intergenerational transmission of child abuse: Rates, research, and clinical implications. *American Journal of Psychiatry,* 150(9):1315–1324.

Olmsted, M. P., Davis, R., Rockert, W. *et al.* (1991): Efficacy of a brief group psychoeducational intervention for bulimia nervosa. *Behavior Research and Therapy,* 29:71–83.

Olmsted, M. P., Kaplan, A. S., & Rockert, W. (1994): Rate and prediction of relapse in bulimia nervosa. *American Journal of Psychiatry,* 151:738–743.

Opjordsmoen, J. (1988): Hypochondriacal psychoses: A long-term follow-up. *Acta Psychiatrica Scandinavica,* 77:587–597.

Opler, L. A., & Feinberg, S. S. (1991): The role of pimozide in clinical psychiatry: A review. *Journal of Clinical Psychiatry,* 52:221–233.

Ost, L. G., & Westling, B. E. (1995): Applied relaxation vs cognitive behavior therapy in the treatment of panic disorder. *Behavior Research and Therapy,* 33(2):145–158.

Packer, S. (1992): Family planning for women with bipolar disorder. *Hospital and Community Psychiatry,* 43(5):479–482.

Pande, A. C., Haskett, R. F., & Greden, J. F. (1992): Fluoxetine versus phenelzine in atypical depression. *Biological Psychiatry,* 31:186.

Pato, M. T., Pigott, T. A., Hill, J. L., *et al* (1991): Controlled comparison of buspirone and clomipramine in obsessive-compulsive disorder. *American Journal of Psychiatry,* 148:127–129.

Pellicer, X. (1993): Eye movement desensitization treatment of a child's nightmares: A case report. *Journal of Behavioral Therapy and Experimental Psychiatry,* 24(1):73–75.

Perilstein, R. D., Lipper, S., & Friedman, L. J. (1991): Three cases of paraphilias responsive to fluoxetine treatment. *Journal of Clinical Psychiatry,* 52:169–170.

Perris, C. (1994): Cognitive therapy in the treatment of patients with borderline personality disorders. *Acta Psychiatrica Scandinavica,* 379(suppl):69–72.

Petrides, G., Dhossche, D., Fink, M., & Francis, A. (1994): Continuation ECT: Relapse prevention in affective disorders. *Convulsive Therapy,* 10(3):189–194.

Philbrick, K. L., & Rummans, T. A. (1994): Malignant catatonia. *Journal of Neuropsychiatry and Clinical Neuroscience,* 6:1–13.

Phillips, K. A. & Gunderson, J. G. (1994): Personality disorders. In R. E. Hales, S. C. Yudofsky, & J. A. Talbott (Eds.), *American Psychiatric Press Textbook of Psychiatry,* (2nd ed.) Washington, DC: American Psychiatric Press.

Phillips, K. A., McElroy, S. L., Keck, P. E., *et al.* (1993): Body dysmorphic disorder: 30 cases of imagined ugliness. *American Journal of Psychiatry,* 150(2):302–308.

Physicians' Desk Reference, (50th ed.) (1996): Montvale, NJ: Medical Economics.

Piccinelli, M., Pini, S., Bellantuono, C., & Wilkinson, G. (1995): Efficacy of drug treatment in obsessive-compulsive disorder. A meta-analytic review. *British Journal of Psychiatry,* 166(4):424–443.

Pithers, W. D. (1994): Process evaluation of a group therapy component designed to enhance sex offenders' empathy for sexual abuse survivors. *Behavior Research and Therapy,* 32(5):565–570.

Plakun, E. M., Burkhardt, T. E., & Muller, J. T. (1985): Fourteen-year follow-up of borderline and schizotypal personality disorders. *Comprehensive Psychiatry,* 26(5):448–455.

Plassmann, R. (1994): Inpatient and outpatient long-term psychotherapy of patients suffering from factitious disorders. *Psychotherapy Psychosomatics,* 62(1–2):96–107.

Poldrugo, F., & Forti, B. (1988): Personality disorders and alcoholism treatment outcome. *Drug and Alcohol Dependence,* 21:171–176.

Pollard, C. A., Ibe, I. O., Krojanker, D. N., *et al.* (1991): Clomipramine treatment of trichotillomania: A follow-up report on four cases. *Journal of Clinical Psychiatry,* 52:128–130.

Ponticas, Y. (1992): Sexual aversion versus hypoactive sexual desire: A diagnostic challenge. *Psychiatric Medicine,* 10(2):273–281.

Pope, H. G., Jr., Hudson, J. I., Jonas, J. M., & Yurgelun-Todd, D. (1983): Bulimia treated with imipramine: A placebo-controlled, double-blind study. *American Journal of Psychiatry,* 140:554–558.

Pope, H. G., Jr., Keck, P. E., Jr., McElroy, S. L., & Hudson, J. I. (1989): A placebo-controlled study of trazodone in bulimia nervosa. *Journal of Clinical Psychopharmacology,* 9:254–259.

Powell, F. C., Hanigan, W. C., & Olivero, W. C. (1993): A risk/benefit analysis of spinal manipulation therapy for relief of lumbar or cervical pain. *Neurosurgery,* 33(1):73–79.

Primac, D. W. (1993): Measuring change in a brief therapy of a compulsive personality. *Psychological Reports,* 72(1):309–310.

Quality Assurance Project (1985): Treatment outlines for the management of obsessive-compulsive disorders. *Australian-New Zealand Journal of Psychiatry,* 19(3):240–253.

Quality Assurance Project (1990): Treatment outlines for paranoid, schizotypal and schizoid personality disorders. *Australian-New Zealand Journal of Psychiatry,* 24(3):339–350.

Quality Assurance Project (1991): Treatment outlines for antisocial personality disorder. *Australian-New Zealand Journal of Psychiatry,* 25(4):541–547.

Quinlivan, R., Hough, R., Crowell, A., *et al.* (1995): Service utilization and costs of care for severely mentally ill clients in an intensive case management program. *Psychiatric Services,* 46(4):365–371.

Ratey, J., Sovner, R., Parks, A., *et al.* (1991): Buspirone treatment of aggression and anxiety in mentally retarded patients: A multiple-baseline, placebo lead-in study. *Journal of Clinical Psychiatry,* 52:159–162.

Ravizza, L., Barzega, G., Bellino, S., *et al.* (1995): Predictors of drug treatment response in obsessive-compulsive disorder. *Journal of Clinical Psychiatry,* 56(8):368–73.

Reid, W. H. (1978): The sadness of the psychopath. *American Journal of Psychotherapy,* 32(4):496–509.

Reid, W. H. (1985): The antisocial personality: A review. *Hospital and Community Psychiatry,* 36(8), 831–837.

Reid, W. H. (in press). Antisocial character and behavior: Threats and solutions. In T. Millon (Ed.), *Selected Papers from the International Symposium on Psychotherapy.* New York: Guilford Press.

Reid, W. H., Ahmed, I., & Levie, C. A. (1981): Treatment of sleepwalking: A controlled study. *American Journal of Psychotherapy* 35:27–37.

Reid, W. H., Blouin, P., & Schermer, M.(1976): A review of psychotropic medications and the glaucomas. *International Pharmacopsychiatry,* 11(3):163–174.

Reid, W. H., & Mason, M. (1995): Cost-effectiveness in the treatment of refractory schizophrenia: Clozapine data at 4.5 years. Abstract and manuscript available from the authors.

Reid, W. H., Mason, M., & Toprac, M. (1994): Savings in hospital bed-days related to treatment with clozapine. *Hospital and Community Psychiatry,* 45(3):261–264.

Reid, W. H., Matthews, W. (1980): A wilderness experience treatment program for antisocial offenders. *International Journal of Offender Therapy and Comparative Criminology,* 24(2):171–178.

Reid, W. H., & Solomon, G. H. (1981): Community-based offender programs. In W. H. Reid, (Ed.), *The Treatment of Antisocial Syndromes*. New York: Van Nostrand Reinhold.

Reite, M., Higgs, L., Lebet, J. P., *et al.* (1994): Sleep inducing effect of low energy emission therapy. *Bioelectromagnetics*, 15(1):67–75.

Reite, M. L., Nagel, K. E., & Ruddy, J. R. (1990): *The Evaluation and Management of Sleep Disorders*. Washington, DC: American Psychiatric Press.

Renfrey, G., & Spates, C. R. (1994): Eye movement desensitization: A partial dismantling study. *Journal of Behavioral Therapy and Experimental Psychiatry*, 25(3):231–239.

Renvoize, E. B., Kent, J., Klar, H. M. (1987): Delusional infestation and dementia: A case report. *British Journal of Psychiatry*, 150:403–405.

Rice, K. M., Blanchard, E. B., & Purcell, M. (1993): Biofeedback treatments of generalized anxiety disorder: Preliminary results. *Biofeedback Self Regulation*, 18(2):93–105.

Richardson, G. S., Carskadon, M. A., Flagg, W. *et al.* (1978): Excessive daytime sleepiness in man: Multiple sleep latency measurement in narcoleptic and control subjects. *Electroencephalography and Clinical Neurophysiology*, 45:621–627.

Richer, M., & Crismon, M. L. (1993): Pharmacotherapy of sexual offenders. *Annals of Pharmacotherapy*, 27(3):316–320.

Rickels, K., Downing, R., Schweizer, E., & Hassman, H. (1993): Antidepressants for the treatment of generalized anxiety disorder: A placebo-controlled comparison of imipramine, trazodone, and diazepam. *Archives of General Psychiatry*, 50:884–895.

Rief, W., Hiller, W., Geissner, E., & Fichter, M. M. (1995): A two-year follow-up study of patients with somatoform disorders. *Psychosomatics*, 36(4):376–386.

Riegel, B., Warmoth, J. E., Middaugh, S. J., *et al.* (1995): Psychogenic cough treated with biofeedback and psychotherapy: A review and case report. *American Journal of Physical Medicine and Rehabilitation*, 74(2):155–158.

Rifkin, A., Doddi, S., Karajgi, B., *et al.* (1991): Dosage of haloperidol for schizophrenia. *Archives of General Psychiatry*, 48:166–170.

Risen, C. B. (1995): A guide to taking a sexual history. *Psychiatric Clinics of North America*, 18(1):39–53.

Roback, H. B., & Shelton, M. (1995): Effects of confidentiality limitations on the psychotherapeutic process. *Journal of Psychotherapy Practice and Research*, 4(3):185–193.

Rocha, F. L., & Rocha, M. E. (1992): Kleptomania, mood disorder and lithium. *Arq Neuropsiquiatr* (Brazil), 50(4):543–546.

Rockwell, E., Krull, A. J., Dimsdale, J., & Jeste, D. V. (1994): Late-onset psychosis with somatic delusions. *Psychosomatics*, 35(1):66–72.

Roesler, T. A., Barry, P. C., & Bock, S. A. (1994): Factitious food allergy and failure to thrive. *Archives of Pediatric Adolescent Medicine*, 148(11):1150–115.

Roose, S. P., Glassman, A. H., Attia, E., Woodring, S. (1994): Comparative efficacy of selective serotonin reuptake inhibitors and tricyclics in the treatment of melancholia. *American Journal of Psychiatry*, 151(12):1735–1739.

Rosen, G. M. (1995): On the origin of eye movement desensitization. *Journal of Behavioral Therapy and Experimental Psychiatry*, 26(2):121–122.

Rosen, R. C., & Leiblum, S. R. (1995): Hypoactive sexual desire. *Psychiatric Clinics of North America*, 18(1):107–121.

Rosenbaum, J. F., Quitkin, F. M., Fava, M., *et al.* (1993): Fluoxetine vs. placebo: Long-term treatment of MDD. *Proceedings*, American College of Neuropsychopharmacology 32nd Annual Meeting.

Rosenbaum, M.B. (1995): Female sexual arousal disorder and female orgasmic disorder. In G. O. Gabbard (Ed.), *Treatments of Psychiatric Disorders* (2nd ed.), Washington, DC: American Psychiatric Press.

Rosenberg, N. K., & Rosenberg, R. (1994): Three years follow-up of panic disorder patients: A naturalistic study. *Scandinavian Journal of Psychology*, 35(3):254–262.

Rosenheck, R., Neale, M., Leaf, P., *et al.* (1995): Multisite experimental cost study of intensive psychiatric community care. *Schizophrenia Bulletin*, 21(1):129–140.

Rosenthal, R. J., & Lorenz, V. C. (1992): The pathological gambler as criminal offender: Comments on evaluation and treatment. *Psychiatric Clinics of North America*, 15:647–660.

Rosowsky, E., & Gurian, B. (1992): The impact of borderline personality disorder in late life on systems of care. *Hospital and Community Psychiatry*, 43(4):386–389.

Rothbaum, B. O., Hodges, L. F., Kooper, R., *et al.* (1995): Effectiveness of computer-generated (virtual reality) graded exposure in the treatment of acrophobia. *American Journal of Psychiatry*, 152(4):626–628.

Rothschild, R., Quitkin, H. M., Quitkin, F. M., *et al.* (1994): A double-blind placebo-controlled comparison of phenelzine and imipramine in the treatment of bulimia in atypical depressives. *International Journal of Eating Disorders*, 15(1):1–9.

Roy, A., Cole, K., Goldman, Z., & Barris, M. (1993): Fluoxetine treatment of postpartum depression (letter). *American Journal of Psychiatry*, 150(8):1273.

Rubin, S. O. (1993): Sex-reassignment surgery male-to-female. Review, own results and report of a new technique using the glans penis as a pseudoclitoris. *Scandinavian Journal of Urology and Nephrology*, 154(suppl):1–28.

Russell, G. F. M., Szmukler, G., Dare, C., & Eisler, I. (1987): An evaluation of family therapy in anorexia nervosa and bulimia nervosa. *Archives of General Psychiatry*, 44:1047–1056.

Sabo, A. N., Gunderson, J. G., Najavits, L. M., *et al.* (1995): Changes in self-destructiveness of borderline patients in psychotherapy. A prospective follow-up. *Journal of Nervous and Mental Diseases*, 183(6):370–376.

Sandoz Pharmaceuticals Corp. (1993): *Management of Adverse Events (Clozaril)*, East Hanover, NJ: Sandoz.

Sands, R. G., & Canaan, R. A. (1994): Two modes of case management: Assessing their impact. *Community Mental Health Journal*, 30(5):441–457.

Saper, J. R., Silberstein, S. D., Lake, A. E., *et al.* (1994): A double-blind trial of fluoxetine: Chronic daily headache and migraine. *Headache*, 34:497–502.

Sarkar, P., Andrade, C., Kapur, B., *et al.* (1994): An exploratory evaluation of ECT in haloperidol-treated DSM-IIIR schizophreniform disorder. *Convulsive Therapy*, 10(4):271–278.

Satlin, A., Volicer, L., Ross, V., *et al.* (1992): Bright light treatment of behavioral and sleep disturbances in patients with Alzheimer's disease. *American Journal of Psychiatry*, 149(8):1028–1032.

Schaefer, L. C, Wheeler, C. C., & Futterweit, W. (1995): Gender identity disorders (transexualism). In G. O. Gabbard (Ed.), *Treatments of Psychiatric Disorders*, Washington, DC: American Psychiatric Press.

Schneider-Helmert, D., & Spinweber, C. L. (1986): Evaluation of *l*-tryptophan for treatment of insomnia: A review. *Psychopharmacology* (Berlin), 89:1–7.

Schneier, F. R., Liebowitz, M. R., Davies, S. O., *et al.* (1990): Fluoxetine in panic disorder. *Journal of Clinical Psychopharmacology,* 10:119–121.

Schneier, F. R., Marshall, R. D., Street L., *et al.* (1995): Social phobia and specific phobias. In G. O. Gabbard (Ed.), *Treatments of Psychiatric Disorders* (2nd ed.). Washington, DC: American Psychiatric Press.

Schneier, F. R., Saoud, J. B., Campeas, R., *et al.* (1993): Buspirone in social phobia. *Journal of Clinical Psychopharmacology,* 13:251–256.

Schreter, R. K. (1980): Treating the untreatables: A group experience with somaticizing borderline patients. *International Journal of Psychiatry and Medicine,* 10:205–215.

Schuckit, M. (1985): The clinical implications of primary diagnostic groups among alcoholics. *Archives of General Psychiatry,* 42:1043–1049.

Schwartz, K., Harding, R., Harrington, D., & Farr, B. (1993): Hospital management of a patient with intractable factitious disorder. *Psychosomatics,* 34:265–267.

Schweizer, E., Patterson, W., Rickels, K., & Rosenthal, M. (1993): Double-blind, placebo-controlled study of a once-a-day, sustained-release preparation of alprazolam for the treatment of panic disorder. *American Journal of Psychiatry,* 150:1210–1215.

Scott, E. M. (1989): Hypnosis: Emotions for the tin man (the schizoid personality). *American Journal of Clinical Hypnosis,* 31(3):204–208.

Scott, J. (1995): Psychotherapy for bipolar disorder. *British Journal of Psychiatry,* 167(5):581–588.

Segraves, R. T., Saran, A., Segraves, K., & Maguire, E. (1993): Clomipramine versus placebo in the treatment of premature ejaculation: A pilot study. *Journal of Sex and Marital Therapy,* 19(3):198–200.

Selden, B. S. (1989): Adolescent epidemic hysteria presenting as a mass casualty, toxic exposure incident. *Annals of Emergency Medicine,* 18:892–895.

Sewell, D. D., & Jeste, D. V. (1992): Distinguishing neuroleptic malignant syndrome (NMS) from NMS-like acute medical illnesses: A study of 34 cases. *Journal of Neuropsychiatry and Clinical Neuroscience,* 4(3):265–269.

Shader, R. I., & Greenblatt, D. (1993): Use of benzodiazepines in anxiety disorders. *New England Journal of Medicine,* 328:1398–1405.

Shader, R. I., & Sharfman, E. L. (1989): Depersonalization disorder. In *Treatments of Psychiatric Disorders.* Washington, DC: American Psychiatric Press.

Shaw, J. (1994): Treatment of primary vaginismus: A new perspective. *Journal of Sex and Marital Therapy,* 20(1):46–55.

Shear, M. K., Leon, A. C., Pollack, M. H., *et al.* (1995): Pattern of placebo response in panic disorder. *Psychopharmacology Bulletin,* 31(2):273–278.

Sheard, M. H., Marini, J. L., Bridges, C. I., *et al.* (1976): The effect of lithium on impulsive aggressive behavior in man. *American Journal of Psychiatry,* 133:1409–1413.

Shearin, E. N., & Linehan, M. M. (1994): Dialectical behavior therapy for borderline personality disorder: Theoretical and empirical foundations. *Acta Psychiatrica Scandinavica,* 379(suppl):61–68.

Shorter, E., Abbey, S. E., Gillies, L. A., *et al.* (1992): Inpatient treatment of persistent somatization. *Psychosomatics,* 33(3):295–301.

Shvartzman, P., & Abelson, A. (1988): Complications of chiropractic treatment for back pain. *Postgraduate Medicine,* 83(7):57–58, 61.

Sifneos, P. E. (1984): Short-term dynamic psychotherapy for patients with physical symptomatology. *Psychotherapy and Psychosomatics,* 42(1–4):48–51.

Silver, S. M., Brooks, A., & Obenchain, J. (1995): Treatment of Vietnam War veterans with PTSD: A comparison of eye movement desensitization and reprocessing, biofeedback, and relaxation training. *Journal of Traumatic Stress,* 8(2):337–342.

Silver, J. A., & Yudofsky, S. C. (1995): Organic mental disorders and impulsive aggression. In E. Hollander & D. J. Stein (Eds.), *Impulsivity and Aggression.* New York: Wiley.

Simeon, D., Stein, D. J., & Hollander, E. (1995): Depersonalization disorder and self-injurious behavior. *Journal of Clinical Psychiatry,* 56(suppl 4):36–40.

Simmons, D. A., Daamen, M. J., Harrison, J. W., *et al.* (1987): Hospital management of a patient with factitial dermatitis. *General Hospital Psychiatry,* 9(2):147–150.

Simms, R. W. (1994): Controlled trials of therapy in fibromyalgia syndrome. *Baillieres Clinical Rheumatology,* 8(4):917–934.

Simpson, G. M., Yadalam, K. G., & Stephanos, M. J. (1988): Double-blind carbidopa/levodopa and placebo study in tardive dyskinesia. *Journal of Clinical Psychopharmacology,* 8(suppl):49–51.

Sindrup, S. H., Gram, L. F., Brosen, K., *et al.* (1990): The selective serotonin reuptake inhibitor paroxetine is effective in the treatment of diabetic neuropathy symptoms. *Pain,* 42:135–144.

Small, J. G., Klapper, M. H., Kellams, J. J., *et al.* (1988): Electroconvulsive therapy compared with lithium, in the management of manic states. *Archives of General Psychiatry,* 45:727–732.

Small, J. G., Klapper, M. H., Milstein, V., *et al.* (1991): Carbamazepine compared with lithium in the treatment of mania. *Archives of General Psychiatry,* 48:915–921.

Smith, G. R., Jr. (1992): The epidemiology and treatment of depression when it coexists with somatoform disorders, somatization, or pain. *General Hospital Psychiatry,* 14:265–272.

Smith, G. R., Jr., Rost, K., & Kashner, T. M. (1995): A trial of the effect of a standardized psychiatric consultation on health outcomes and costs in somatizing patients. *Archives of General Psychiatry,* 52(3):238–243.

Smith, W. H. (1993): Incorporating hypnosis into the psychotherapy of patients with multiple personality disorder. *Bulletin of the Menninger Clinic,* 57(3):344–354.

Snaith, R. P., & Collins, S. A. (1981): Five exhibitionists and a method of treatment. *British Journal of Psychiatry,* 138:126–130.

Soloff, P. H., Cornelius, J., George, A., *et al.* (1993): Efficacy of phenelzine and haloperidol in borderline personality disorder. *Archives of General Psychiatry,* 50:377–385.

Soloff, P. H., George, A., Nathan, S., *et al.* (1986): Amitriptyline and haloperidol in unstable and schizotypal borderline disorders. *Psychopharmacology Bulletin,* 22(1):177–182.

Solomon, D. A., Keitner, G. I., Miller, I. W., *et al.* (1995): Course of illness and maintenance treatments for patients with bipolar disorder. *Journal of Clinical Psychiatry,* 56(1):5–13.

Solomon, S. S., Lipton, R. B., & Newman, L. C. (1991): Prophylactic therapy of cluster headaches. *Clinical Neuropharmacology,* 14:116–130.

Solyom, C., & Solyom, L. (1990): A treatment program for functional paraplegia/ Munchausen syndrome. *Journal of Behavioral Therapy and Experimental Psychiatry,* 21:225–230.

Solyom, C., Solyom, L., LaPierre, Y., *et al.* (1981): Phenelzine and exposure in the treatment of phobias. *Biological Psychiatry,* 16:239–247.

Somer, E. (1995): Biofeedback-aided hypnotherapy for intractable phobic anxiety. *American Journal of Clinical Hypnosis,* 37(3):54–64.

Spates, C. R., & Burnette, M. M. (1995): Eye movement desensitization: Three unusual cases. *Journal of Behavioral Therapy and Experimental Psychiatry,* 26(1):51–55.

Spencer, T., Wilens, T., Biederman, J., *et al.* (1995): A double-blind, crossover comparison of methylphenidate and placebo in adults with childhood-onset attention-deficit hyperactivity disorder. *Archives of General Psychiatry,* 52(6):434–443.

Spiegel, D. (1994): Dissociative disorders. In R. E. Hales, S. C. Yudofsky, & J. A. Talbott (Eds.): *American Psychiatric Association Textbook of Psychiatry.* (2nd ed.). Washington, DC: American Psychiatric Press.

Spielman, A. J., Saskin, P., & Thorpy, M. J. (1987): Treatment of chronic insomnia by restriction of time in bed. *Sleep,* 10:45–56.

Spivak, H., Rodin, G., & Sutherland, A. (1994): The psychology of factitious disorders: A reconsideration. *Psychosomatics,* 35(1):25–34.

Sranek, J. J., Simpson, G. M., Morrison, R. L., *et al.* (1986): A prospective study of anticholinergic agents for prophylaxis of neuroleptic-induced dystonic reactions. *Journal of Clinical Psychiatry,* 47:305–309.

Stein, D. J., & Hollander, E. (1992): Low-dose pimozide augmentation of serotonin reuptake blockers in the treatment of trichotillomania. *Journal of Clinical Psychiatry,* 53:123–126.

Stein, D. J., Hollander, E., Anthony, D. T., *et al.* (1992): Serotonergic medications for sexual obsessions, sexual addictions, and paraphilias. *Journal of Clinical Psychiatry,* 53:267–271.

Stein, D. J., Hollander, E., & Josephson, S. C. (1994): Serotonin reuptake blockers for the treatment of obsessional jealousy. *Journal of Clinical Psychiatry,* 55(1):30–33.

Stein, D. J., & Hollander, E. (1993): The spectrum of obsessive-compulsive-related disorders. In E. Hollander (Ed.)., *Obsessive-Compulsive Disorders.* Washington, DC: American Psychiatric Press.

Stevenson, J., & Meares, R. (1992): An outcome study of psychotherapy for patients with borderline personality disorder. *American Journal of Psychiatry,* 149(3):358–362.

Sticher, M., Abramovits, W., & Newcomer, V. V. (1980): Trichotillomania in adults. *Cutis,* 26(1):90, 97–101.

Stiebel, V. G. (1995): Maintenance electroconvulsive therapy for chronic mentally ill patients: A case series. *Psychiatric Services,* 46(3):265–268.

Stone, M. H. (1985a): Schizotypal personality: Psychotherapeutic aspects. *Schizophrenia Bulletin,* 11(4):576–589.

Stone, M. H. (1985b): Analytically oriented psychotherapy in schizotypal and borderline patients: At the border of treatability. *Yale Journal of Biological Medicine,* 58(3):275–288.

Stone, M. H. (1993): Long-term outcome in personality disorders. *British Journal of Psychiatry,* 162:299–313.

Stone, M. H. (1994): Characterologic subtypes of the borderline personality disorder, with a note on prognostic factors. *Psychiatric Clinics of North America,* 17(4):773–784.

Strain, J. J. (1995): Adjustment disorders. In G. O. Gabbard (Ed.), *Treatments of Psychiatric Disorders* (2nd ed.). Washington, DC: American Psychiatric Press.

Stravynski, A., Belisle, M., Marcouiller, M., *et al.* (1994): The treatment of avoidant personality disorder by social skills training in the clinic or in real-life settings. *Canadian Journal of Psychiatry,* 39(8):377–383.

Streichenwein, S. M., & Thornby, J. I. (1995): A long-term, double-blind, placebo-controlled crossover trial of the efficacy of fluoxetine for trichotillomania. *American Journal of Psychiatry,* 152:1192–1196.

Strider, F. D., & Menolascino, F. J. (1981): Treatment of antisocial syndromes in the mentally retarded. In W.H. Reid (Ed.), *The Treatment of Antisocial Syndromes.* New York: Van Nostrand Reinhold.

Strober, M., Schmidt-Lackner, S., Freeman, R., *et al.* (1995): Recovery and relapse in adolescents with bipolar affective illness: A five-year naturalistic, prospective follow-up. *Journal of the American Academy of Child and Adolescent Psychiatry,* 34(6):724–731.

Stuart, S., & O'Hara, M. W. (1995): Interpersonal psychotherapy for postpartum depression. *Journal of Psychotherapy Practice and Research,* 4(1):18–29.

Stürup, G. K. (1968a): Treatment of sexual offenders in Herstedvester, Denmark: The rapists. *Acta Psychiatrica Scandinavica,* 204(suppl):5–62.

Stürup, G. K. (1968b): *Treating the "Untreatable": Chronic Criminals at Herstedvester.* Baltimore: Johns Hopkins Press.

Stürup, G. K., & Reid, W. H. (1981): Herstedvester: An historical overview of institutional treatment. In W.H. Reid (Ed.), *The Treatment of Antisocial Syndromes.* New York: Van Nostrand Reinhold.

Sullivan, M. D. (1993): Psychosomatic clinic or pain clinic: Which is more viable? *General Hospital Psychiatry,* 15(6):375–380.

Swann, A. C. (1995): Mixed or dysphoric manic states: Psychopathology and treatment. *Journal of Clinical Psychiatry,* 56(suppl 3):6–10.

Swedo, S. E., Leonard, H. L., Rapoport, J. L., *et al.* (1989): A double-blind comparison of clomipramine and desipramine in the treatment of trichotillomania (hair pulling). *New England Journal of Medicine,* 321:497–501.

Swift, W. J., Ritholz, M., Kalin, N. H., & Kaslow, N. (1987): A follow-up study of thirty hospitalized bulimics. *Psychosomatic Medicine,* 49:45–55.

Taber, J. I., McCormick, R. A., Russo, A. M., *et al.* (1987): Follow-up of pathological gamblers after treatment. *American Journal of Psychiatry,* 144:757–761.

Tardiff, K. (1992): The current state of psychiatry in the treatment of violent patients. *Archives of General Psychiatry,* 49:493–499.

Tarrier, N., Barrowclough, C., Porceddu, K., & Fitzpatrick, E. (1994): The Salford Family Intervention Project: Relapse rates of schizophrenia at five and eight years. *British Journal of Psychiatry,* 165(6):829–832.

Teicher, M. H., Glod, C. A., Oren, D. A., *et al.* (1995): The phototherapy light visor: More to it than meets the eye. *American Journal of Psychiatry,* 152:1197–1202.

Teichman, Y., Bar-el, Z., Shor, H., *et al.* (1995): A comparison of two modalities of cognitive therapy (individual and marital) in treating depression. *Psychiatry,* 58(2):136–148.

Telch, M. J., Lucas, J. A., Schmidt, N. B. *et al.* (1993): Group cognitive-behavioral treatment of panic disorder. *Behavior Research and Therapy,* 31:279–287.

Thase, M. E., Mallinger, A. G., McKnight, D., & Himmelhoch, J. M. (1992): Treatment of imipramine-resistant recurrent depression, IV: A double-blind crossover study of tranylcypromine for anergic bipolar depression. *American Journal of Psychiatry,* 149(2):195–198.

Thase M. E., Reynolds, C. F., III, Frank, E., *et al.* (1994): Response to cognitive-behavioral therapy in chronic depression. *Journal of Psychotherapy Practice and Research,* 3(3):204–214.

Thase, M. E., Wright, J. H. (1991): Cognitive behavioral therapy manual for depressed inpatients: A treatment protocol outline. *Behavior Therapy,* 22:571–595.

Thienemann M., & Koran, L. M. (1995): Do soft signs predict treatment outcome in obsessive-compulsive disorder? *Journal of Neuropsychiatry and Clinical Neuroscience,* 7(2):218–222.

Thigpen, C. H., & Cleckley, H. H. (1957): *The Three Faces of Eve.* New York: McGraw-Hill.

Thomsen, P. H. (1995): Obsessive-compulsive disorder in children and adolescents: A 6-22 year follow-up study of social outcome. *European Child and Adolescent Psychiatry,* 4(2):112–122.

Thomsen, P. H., & Mikkelsen, H. U. (1995): Course of obsessive-compulsive disorder in children and adolescents: A prospective follow-up study of 23 Danish cases. *Journal of the American Academy of Child and Adolescent Psychiatry,* 34(11):1432–1440.

Tobin, J. D. (1993): Treatment of somnambulism with anticipatory awakening. *Journal of Pediatrics,* 122(3):426–427.

Tollefson, G. D., Birkett, M. Koran, L., & Genduso, L. (1994): Continuation treatment of OCD: Double-blind and open-label experience with fluoxetine. *Journal of Clinical Psychiatry,* 55(suppl):69–76, 77–78.

Tomasovic, J. J. (1989): Sleep disorders. In W. H. Reid, *The Treatment of Psychiatric Disorders* (2nd ed.). New York: Brunner/Mazel.

Treasure, J., Schmidt, U., Troop, N., *et al.* (1994): First step in managing bulimia nervosa: Controlled trial of therapeutic manual. *British Medical Journal,* 308(6930):686–689.

True, P. K., & Benway, M. W. (1992): Treatment of stress reaction prior to combat using the "BICEPS" model. *Military Medicine,* 157(7):380–381.

Trull, T. J., Nietzel, M. T., Main, A., *et al.* (1988): The use of meta-analysis to assess the clinical significance of behavior therapy for agoraphobia. *Behavior Therapy,* 19:527–538.

Tupin, J. P., Smith, D. B., Clanon, T. L., (1973): The long-term use of lithium in aggressive prisoners. *Comprehensive Psychiatry,* 14:311–317.

Turner, S. M., Beidel, D. C., & Cooley-Quille, M. R. (1995): Two-year follow-up of social phobias treated with Social Effectiveness Therapy. *Behavior Research and Therapy,* 33(5):553–555.

Tyrer, P., Morgan, J., Van Horn, E., *et al.* (1995): A randomised controlled study of close monitoring of vulnerable psychiatric patients. *Lancet,* 345(8952):756–759.

Uhlenhuth, E. H., Matuzas, W., Glass, R. M., & Easton, C. (1989): Response of panic disorder to fixed doses of alprazolam or imipramine. *Journal of Affective Disorders*, 17:261–270.

Ungvari, G., & Vladar, K. (1986): Pimozide treatment for delusion of infestation. *Act Nerv Super* (Prague), 28(2):103–107.

Vallejo, J., Olivares, J., Marcos, T., *et al.* (1992): Clomipramine versus phenelzine in obsessive-compulsive disorder: A controlled clinical trial. *British Journal of Psychiatry*, 161:665–670.

van Ameringen, M., Mancini, C., & Streiner, D. L. (1993): Fluoxetine efficacy in social phobia. *Journal of Clinical Psychiatry*, 54:27–32.

van der Kolk, B. A., Dreyfuss, D., Michaels, M., *et al.* (1994): Fluoxetine in posttraumatic stress disorder. *Journal of Clinical Psychiatry*, 55(12):517–522.

van Oppen, P., de Haan, E., van Balkom, A. J., *et al.* (1995): Cognitive therapy and exposure in vivo in the treatment of obsessive-compulsive disorder. *Behavior Research and Therapy*, 33(4):379–390.

Van Putten, T., Marder, S. R., & Mintz, J. (1990): A controlled dose comparison of haloperidol in newly admitted schizophrenic patients. *Archives of General Psychiatry*, 47:754–758.

van Vliet, I. M., den Boer, J. A., & Westenberg, H. G. (1994): Psychopharmacological treatment of social phobia: A double blind placebo controlled study with fluvoxamine. *Psychopharmacology* (Berlin), 115(1–2):128–134.

Vanelle, J. M., Loo, H., Galinowski, A., *et al.* (1994): Maintenance ECT in intractable manic-depressive disorders. *Convulsive Therapy*, 10(3):195–205.

Vaughan, K., Armstrong, M.S., Gold, R., *et al.* (1994): A trial of eye movement desensitization compared to image habituation training and applied muscle relaxation in post-traumatic stress disorder. *Journal of Behavioral Therapy and Experimental Psychiatry*, 25(4):283–291.

Velikova, G., Selby, P. J., Snaith, P. R., & Kirby, P. G. (1995): The relationship of cancer pain to anxiety. *Psychotherapy and Psychosomatics*, 63(3–4):181–184.

Versiani, M., Nardi, A.E., Mundim, F. D., *et al.* (1992): Pharmacotherapy of social phobia: A controlled study with moclobemide and phenelzine. *British Journal of Psychiatry*, 161:353–360.

Vogel, G. W., & Morris, D. (1992): The effects of estazolam on sleep, performance, and memory: A long-term sleep laboratory study of elderly insomniacs. *Journal of Clinical Pharmacology*, 32:647–651.

Waldinger, M. D., Hengeveld, M. W., & Zwinderman, A. H. (1994): Paroxetine treatment of premature ejaculation: A double-blind, randomized, placebo controlled study. *American Journal of Psychiatry*, 151(9):1377–1379.

Walker, P. A., Berger, J. C., Green, R., *et al.* (1990): *Standards of Care* (rev. draft). Sonoma, CA: Harry Benjamin International Gender Dysphoria Association. (See also Walker, P. A., *et al.* (1985): Standards of care: The hormonal and surgical sex reassignment of gender dysphoric persons. *Archives of Sexual Behavior*, 14:79–90.)

Walling, M. K., O'Hara, M. W., Reiter, R. C., *et al.* (1994): Abuse history and chronic pain in women: II. A multivariate analysis of abuse and psychological morbidity. *Obstetrics and Gynecology*, 84(2):200–206.

Walsh, B. T., Stewart, J. W., Roose, S. P., *et al.* (1984): Treatment of bulimia with phenelzine: A double-blind, placebo-controlled study. *Archives of General Psychiatry,* 41:1105–1109.

Wardle, J., Hayward, P., Higgitt, A., *et al.* (1994): Effects of concurrent diazepam treatment on the outcome of exposure therapy in agoraphobia. *Behavior Research and Therapy,* 32(2):203–215.

Warnock, J. K. (1993): Selective serotonin reuptake inhibitors in treatment of skin picking in Prader-Willi syndrome. In *Proceedings,* American Psychiatric Association Annual Meeting (New Research). Washington, DC: American Psychiatric Association.

Webb, N. B., Sakheim, G. A., Towns-Miranda, L., & Wagner, C. R. (1990): Collaborative treatment of juvenile firesetters: Assessment and outreach. *American Journal of Orthopsychiatry,* 60(2):305–310.

Wehr, T. A., Sack, D. A., Rosenenthal, J. E., *et al.* (1988): Rapid cycling affective disorder: Contributing factors and treatment responses in 51 patients. *American Journal of Psychiatry,* 145:179–184.

Weiner, R. D. (1995): Electroconvulsive Therapy. In G. O. Gabbard (Ed.), *Treatments of Psychiatric Disorders.* Washington, DC: American Psychiatric Press.

Weintraub, M. I. (1995): Chronic pain in litigation: What is the relationship? *Neurology Clinics,* 13(2):341–349.

Werder, S. F. (1995): An update on the diagnosis and treatment of mania in bipolar disorder. *American Family Physician,* 51(5):1126–1136.

Wheadon, D. E., Bushnell, W. D., & Steiner, M. (1993, December): A fixed dose comparison of 20, 40 or 60 mg of paroxetine to placebo in the treatment of obsessive-compulsive disorder. *Proceedings of the American College Neuropsychopharmacology,* Maui, Hawaii.

White, W., & Boskind-White, M. (1981): An experiential-behavioral approach to the treatment of bulimarexia. *Psychotherapy Theory, Research and Practice,* 18:501–507.

Wilens, T. E., Biederman, J., & Spencer, T. J. (1995): Venlafaxine for adult ADHD (letter). *American Journal of Psychiatry,* 152(7):1099–1100.

Wilson, G. T., Rossiter, E., Kleifield, E., *et al.* (1986): Cognitive-behavioral treatment of bulimia nervosa: A controlled evaluation. *Behavior Research and Therapy,* 24:277–288.

Wilson, K. C., Scott, M., Abou-Saleh, M., *et al.* (1995): Long-term effects of cognitive-behavioural therapy and lithium therapy on depression in the elderly. *British Journal of Psychiatry,* 167(5):653–658.

Wilson, S. A., Becker, L. A., & Tinker, R. H. (1995): Eye movement desensitization and reprocessing (EMDR) treatment for psychologically traumatized individuals. *Journal of Consulting Clinical Psychology,* 63(6):928–937.

Winchel, R. M., Jones, J. S., Stanley, B., *et al.* (1992): Clinical characteristics of trichotillomania and its response to fluoxetine. *Journal of Clinical Psychiatry,* 53(9):304–308.

Wincze, J. P., Banasal, S., & Malmuc, M. (1986): Effects of medroxyprogesterone acetate on subjective arousal, arousal to erotic stimulation, and nocturnal penile tumescence in male offenders. *Archives of Sexual Behavior,* 15:293–305.

Winston, A., Laikin, M., Pollack, J., *et al.* (1994): Short-term psychotherapy of personality disorders. *American Journal of Psychiatry,* 151:190–194.

Wirz-Justice, A., Graw, P., Kräuchi, K., *et al.* (1993): Light therapy in seasonal affective disorder is independent of time of day or circadian phase. *Archives of General Psychiatry*, 50(12):929–937.

Wise, T. N. (1995): Fetishism: Etiology and treatment: A review from multiple perspectives. *Comprehensive Psychiatry*, 26:249–257.

Wise, T. N., Epstein, S., & Ross, R. (1992): Sexual issues in the medically ill and aging. *Psychiatric Medicine*, 10(2):169–180.

Wisner, K. L., Wheeler, S. B. (1994): Prevention of recurrent postpartum major depression. *Hospital and Community Psychiatry*, 45(12):1191–1196.

Wolff, R. (1984): Satiation in the treatment of inappropriate fire setting. *Journal of Behavioral Therapy and Experimental Psychiatry*, 15(4):337–340.

Wolpe, J. (1973): *The Practice of Behavior Therapy* (2nd ed.). New York: Pergamon.

Wonderlich, S. A., Fullerton, D., Swift, W. J., & Klein, M. H. (1994): Five-year outcome from eating disorders: Relevance of personality disorders. *International Journal of Eating Disorders*, 15(3):233–243.

Wong, S. E., Martinez-Diaz, J. A., Massel, H. K., *et al.* (1993): Conversational skills training with schizophrenic inpatients: A study of generalization across settings and conversants. *Behavior Therapy*, 24:285–304.

Wright, J. H., Thase, M. E., Bec, A. T., *et al.* (Eds.) (1992): *Cognitive Therapy With Inpatients: Developing a Cognitive Milieu.* New York: Guilford.

Xie, L., & Dong, X. (1994): 124 cases of dyssomnia treated with acupuncture at sishencong points. *Journal of Traditional Chinese Medicine*, 14(3):171–173.

Yager, J. (1994): Psychosocial treatments for eating disorders. *Psychiatry*, 57(2):153–164.

Yamashita, S., Oishi, R., & Gomita, Y. (1995): Anticonflict effects of acute and chronic treatments with buspirone and gepirone in rats. *Pharmacology and Biochemistry of Behavior*, 50(3):477–479.

Young, W. C. (1986): Restraints in the treatment of a patient with multiple personality. *American Journal of Psychotherapy*, 40(4):601–606.

Yudofsky, S. C., Silver, J. M., & Schneider, S. C. (1987): Pharmacologic treatment of aggression. *Psychiatric Annals*, 17:397–407.

Zarate, C. A. Jr., Tohen, M., & Baldessarini, R. J. (1995a): Clozapine in severe mood disorders. *Journal of Clinical Psychiatry*, 56(9):411–417.

Zarate, C. A., Jr., Tohen, M., Banov, M. D. *et al.* (1995b): Is clozapine a mood stabilizer? *Journal of Clinical Psychiatry*, 56(3):108–112.

Zarate, R., & Agras, W. S. (1994): Psychosocial treatment of phobia and panic disorders. *Psychiatry*, 57(2):133–141.

Part IV

DISORDERS USUALLY FIRST DIAGNOSED IN INFANCY, CHILDHOOD, OR ADOLESCENCE

Beverly J. Sutton, M.D.

INTRODUCTION

The developmental level of the child has a major impact on how a disorder will be expressed and what treatments will be effective. Some behaviors are part of normal development at one age and evidence of disorder at another age. At this point in our clinical development, we are still refining the dimensions of a disorder. The American Academy of Child and Adolescent Psychiatry regularly publishes practice parameters based on diagnosis. When the precise etiology of each disorder is known, treatment may be available to correct the basic problems. In the meantime, many of our treatment plans will be based on symptoms, theories, and treatment-outcome research.

Therapeutic changes in the environment can be helpful for any patient, but these modifications are often critical for child and adolescent patients. Children depend on their parents and other adults to ensure their survival and the quality of life we consider adequate for normal development. Therefore, psychosocial programs are frequently used and may have more impact on the child than comparable programs have on an adult patient. The clinician who is generally familiar with the various psychosocial modalities will need to collaborate with others who specialize in specific programs to ensure adequate implementation. Youths require more comprehensive care than do adults with similar problems because attention must be given both to treating the psychopathology and to supporting the developmental process. The accepted fiscal formula states that a child requires three to five times the treatment resources of the adult patient in order to receive the same standard of care.

The pharmacokinetics and pharmacodynamics of medication in children and adolescents must be remembered when considering the use of medication. Generally, the younger the child, the shorter is the half-life of medication. Thus, the daily dose of medication is usually divided so that it remains at therapeutic levels rather than peak, sometimes reaching toxic levels after a single large dose, and then plummet to ineffective levels for the remainder of the day. Five to six times the half-life of medication is the general formula used for steady state or washout. When ordering medication, the general guidelines discussed by Popper and Frazier (1990) are basic to good practice. The *USP DI, Drug Information for the Health Care Professional* is recommended as a medication information resource.

Pharmaceutical companies tend to support research on adult patients. When the federal government approves the medication for clinical use, companies often slow their support of rigorous and expensive studies on children and adolescents. This results in the practice by clinicians of using medication in youths for the same indicators that would be appropriate for adults, whether or not there is research to support this assumption. Although open treatment trials and case studies provide only enough information to set up more definitive studies, it is not unusual for a medication to become a standard for treating certain symptoms in a youngster when the only support for its use in this age group is an open trial involving a small number of patients or a case report.

Finally, for clinicians who work with deaf patients, suprasegmental communication may be confused with the abnormal involuntary movements of tardive dyskinesia. Three to five rapid movements of the lower lip to meet the upper lip mean, "Oh, I understand." Tweaking one side of the nose means, "I know that," and tweaking both sides means, "I know that, but don't like it." These movements are designed for communication and are not involuntary or out of context. It is impolite to interrupt the person signing, and so the suprasegmental communication provides feedback without interruption. For those assessing involuntary movements secondary to neuroleptics, this is disconcerting unless the communication form is understood.

CHAPTER 29

MENTAL RETARDATION
317, 318.X, 319

GENERAL THERAPY AND EDUCATION

For the past 20 years, behavioral therapy has been the dominant form of treatment for the mentally retarded person. Behavioral interventions must match the child's ability. If the child can take part in building the treatment plan, treatment maintenance and generalization effects are enhanced. Applied behavioral analysis is usually used to develop and maintain behavior-modification programs, cognitive-behavioral treatment, and behavioral family therapy. Cognitive-behavioral treatment examples include self-instruction training (providing the child with problem-solving skills while giving prompts to help complete the task) and correspondence training (reinforcing children for doing what they said they would do). Behavioral family therapy includes education on child development, styles of interaction, and behavior modification techniques, along with discussions about feelings and goals. Early intervention programs may alter outcomes by decreasing adverse stimuli on the child and family. Procedures using aversive consequences may be used as one part of a skill-building therapy program when there is a severe problem that has not responded to other procedures. Objective behavioral data (including notation of side effects) must be monitored and the aversive component removed expeditiously when it is no longer required.

Psychotherapeutic interventions may be needed for crisis care, depression, low self-esteem, or other problems. Psychotherapy for persons with mental retardation should set specific goals and use brief, clear verbalizations. The focus should be on current events and feelings, reality testing, helpful limit setting, and education about the meaning of problems.

At the first interview regarding their mentally retarded child, the parents need to hear the essentials and then be encouraged to talk about feelings. Later on, they wish to know how to plan for their retarded child, not only during childhood, but also in adult life. The family members are at risk for encountering problems, and these problems influence the functioning of the retarded person as well. Although the severely retarded child will need continuous direction and supervision as an adult, the moderately retarded adult can, with proper training and orientation, travel alone in familiar places and maintain unskilled or semiskilled occupations. In addition to "sheltered" employment, "supported" or competitive employment is now possible with a survey-train-place-maintain approach. Developing a life plan provides direction and support for the patient and family. The Association of Retarded Citizens has taken an active role in obtaining services for retarded people.

Public Law 94-142, passed in 1975, guarantees all handicapped youngsters 3 to 22 years of age, a free public education appropriate to their needs. The law was extended by PL 99-457 to increase the services. The definition of a "handicapped" person includes those who are blind, visually handicapped, deaf, hard of hearing, deaf/blind, mentally retarded, orthopedically impaired, seriously emotionally disturbed, specifically learning disabled, and speech impaired. Physicians should be familiar with local educational and other resources so that they can assist the family in finding habilitation programs, support groups, and advocacy services.

CONCOMITANT PSYCHIATRIC DISORDERS

Psychiatric disorders are four to five times more frequent in the retarded population than in the general population. Problems are fewer when the children are young, have mild or profound retardation, and live at home. The prognosis is poorer as the degree of retardation increases. An understanding of the handicapped child's development may provide clues to appropriate goals for the child and the behavioral interventions. In general, function improves when more opportunity for pleasurable activities is afforded, needs and preferences are attended to, and personal competence and independence are strengthened. All psychiatric diagnoses can be seen. About half of children with mental retardation have a psychiatric diagnosis.

Parent training is necessary for dealing with oppositional behavior in younger children. Teaching prosocial skills (independent play, positive peer interaction, and assertive verbal communication of needs and desires) is also useful. Social skills training includes instruction, modeling, role playing, and practice. Generalization may be supported by shifting the child pairs and the trainer-child interaction during training. Rituals, preoccupation with sameness, and bullying behavior may respond to programming, especially out of the home.

Feeding skills are taught with guidance and/or "chaining." It is faster to teach these skills outside of regular mealtimes. Self-care skills can be taught individually and then chained. Toileting intervention may involve signal devices, time out for accidents, and "overcorrection." (Overcorrection provides consequences beyond restitution for the behavior. For example, a boy who soils his pants is made to wash, get clean clothes, and do other cleaning chores.) Telephone-dialing skill can be taught with color coding, and this can be extremely important for emergency situations. Telling time is necessary for scheduling appointments or work and can usually be learned with special equipment and training.

Behaviors frequently seen in retarded persons include self-injurious behavior, stereotypy, rumination, pica, and autistic mannerisms. An intolerant environment may produce many kinds of behavior problems. Brain injury and certain types of seizures are sometimes associated with aggression and rage states. Some mentally retarded/mentally ill persons are in need of physical care, but cannot express their physical needs, except through irritability, anger, or other attention-gaining behaviors. Some have a high threshold for pain and may become extremely sick before someone notices other symptoms (e.g., pallor, anorexia). Some mentally retarded persons with behavior problems benefit from tension-reduction programs, such as swimming or other physical exercise.

SELF-INJURIOUS BEHAVIOR

The initial goals of therapy are usually practical ones, such as altering self-injurious behavior (SIB) or extreme aggressiveness. Treatment of SIB requires an understanding of what led to the behavior; attention to these conditions is necessary before implementing intervention programs. Additional factors that increase compliance include insisting on eye contact, making requests in a firm manner, and following requests with reinforcement or punishment.

Self-injuries behavior is usually treated with behavior modification programs similar to those used for noninjurious stereotypies. Differential reinforcement of incompatible behaviors may be more effective than differential reinforcement of other behaviors in decreasing self-injury. Differential reinforcement of other, more appropriate behaviors, such as smiling, with time-out procedures has been helpful in decreasing aggressive behaviors. Treatment plans should attend to the maintenance and generalization of the desired behaviors.

Punishment is very effective in decreasing severe behavior problems but is an ethical issue for some staff members. Facial screening is often more acceptable in this regard, for both infants and older children (Rojahn & Marshburn, 1992). A bib is tied around the neck and left on the chest until SIB occurs. At the time of unwanted behavior, the bib is pulled in front of the face and held for one minute. With facial screening, there is usually a 50% or greater decrease in behavior in the first session, then a gradual drop to almost zero in 5 to 10 sessions. Positive effects may last for months, or even years. The facial screening procedure may not be a wise choice for a physically strong and combative patient. The procedure is quite benign, with no serious side effects. Restraint is a last-resort procedure; some patients prefer restraint to being released and then required to behave appropriately or participate in a program.

Thioridazine in low doses decreases SIB and in higher doses decreases aggressive behavior (Crnic & Reid, 1989). Naltrexone is also used for SIB (Aman, 1993). Carbamazepine is often used for aggression and dyscontrol. Propranolol needs more study but has been used in cases of aggressive behavior and self-injury. Lithium may help in aggressive behavior when there is a family history of bipolar disorder or when the behavior is explosive or severe (Kaplan & Sadock, 1993).

When a mental illness is known to respond to medication, some feel that medication is the treatment of choice, even for patients who may respond to psychosocial interventions alone. To be effective, psychosocial treatments require time and effort by well-trained people. Medication is quick and easy by comparison. Some retarded persons have brain injury or physical problems and may be more sensitive to medication or more prone to side effects than are nonretarded persons. Behavioral and cognitive problems are often associated with anticonvulsant use. One older study found that 42% of children treated with phenobarbital developed behavior problems, compared with only 18% of those who received no treatment (Wolf & Forsythe, 1978). Problems with medication interaction and/or toxic states can occur even at dosages usually considered therapeutic.

Treatment for stereotypies includes relief from excessive stimulation or boredom, behavioral therapy, and, in severe cases, neuroleptic medication. The behavioral program may consist of manipulation of the stimuli site (not generally very effective, but includes removing things that seem to precipitate stereotypic behavior and providing items that may decrease it, such as television), aversive procedures (effective, but may have negative side effects), and positive procedures (effective, but more so when combined with overcorrection, restraint, or introduction of toys). (See stereotypic movement disorder.)

Pica is seen in about half of mentally retarded children at one year and in 10% at four years of age. Inadequate care or supervision may precipitate this problem. Eating problems and drooling restrict social interaction. Physical restraint, blindfolding/facial screening, and overcorrection have proved successful. Rumination occurs in 5 to 10% of the retarded population in institutions, particularly in severely to profoundly retarded persons. Overeating (three to eight times the average amount) has stopped rumination in some studies. Refusal of solid food is often a problem. Gradually changing the texture of food (i.e., from calorie-rich liquid to pureed, chopped, and then solid food) may be of limited value. When only solid food is presented, some children become hungry enough to eat. Oral manipulation techniques may help when there is a neurological problem.

One-third to one-half of mentally retarded children have attention-deficit/ hyperactivity disorder (ADHD). Stimulants can be used effectively for the active, distractible behavior, especially in younger patients who do not have stereotypies. Abdominal pain, insomnia, headaches, and anorexia may occur with stimulant use.

One in six students receiving special education is mentally retarded. Oral instructional modes are emphasized and statements are repeated or stories told. Bright pictures and charts with stick-on stars for desired behaviors ("star charts") help maintain the child's attention. Decreasing inappropriate or disruptive behaviors helps compliance but may not increase learning. A "gentle teaching" program creates opportunities to give rewards but requires great tolerance on the part of the caregiver, particularly when the child is aggressive. The strategies used teach the rewards possible when interacting with another person. Bonding is the goal of this intervention; punishment is not used. The attitude of the caregiver is carefully monitored.

CHAPTER 30

LEARNING, MOTOR SKILLS, AND COMMUNICATION DISORDERS

LEARNING DISORDERS
(ACADEMIC SKILLS DISORDERS)

The type of learning disorder determines the form of therapy. The need for specific forms of therapy may vary over time. Special education; speech and language therapy; sensorimotor integration; occupational therapy; individual, group, and family psychotherapy; and skills training are all considered and woven into the educational plan as needed. Behavior modification programs can encourage on-task behaviors and decrease the inappropriate behaviors often seen in the child or adolescent with learning disorders. Social skills training tends not to generalize but may persist when paired with positive peer experiences. About 40% of those with learning disorders have a parent with a learning disorder; this must be considered when planning family assistance and interventions.

315.00 READING DISORDER

Reading disorder (dyslexia) affects 2 to 8% of children in elementary school. Although boys are said to be at greater risk for this disorder, at least one report indicates that girls are affected almost as frequently as boys. People with specific developmental disorders tend to have relatives who have some form of specific developmental disorder. Developmental reading and articulation disorders seem to "breed true," but the familial incidence of other learning disorders shows much variation. Contrary to general belief, the distribution of hand dominance in dyslexia is similar to that of the general population. Although few dyslexic children

435

have visual-perception problems, most have problems with language or expressive writing. Curiously, one study reports that, in a rather brief period of instruction (2.5 to 5.5 hours), reading-disabled students were taught to read 30 different Chinese characters (Rozin *et al.,* 1970).

Unless treated, dyslexic children continue to increase the discrepancy between their reading levels and those of their peers. Sometimes switching from phonetic to holistic instruction, or the reverse, is effective. Phonologic skills are closely related to the ability to read and spell. Special education with tutoring and small-group instruction is the approved remediation. Instruction is multisensory and long term; the progress is usually slow. More research is needed to determine the benefit of specific remediation.

In one study (Karsh & Repp, 1992), learning-disabled students spent 12% of their time in school on academic tasks. There are several reasons for such limited instruction, but the main one is insufficient resources. Computer-assisted instruction can increase the opportunities for these children to have direct instruction and practice, through academic and nonacademic games, tutoring, simulation, and programming. For regular education students, a combination of teacher instruction and computer-assisted instruction has been found more effective than either method alone (Karsh & Repp, 1992). Computer drill and practice programs are particularly useful. Cognitive-behavioral approaches appear promising (Harris *et al.,* 1992), but additional information on outcome measures is needed.

Several different types of medication have been studied to some extent: stimulants, nootropics, anti-motion-sickness medications, and the major psychotropics. Children with mild learning disorders and ADHD (20 to 40%) are more likely to be helped by stimulants than those without ADHD (Rumsey, 1992; Aman & Rojahn, 1992). Nootropics are chemically related to γ-aminobutyric acid and are thought to enhance higher cortical functions (Aman & Rojahn, 1992). The studies using these compounds are not clear regarding the improvement of the learning-disabled person's skills. The rationale for using anti-motion-sickness medication is that people with dyslexia have a visual oculomotor dysfunction. These medications are not recommended at this time; in fact, some researchers feel that they can be harmful to some children. Benzodiazepines tend to decrease learning in persons without learning disabilities, so there is reluctance to use them for those who have learning problems. Antianxiety medications, antidepressants, and neuroleptics remain research medications for children with learning disorders. The American Academy of Pediatrics reported that the use of megavitamin therapy for learning disabilities is not helpful, and it may damage the nervous system (Barness, 1993). Parents who read to their children are models for an appreciation of reading, and provide additional information for the child.

315.1 MATHEMATICS DISORDER

Mathematics skills begin to develop as early as 4 months of age, according to a study by Wynn (1992). Children with this disorder may have trouble with terminology and concepts, difficulty recognizing symbols or organizing things into groups, attention problems with accurate copying or carrying, and/or problems involving sequential math procedures. Achievement is highly dependent on the quality of instruction; many people who have problems with math have not had appropriate instruction. Focused and systematic instruction improves skills, but some students need more intensive interventions. Missing class periods or having inconsistent instruction can result in confusion for the student. The drill and practice programs in computer-assisted instruction help these children develop rapid recall of basic math facts. A strong, consistent, well-planned instructional program is essential. Teacher instruction before computer-assisted instruction is necessary to the success of the latter. The research on computer-assisted instruction is insufficient to draw conclusions about outcome effectiveness at this time. Some suggest that the computer be used primarily for drill and practice.

315.2 DISORDER OF WRITTEN EXPRESSION

Children with expressive writing disorder have difficulty with spelling, grammar, organization, and punctuation. (For poor penmanship, see "developmental coordination disorder.") Letter reversals and mirror writing are features of low reading levels and are not part of this disorder. Education begins with letter-sound associations for reading, spelling, and writing, followed by blending and combinations of letters for word production in reading and spelling. Sentence writing and story writing come next. Spelling assessment and instruction are available in computer-assisted programs. The "holistic" approach starts with the student's ideas, provides structure for a topic, and refines language and organization, and eventually a paper is produced. This affords an opportunity for the creative communication of ideas before attention to the mechanics of writing is required. With effective remediation, writing-disordered persons compensate to some degree, but still require more effort and time to complete writing projects than do their peers.

MOTOR SKILLS DISORDER

315.4 DEVELOPMENTAL COORDINATION DISORDER

In developmental coordination disorder, the problem is speed and dexterity of movement. Measures of motor performance in aiming and timing are good indicators of the impairment. On neurological examination, this condition is more likely to be found than dyspraxia (problems with planned movement), but it is often called a "soft sign" and attributed to other diagnoses (e.g., attention-deficit/ hyperactivity disorder).

If clumsiness is not causing the child a problem, some clinicians advise parents to avoid direct remediation and to concentrate on the child's emotional state. In an absence of other problems, motor deficits are a low priority for referral and the remedial assistance available is limited in many areas. Teachers who notice poor penmanship or poor performance in physical education classes can refer these children before a pattern of failure is established. Without treatment, coordination difficulties persist in many children, sometimes causing academic lags and emotional problems.

Practice is a very effective remediation, but the child must be given extra time to complete motor tasks. Sensorimotor approaches and adaptive physical education classes provide specific help. Assistive approaches are also very helpful (e.g., Velcro instead of laces for shoes, zippers instead of snaps or buttons).

Some clinicians believe that poor visuospatial perceptual judgment may contribute to problems with movement in the clumsy child. They recommend that occupational therapists give more emphasis to perceptual training programs (Lord & Hulme, 1987).

COMMUNICATION DISORDERS

315.31 EXPRESSIVE LANGUAGE DISORDER
315.31 MIXED RECEPTIVE/EXPRESSIVE LANGUAGE DISORDER

Nonverbal communication usually remains intact in language-disordered children. Fifty percent of expressive language-disordered children catch up without therapy by school age. More severe conditions usually normalize by late adolescence, although academic underachievement is common. Receptive language disorder is the most disabling; severely affected children almost never reach normal language levels.

Language-disordered children require special academic programs. Language assessment provides the information needed for specific interventions. Speech/language therapy is indicated, along with social skills training. Some children who need speech/language classes function too well for their school district's arbitrary cutoff scores, and are returned to regular classes in spite of their poor performance. The emphasis of treatment should be on comprehension rather than on verbal output. Going from the concrete to the abstract, then to syntax as the child can manage it, appears to be a helpful sequence. Little is known about the efficacy of speech/language therapy, but it may prevent behavior disorders to some extent. Parental guidance is needed to help keep the child motivated. Home training emphasizes communication, not correction.

About one-fourth of children with communication disorders have psychiatric disorders, most commonly, a behavioral disturbance. Behavior problems are best approached through prevention and by teaching the child self-control. When this does not work, behavior modification programs are needed. Psychotherapy may be indicated for depression or other problems related to coping with the communication disorder. Children with receptive and expressive language disability may be able to use therapy that does not rely on listening and talking.

315.39 PHONOLOGICAL DISORDER

Phonological disorder (developmental articulation disorder) is the most benign developmental disorder, affecting about 10% of children under 8 and 5% over eight years of age. Mild articulation disorders usually stop by the age of eight. With adequate speech therapy, more severely involved articulation-disordered children have almost 100% remission. Problems with vowel sounds are usually organic in origin, and should not be diagnosed as articulation disorders.

307.0 STUTTERING

Stuttering is common between two and six years of age. Rarely, it is a side effect of medication, such as tricyclic antidepressants, neuroleptics, lithium, or alprazolam.

Children who feel pressured tend to respond to a clinician who makes simple, quiet statements in a fluent fashion. Training parents to talk slowly helps a stuttering child to speak normally; children tend to imitate adults. A child who stutters occasionally probably will not stutter as an adult.

Operant conditioning, systematic desensitization, and artificial speech patterns were highly touted treatment programs at various times (Bloodstein, 1993). Operant conditioning uses reward and punishment to shape both fluency and body tension. Systematic desensitization involves gradual exposure to anxiety-provoking situations, with the focus on relaxing to counteract the tension and stress that aggravate stuttering. Introducing artificial speech patterns is a deliberate attempt to change the rate and rhythm of speech (e.g., creating drawls and recitatives). Speech therapy involves speech skills, comfort with attempts to speak, relaxation, adjustment of body movements, rhythm control, and practice in speaking. About one-third to one-half of stutterers gain lasting fluency.

Most people who stutter have normal speech when singing or reading poetry, and when listening to white noise through headphones. The Edinburgh Master device provides white noise when the person is speaking, and then ceases when the speaking stops. Many patients dislike listening to the sound, but it is effective for those with severe stuttering.

Delayed audio feedback, in which the patient's own voice is played back through headphones after a very brief pause, is effective, but the feedback device is cumbersome and patients are not easily weaned from it. The therapeutic effect may be a result of forcing the patient to slow his or her speech, which may be helpful even without delayed audio feedback.

Stutterers' support groups include the National Stuttering Project, 2151 Irving Street, Suite 208, San Francisco, CA 94122; the National Council on Stuttering, 558 Russell Road, DeKalb, IL 60115; and Speak Easy International, 233 Concord Drive, Paramus, NJ 07652. The Stuttering Foundation of America, P.O. Box 11749, Memphis, TN 38111-0749 has literature available, and the Stuttering Resource Foundation, 123 Oxford Road, New Rochelle, NY 10804 has public service announcements and directories for speech clinics.

CHAPTER 31

PERVASIVE DEVELOPMENTAL DISORDERS

Children with pervasive developmental disorders (PDD) have impairment of social interaction and communication, along with unusual behavior or interests. Mental retardation is frequently seen. Comprehensive assessment in all functional domains is necessary before overall treatment planning and habilitation can be expected to succeed. Special education, speech and language training, skills training, vocational education, medication, and family education may all be useful. With the exception of Asperger's disorder, parents receive few cues to help them intuitively care for their child. Parent education can replace some of the missing emotional and social feedback ordinarily obtained from a normal infant. This feedback shapes the parents' behavior to fit the needs of the child. In addition, once parents learn they can teach their preschool child to respond to praise, they feel more competent and needed. Without such early training, the autistic child, for example, is unresponsive to this common social reinforcer. Since most PDD children require long-term care, parents should receive extended support from treatment personnel and support groups, along with assistance in preparing a life plan for their child.

299.00 AUTISTIC DISORDER

Clinicians were fascinated by the autistic child long before Kanner's classic description appeared in the literature. At one time, it was thought that there were more people studying autism than people meeting the diagnostic criteria for the disorder. Treatment tended to focus on the affective deficit, the cognitive deficit, or the organic brain disorder, depending on the orientation of the clinician. Now, the comprehensive individualized treatment plan addresses all areas of weakness and builds on the strengths of the child. The autistic child's cognitive strengths tend to be memory and visuospatial tasks; weaknesses are in symbol formation, abstractions, and concepts. When and if an autistic child begins to speak, the language is abnormal; the child does not use it for social communication. Social development is slow and lacks responsiveness to others. Unusual attachment to objects and rituals may interfere with learning new tasks, as do the stereotypies of finger flicking, whirling objects, and body twirling. Some children are overactive, disruptive, fearful, and aggressive; have temper tantrums; and exhibit self-injurious behavior.

A structured program is needed so that planned interaction can be established along with individual teaching. The child's behavior deteriorates when the environment is not structured. Preschool children can be taught to respond to praise; older children who have not been so taught do not respond to praise. Tasks are broken down into a few attainable steps and short, simple sentences are used.

For severely to profoundly retarded autistic children, treatment programs emphasize self-care, reasonable compliance, basic social behaviors, reduction of harmful behavior, communication of needs, and appropriate recreational behavior. For autistic children with intelligence ranging from normal to moderately retarded, age-appropriate communication and social/behavioral skills are emphasized.

Initial treatment should minimize inappropriate behaviors, such as aggression and noncompliance. Intrusion into the child's solitary activity may be needed, but this should be done in a way that is pleasant to the child. Basic skills, such as sitting in a chair and attending to the teacher (eye contact) and task, are taught.

Compliant behaviors and disruptive behaviors appear to be inversely related; that is, an increase in one automatically reduces the other. Thus, stereotyped behaviors can often be decreased by introducing incompatible alternative behaviors. Understanding disruptive or noncompliant behaviors as "escape" behaviors provides additional information for the behavior program format. Aversive programs to reduce disruptive behaviors may be necessary at times.

Once the child can sit and attend for 15 to 20 minutes, basic social and communication skills, self-help skills, and play are addressed. The building of social behavior can be supported by imitating toy manipulations (which increases eye contact and vocalization), prompting the child to play with a preferred toy (decreasing social avoidance), and helping the child with homework (increasing positive verbal interaction with parents). Several behavioral techniques have been useful in increasing social behaviors (Newsom & Rincover, 1989).

All forms of communication should be supported. Language training is more effective when there is already some evidence of language skills. Communication skills programs mainly emphasize operant speech training or total communication. For operant speech training, the basic skills are needed, and then verbal imitation, receptive labeling (the child picks items as requested), and expressive labeling (the child identifies objects) are introduced. If the child remains mute, sign language can be tried. If efforts in sign language meet similar blocks, picture boards or cards can be used.

"Facilitated communication" (supporting the patient's arms or hands while he or she uses a typewriter or computer) is not considered a valid technique for communicating with autistic or mentally retarded people. Some advocates insist that it be available for those patients who cannot use speech, sign language, or picture boards. In the past, information obtained with facilitated communication was used to create treatment plans and support allegations of patient abuse. The American Academy of Pediatrics (1993) has published a policy statement indicating that the absence of scientific validation for (and citing some studies specifically refuting) the technique makes information obtained in this way questionable.

Treatment gains do not readily transfer to another situation. Therapeutic efforts need to be focused on the child's home as well as the school. Parent education and support are extremely important. Parents tend to stop the structured teaching sessions for a variety of reasons: they need help with community resources, nonresponsive agencies, personal feelings, marital problems, and patient-sibling issues. Showing normal siblings how to teach their autistic brother or sister to play appears to be very helpful to the normal siblings.

Parents often wish to try unproved treatment regimens to find help for the autistic child and relief for the family. Megavitamin therapy and many other regimens lack evidence of effectiveness, and may be harmful (Dulcan & Popper, 1991; Rutter, 1985). Clinicians and support groups can help the family avoid these sometimes costly ventures.

An interesting new study suggests that the prognosis for the autistic child may be improved by intensive early behavioral intervention. McEachin *et al.* (1993) reported on a behavioral program consisting of about 40 hours per week of one-to-one training with 19 autistic children under four years of age. Treatment was based on developing language, social behavior, and play, while suppressing rituals, tantrums, and aggression. The treatment lasted two or more years and included academic mainstreaming and parent training. The control children consisted of 19 autistic children who received 10 hours or less per week of behavioral treatment and special education and whose parents received training, and another group of 21 autistic children not referred to the study but followed by another agency. At a mean age of seven years, the experimental group had made major educational advances and gained an average of 20 IQ points. Only 2.5% of the control subjects reached normal levels of functioning. At a mean age of 11.5 years, members of the experimental group had maintained their gains over the controls. Although small, this study is one of only a few that indicate very positive outcomes for autistic children, in marked contrast to the consistently documented poor prognosis for normal outcome in adulthood (less than 2% according to Rutter, cited in McEachin *et al.* [1993]).

Seizures occur in 35 to 50% of autistic patients by 20 years of age. Anticonvulsants and seizure precautions are part of the treatment plan.

Several studies have shown that haloperidol decreases hyperactivity, social withdrawal, stereotypies, abnormal object preoccupation, negativism, and angry affect, while increasing learning. This effect does not appear to decrease with time. The usual dose of haloperidol for autistic children is low (0.5 to 4.0 mg/day in divided doses) and provides its effect with minimal sedation (Teicher & Glod, 1990). In one study, almost one-third of children being treated with or withdrawing from haloperidol developed dyskinesias that eventually (over 1 to 30 weeks) resolved without additional medication. These drug-related dyskinesias may mimic Tourette's disorder or stereotypy (Campbell & Cueva, 1995). Fenfluramine has not been very effective in autistic children, but may help some who have agitation and an IQ over 40; controlled studies with fenfluramine do not show efficacy of the medication over placebo (Campbell & Cueva, 1995). There are no reports of controlled studies of children treated with fluvoxamine.

In a double-blind, placebo-controlled study by Campbell *et al.* (1993), naltrexone reduced hyperactivity in young autistic children and had no serious side effects or effects on discrimination learning. Naltrexone was not superior to placebo in reducing SIB, which was slightly increased on withdrawal from the drug. Kolmen *et al.* (1995) found "modest improvement" in 8 of 13 children using naltrexone in a double-blind, placebo-crossover study.

Stimulant medication may increase attention span while decreasing hyperactivity and impulsivity in some autistic children (Dulcan & Popper, 1991. A double-blind study of antidepressant medication showed that clomipramine was better than placebo or desipramine for stereotypies, anger, and compulsive behaviors (Gordon *et al.*, 1993). Clomipramine and desipramine were equally superior to placebo in decreasing hyperactivity for these patients. Sanchez *et al.* (1996) in a study of eight children, 3.5 to 8.7 years, receiving 2.5 to 4.64 mg/kg of clomipramine found one child improved moderately, and six were worse. One child was dropped out of the study after two episodes of urinary retention. Hyperarousal may be decreased with β-blockers, but controlled studies are needed.

ORG 2766, an adrenocorticotrophic hormone (4-9) analog, shows some promise. In animal and human studies, it improved social behavior, adaptation, and information processing. A recently expanded double-blind, placebo-crossover study of autistic children indicated that after eight weeks on a dose of 40 mg/day, play behavior and social interaction increased significantly (Buitellar *et al.*, 1992).

299.80 Asperger's Disorder

Children with Asperger's disorder (AD) show abnormal social behavior that cannot be attributed to other factors. Their communication is off the point and they seem not to be able to use social context to achieve understanding. Although most normal children may become preoccupied with a hobby, AD children obsess over an interest and prefer this activity to all others. Play is repetitive.

Attention deficit and impulsivity are commonly seen in the latency-aged child with AD, as are social phobias, generalized anxiety disorders, and depression. Learning disabilities and fine motor coordination problems also may need to be addressed in the treatment plan. Tourette's disorder and unusual antisocial behavior may occasionally be seen.

Treatment is similar to that for a child with autism who is not retarded. The AD child performs better when in a regular classroom. Interventions may include training in socialization, communication, play, adaptive skills, and behavior control. Trying to convert the patient's unusual interests into strengths may be possible at times. Early speech and language training to support functional communication is necessary. There may be problems with academic development and early vocational training is recommended, particularly for jobs that require few social skills.

Older children can benefit from group therapy and social skills training. Such children often enjoy sports and camping, and learning new skills. Brief psychotherapy may bolster a child's low self-esteem. Some patients like to read about AD or talk with other people who have the same condition. Parents also need education and support. Stimulants, antidepressants, or other medication may be useful for distractibility, depression, anxiety, and obsessive-compulsive symptoms when these symptoms interfere with function. If there is great anxiety or high levels of arousal, neuroleptics can be helpful.

299.80 RETT'S DISORDER

Girls with Rett syndrome have autism, dementia, ataxia, and persistent hand-wringing. They appear normal during the first 7 to 18 months of life, and then rapidly deteriorate in social, motor, and cognitive functions, until reaching a static state at about four years of age. After the second year of life, a small head and hand-wringing differentiate Rett syndrome from autism. Some 75 to 80% develop seizures during this time, which may be difficult to control. The most common seizures are minor motor seizures (blackout spells, eye rolling and staring); the next most common are tonic-clonic type. Three-quarters of patients are bedridden or use a wheelchair by adolescence; all have severe scoliosis.

Feeding problems may require pureed foods and thickened drinks and the avoidance of thin liquids. Weight gain can be achieved with a high-calorie, low-carbohydrate, high-fat diet with supplements. The caregiver must monitor for, and promptly treat, constipation.

Music with a heavy beat (rock and roll, German "oom-pah" music) seems to decrease these patients' fidgeting and noisy behavior. Headphones can provide this soothing influence for the child at home or in public without interfering with other activities. Car rides, rocking, and warm baths can also be calming.

A stimulating environment, medication, and psychosocial interventions have been tried in these girls without benefit (Tuten & Miedaner, 1989). Behavior modification does not appear to be very effective in altering behavior or interrupting SIB (Perry, 1991). Music therapy supports social communication, attention, and hand use. Sufficient sleep and diet appear to decrease irritability and tantrums.

A study using tyrosine and tryptophan showed no improvement (Nielson *et al.*, 1990), although some improvement in behavior and motor function has been noted on a ketogenic diet (Perry, 1991; Haas *et al.*, 1986). In a double-blind, placebo-controlled study of 25 Rett syndrome patients, naltrexone improved awake respiratory patterns but had a negative effect on motor development and progression of the disorder (Percy, *et al.*, 1994). Studies of bromocriptine are varied, with some reporting improvement in hand activity, communication, hyperpnea, and bruxism (Zappella, 1990), and others showing little or no change. No positive response has been shown with antiparkinsonian agents (Percy, *et al.*, 1990). Short-term use of chloral hydrate, diphenhydramine, or chlorazepate may help establish appropriate sleep patterns.

Physical therapy helps to maintain motion and supports ambulation. Good positioning is necessary; all support furniture must fit properly and keep the body upright.

Hydrotherapy also improves range of motion and comfort. The training sessions must fit the child's tolerance, and may last up to two hours, depending on the child's response. Treatment of scoliosis can prevent problems with heart and lung function. For the treatment of apraxia-ataxia, a therapy ball, floor activities stimulating balance skills, segmental rolling, and weight-shifting activities are useful. Overcorrection of inappropriate hand and foot movements stopped this behavior in two schizophrenic children studied by Epstein *et al.* (1974), but when the intervention stopped, the abnormal movements returned (more severe than at the beginning of the study). Tuten and Miedaner (1989) got conflicting results when using hand splints to increase purposeful hand movements. This lack of results may have been attributable to differences in the patients' ages or functional levels.

Carbamazepine is the medication of choice for seizure control, especially in blood levels of 10 to 15 mg/ml. In a small study of valproate, half the children were helped but developed elevated ammonia levels and liver enzymes. Philippart (1986) found little effect with ethosuximide, clonazepam, and metharbital in a small study. ACTH or a ketogenic diet may help for a short time. Haas *et al.* (1986) found improved seizure control in five of seven children on a ketogenic diet using medium-chain triglyceride oil. Phenobarbital, phenytoin, and clorazepate may also be helpful in more difficult cases (Thompson & Thompson, 1987; Philippart, 1986). Apneic spells while awake may precipitate the seizures.

Support for these children and their parents can be obtained through the International Rett's Syndrome Association, 10900 Bolton Drive, Potomac, MD 20854.

299.10 CHILDHOOD DISINTEGRATIVE DISORDER

Also known by a variety of other names, including Heller syndrome, this disorder is characterized by a longer period of normal development than is Rett syndrome; it affects boys more often than girls and involves intellectual and social deterioration, with motor or basal ganglia dysfunction. There is a single episode of deterioration lasting six to nine months, and then slight improvement. The children have excessive anxiety.

Treatment consists of parent education, behavior modification, and special education for the child. Because of multiple health problems, physical care must be carefully monitored. Haloperidol, benzodiazepines, and anticonvulsants have been used for behavior control but are usually not helpful. These children remain severely retarded and completely dependent on others.

299.80 PERVASIVE DEVELOPMENTAL DISORDER NOS

For this diagnosis to be used, most of the symptoms of a pervasive developmental disorder must be present but not meet both behavioral and onset criteria. Treatment is based primarily in an educational setting with a focus on social skills development. Although insight-based psychotherapy has little utility for this group, a therapeutic relationship can offer support, structure, and information for the child. Family or parent therapy can be helpful, and may include support for the family upon making a decision to place the child in residential treatment or a group home. While support for the child is important, the needs of other family members should not be ignored.

Medication may be used for target symptoms. Neuroleptics may be effective for aggression, disorganization, and SIB. Antidepressants can assist with depression, hyperactivity, and obsessive-compulsive behavior. Carbamazepine and lithium may decrease aggression and SIB. Naltrexone may be used for severe SIB. It must be noted that response of a target behavior or symptom to medication does not, in itself, confirm a specific diagnosis.

CHAPTER 32

ATTENTION-DEFICIT AND DISRUPTIVE BEHAVIOR DISORDERS

314.00, 314.01, 314.9 ATTENTION-DEFICIT/ HYPERACTIVITY DISORDER

The hyperactivity and short attention span behavior of children with attention-deficit/hyperactivity disorder (ADHD) is readily apparent in a busy classroom but may not be obvious in the physician's office. In low-demand settings, ADHD children may look like normal children. However, they have difficulty modulating their level of arousal and are usually over- or underaroused. Often, physicians do not agree on how to treat ADHD because the children are "presorted." Children with ADHD, seizures, and mental retardation go to a neurologist; those with ADHD, learning disorders, and other behavior problems go to a child psychiatrist; and children with uncomplicated ADHD go to a primary care physician.

Five percent of ADHD children have neurological disorders, particularly seizures and cerebral palsy. In children, ADHD is commonly associated with conduct disorder, oppositional defiant disorder, and mood disorders. It is also increased in children with mental retardation, Tourette's disorder, and specific learning disorders. Children with hyperthyroidism and those taking such medications as theophylline, carbamazepine, benzodiazepines, and phenobarbital can present symptoms very similar to those of ADHD. Hyperactivity usually decreases in early adolescence. About one-fourth of ADHD children have severe antisocial behavior in adulthood.

Parent education about the disorder is essential and may prevent unnecessarily harsh consequences for the child's behavior. The child will be more compliant if the father becomes involved in the child's behavior control. Children respond better to repeated prompts, immediate reinforcement for compliance, and rapid punishment (time out, response cost) for noncompliance. Treatment does not cure ADHD, but can reduce conduct problems, low academic achievement, and depression. Symptoms often appear again when treatment stops; long periods of therapy may be required. Support groups become very important during this sustained effort for the ADHD patient and family. Parent support groups include Children with Attention Deficit Disorders (CHADD), Suite 185, 1859 North Pine Island Road, Plantation, FL 33322; and Attention Deficit Disorders Association (ADDA), 4300 West Park Boulevard, Plano, TX 75093.

Environmental adjustment may be adequate treatment for some children with ADHD. Others require more intensive interventions, including special education classes, medication, stimulus-control procedures (both to increase and to decrease stimulation), and remediation of coexisting psychiatric problems. Children with ADHD may qualify for public special education programs, which can be specified in individualized educational plans. Teachers are given help with classroom management and fill out "report cards" for the parents each day. Scoring of attention and activity is easily done with the Child Attention Problems (CAP) Rating Scale. Contingency management programs often consist of token economy, time out, and response-cost programs. Negative consequences are more effective when they are part of the initial program in the classroom rather than added later. With treatment, social interactions at school may be sustained, but incomplete schoolwork usually remains a problem.

Medication

About 75% of ADHD children respond to stimulants, such as methylphenidate, dextroamphetamine, or pemoline. Stimulants help productivity and accuracy in academics but probably not final achievement. Methylphenidate and dextroamphetamine are equally effective in studies. Pemoline, which is longer acting, is usually somewhat less effective for symptom control (Kaplan & Sadock, 1993). By the age of three years, stimulant pharmacokinetics in these children are similar to those in adults. It is difficult to determine which stimulant is best for a child, but the usual practice is to start with methylphenidate, unless the long-acting pemoline is desired. There is controversy about whether or not long-acting methylphenidate is as effective as the short-acting form (Greenhill, 1992). Failure to respond to one stimulant does not mean that the child will not respond to another.

The dose of methylphenidate is individually adjusted, beginning with about 5 mg/day. If the child weighs more than 30 kg, the starting dose is usually 10 mg. After a few days of morning medication, a second dose is added at noon. In some cases, a smaller dose is added around 4:00 P.M. The morning or noon dose may then be increased every 5 to 14 days until symptoms are controlled. The therapeutic dose is usually 0.3 to 0.7 mg/kg twice a day. Single doses over 20 mg are unusual; the total daily dose is rarely more than 60 mg, even for adolescents

(Dulcan, 1990). Methylphenidate may have more effect on hyperactivity than dextroamphetamine; it can impair cognitive function in high doses (more than 1 mg/kg per dose), and some children show this deficit at lower doses.

Pemoline is started at 18.75 mg in a single morning dose, then increased by 0.5 to 3.0 mg/kg per day. The usual daily maximum is 112.5 mg; however, older adolescents and adults may require up to 2.2 mg/kg (Dulcan, 1990). Pemoline shows its strongest action after about three weeks. Liver function should be monitored as chemical hepatitis may develop. It has also been associated with night terrors and choreiform movements (Dulcan & Popper, 1991). Pemoline has little street value because it lacks the euphoric "rush" seen with methylphenidate or dextroamphetamine. If there is a danger that others may acquire the patient's medication, it is lessened by prescribing pemoline.

In usual doses, stimulants have a wider margin of cardiovascular safety than do the tricyclic antidepressants. Some 1 to 2% of ADHD children receiving stimulants develop motor or vocal tics. One-fourth to one-half of patients with Tourette's disorder have more tics with stimulant medication. Contrary to information available a few years ago, ADHD symptoms continue to respond to stimulants as the child passes through adolescence. Many patients continue to need medication even in young adulthood (Hechtman, 1992).

Giving stimulants with tricyclic or tetracyclic antidepressants and some anticonvulsants (primidone, phenobarbital, and phenytoin) decreases the metabolism of both medications, resulting in elevated plasma levels. In the past, imipramine was often added to methylphenidate when the child had both ADHD and depression. This combination can produce confusion, labile affect, marked aggression, and agitation. Amphetamines should not be used within two weeks of taking monoamine oxidase inhibitors (MAOIs). Using other psychotropic medications with stimulants is not usually recommended.

After stimulants, tricyclic antidepressants are the next most effective medication for ADHD, particularly in preadolescents. Imipramine and desipramine are the most often used. If stimulants produce severe rebound or dysphoria, tics are present, or there is a drug problem in the home or classroom, antidepressants can often be very effective. Quinn and Rappaport (1975) compared imipramine with stimulants in a long-term study. They were both effective, but side effects were twice as common with imipramine and twice as many imipramine-treated children dropped out of treatment. Nortriptyline, amitriptyline, and clomipramine are also helpful. Desipramine has a lower risk of side effects (Green, 1992); however, six cases of sudden death have been reported, so parents are usually reluctant to accept this medication. The (generally remote) possibility of cardiotoxicity with tricyclics should be communicated to parents. Long-acting tricyclics, such as imipramine pamoate, are not recommended for children or young adolescents. Dry mouth may increase dental caries, and some patients have difficulty with dry contact lenses.

Most clinicians report tricyclic antidepressants to be ineffective in adolescents (Wender, 1990); however, the MAOIs produce good results in those willing to follow the low-tyramine diet. In a double-blind crossover study, clorgyline (an MAO-A inhibitor no longer available in the United States) and tranylcypromine produced immediate, significant improvement, but selegiline, an MAO-B inhibitor, did not (Zametkin *et al.*, 1985). Some children respond well to bupropion; Barrickman and associates (1995) found bupropion and methylphenidate equally effective for symptom control.

Antipsychotic medications are considered third-rank treatment for ADHD. Thioridazine produces mild to moderate lethargy but only minimal problems for cognitive performance. Similarly, chlorpromazine and low-dose haloperidol (0.5 to 2.0 mg/day) decrease hyperactivity and behavior problems, but have little effect on learning.

Medications not shown helpful in ADHD include fenfluramine, diazepam, lithium, and mianserin (Campbell & Cueva, 1995). Clonidine improves compliance and decreases emotional outbursts but does not increase the attention span (Hunt *et al.*, 1990). Clonidine may be helpful for ADHD children who have tics. Rebound hypertension may be a problem with abrupt discontinuation.

A medication holiday should be attempted each year. Some clinicians advocate timing the holiday for summer vacation when the child's activity level and attention span are less critically monitored. Others suggest that the holiday be during the regular school year so that the need to continue medication can be more accurately assessed. Growth problems with stimulants are not a problem for most children and can be further minimized by medication holidays.

From a purely economic standpoint, medication is much less expensive than behavioral intervention. Behavioral interventions are difficult to implement and require careful training and monitoring. Unfortunately, long-term follow-up using stimulant medication alone does not indicate improvement in outcome for most ADHD children (Pelham & Sams, 1992).

Behavior Therapy

Behavior therapy programs typically consist of the structured use of time out, point systems, and contingency management. Aversive therapy and contingent rewards should be used together for prolonged periods, with mandatory support from parents and teachers. New settings and environmental novelty decrease behavioral problems, as do response cost procedures (e.g., return of earned tokens if unacceptable behavior occurs).

Token rewards may be better than praise in increasing on-task behavior (Barkley, 1989). However, few parents can set up an effective token economy without careful training and follow-up. Group reward that is based on the functioning of only one child is also effective. Skills training for patients may be needed. The use of behavioral programs often allows a decrease in medications. Behavioral techniques that work on the training site must be extended to other settings in which the child functions. Cognitive-behavior therapies, including self-monitoring, self-reinforcement, and self-instruction, are being studied for their effectiveness in generalization and maintenance (behavior control over time). Thus far, they seem not to be effective in ADHD (Pelham & Sams, 1992).

Combining contingency management training with stimulant medication is better than either program alone. The combination of stimulant medication and cognitive-behavioral therapy has provided varied results (Barkley, 1989). There are no psychosocial treatment outcome studies involving adolescent or young adult ADHD patients. Educating the adolescent about ADHD is considered worthwhile.

Dietary treatments have not proved generally effective. Sucrose and aspartame have been reported to cause hyperactivity and other behavior problems; however, a double-blind, controlled study of children 3 to 10 years old showed no behavioral or cognitive effects of these substances, even at levels exceeding the usual dietary intake (Wolraich *et al.*, 1994).

Sometimes a parent will insist on a special diet. As long as the regimen is nutritionally adequate, it can be allowed and emphasis transferred to other treatment strategies without alienating the family.

Up to 30% of adolescents with ADHD do not complete high school; most do not go to college. About 60% of young adults continue to have ADHD; 75% also have interpersonal problems. Many (23 to 45%) have juvenile convictions and develop adult antisocial syndromes (Barkley, 1989). Caring for children with ADHD requires expertise in many types of treatment and the maintenance of therapy and/or surveillance over extended periods.

313.81 OPPOSITIONAL DEFIANT DISORDER

Oppositional defiant behavior is seen in normal children from 18 to 36 months of age, and again in adolescence. It usually does not last more than six months.

The child with oppositional defiant disorder (ODD) takes a self-defeating stand in most arguments. Symptoms are more intense around familiar people. Training the family in behavior management is usually effective. Individual and family psychotherapy are rarely helpful. Therapy for a coexisting psychiatric disorder, if one exists, may improve compliance. Barkley (1989) found up to a 70% overlap of ODD and ADHD symptoms in clinic children, and developed a 10-step program for parents of 2- to 11-year-old ADHD-ODD children. The program finds ways to give positive attention; builds child compliance with brief commands, eliminates question-like commands and competing interests, such as television; establishes a token economy at home; implements effective time-out procedures for noncompliance (immediate, or the parents decide how long); extends time out to other noncompliant behaviors; manages noncompliant behavior in public; makes plans for future behaviors; and provides a review or "booster" therapy session. Barkley recommends problem-solving communication training for such adolescents. Severe family dysfunction limits program success.

312.8 CONDUCT DISORDER

One-third to three-fourths of children referred to mental health clinics present with a conduct disorder. Many disturbances contribute to the final behavioral picture of conduct disorder; the major provocateurs must be teased out and addressed. Family discord, inadequate supervision at home, and lack of a sustaining relationship with a parent contribute to the risk for developing a conduct disorder. The number of problem behaviors decreases with age, but children with severe, inadequately treated conduct disorders often show similar behavior in adulthood. When noncompliant behavior is treated, other behaviors improve as well. The diagnosis of conduct disorder may be a reflection of many different problems. No single treatment modality is universally effective.

Children with conduct disorder, especially boys, are at a significant disadvantage when they start school, in both readiness to learn and social adjustment. Rates of positive teacher attention to prosocial behavior are very low and probably not sufficient to maintain such behavior. Changing the teacher's social behavior does not, by itself, alter extremely disruptive behavior. Adding token reinforcement, concrete rewards, or activity reinforcers promotes behavior change. Learning disabilities often coexist with conduct disorder, and, if present, must be addressed.

For preadolescent children with conduct disorder, parent training and behavioral family therapy appear to be effective, although parental cooperation is a limiting factor. An adequate father-child relationship decreases difficult temperament, especially in girls. Decreased mother-child closeness predicts more difficult temperament for both boys and girls (Bezirganian & Cohen, 1992). Temperamental inflexibility in the child is the most powerful predictor of behavior problems in both boys and girls.

The parents must have clear rules for the child, actively monitor compliance, and apply defined consequences consistently. In older children, legal intervention may be necessary to produce effective limit setting and communicate the seriousness of behavior violations to the child and family.

A parent training program and two play therapy approaches designed specifically for elementary school children with conduct disorder are described by Kernberg and Chazan (1991). Parents are taught effective styles of interacting with their children, and then the intervention is generalized to the community. The goal is to increase the pleasure of family togetherness. "Supportive-expressive" play therapy promotes an alliance between parents and child and the maintenance of a positive but realistic attitude. The goal is to strengthen the child's ego functions through play or verbal communication. "Play group" psychotherapy involves three to six children and two psychotherapists. A safe environment is provided, in which interpersonal behaviors can be studied and rehearsed. The child and therapist choose specific goals (e.g., stopping hitting or yelling, adhering to the rules of a game).

Children in "multimodal day treatment" (Grizenko *et al.*, 1993) improved in both self-perception and disruptive behavior over children on a waiting list. Treatment consisted of 2.5 hours of special education and three hours of therapy and skills training each day. Family therapy took place weekly and medication was prescribed as needed. The staff in this situation must be able to set limits and confront while maintaining compassionate support.

The effect of family home-based programs for conduct-disordered adolescents is less clear. Residential programs, such as the "teaching-family" model,[1] do not show an advantage over nonbehavioral interventions of this type (McMahon & Wells, 1989). Except for some hope for anger-coping programs and problem-solving skills training, the outcome of skills training programs has been disappointing. A study of the family's preconceived ideas and biases helps to focus psychotherapeutic interventions designed to interrupt aggression.

Medications

If conduct disorder is secondary to depression, antidepressants may be helpful. Lithium often decreases the severe impulsive aggression seen with intense affective storms. Children with abnormal electroencephalograms, impulsive aggression, and labile affect may respond to carbamazepine. Cueva *et al.* (1996) in a double-blind, placebo-controlled study of 5- to 12-year-old children with conduct disorder found no advantage of carbamazepine over placebo, and side effects were common. Propranolol may help some patients with rage reactions who show evidence of organicity, although some clinicians do not recommend β-blockers for children. Stimulants may help children with conduct disorder who also have ADHD. Neuroleptics may be helpful for explosive, severely aggressive children; one study showed positive results with haloperidol (Stewart *et al.*, 1990). Phenytoin is probably ineffective for most children.

Unfortunately, most treatment programs are time-limited and do not provide the needed sustained treatment into the young adult years. Ongoing multimodal treatment programs and support linkages must be developed.

312.9 DISRUPTIVE BEHAVIOR DISORDER NOS

Patients with other or mixed disruptive syndromes should first be carefully evaluated to differentiate normal behaviors or other disorders, and then treated using the general principles outlined above.

---

[1]Adolescents, primarily adjudicated delinquents, live in a group home with a married couple using a point system, self-government, social skills training, tutoring, and careful oversight of school functioning.

CHAPTER 33

FEEDING AND EATING DISORDERS

307.52 PICA

Some form of indiscriminate eating is seen in 50% of children 1 1/2 to 3 years of age and 10% of children older that 12. In small children, inadequate supervision may make it a serious problem. Lead poisoning, from old paint or contaminated dirt, is not uncommon. Mentally retarded persons are at higher risk, with the behavior occasionally reaching bizarre and dangerous proportions. Parents frequently need support and education so that they can appropriately attend to their children and decrease the indiscriminate eating.

In children, iron supplements usually stop pica in less than seven days (Blinder *et al.*, 1989); the reason is unclear, since anemia is not always present.

Behavior modification programs are frequently used in treating mentally retarded persons and must be carefully planned and monitored. Not teaching a retarded person to eat with utensils may increase the persistence of finger-to-mouth behavior. Time out, response interruption, overcorrection (e.g., have the patient spit out the material and thoroughly cleanse the mouth and teeth), physical restraint (10 seconds seeming the most effective duration), and facial screening (briefly covering or blocking the child's face with a light cloth) are used.

307.53 RUMINATION DISORDER

Rumination disorder can cause death in 25 to 40% of affected infants (Kanner, 1957). Psychosocial evaluation often reveals multiple stresses in the family in addition to the concern about rumination. Attention given to a child who is receiving inadequate care can be a positive influence; however, a mother's attention to the vomiting may also reinforce and maintain the ruminating behavior. If the infant requires hospitalization, support for attachment behavior is essential. A staff member is chosen to engender a relationship, transfer this attachment back to the mother, monitor and assist the mother while she is feeding her infant, and integrate the mother into the total treatment program. Video recording of the mother-infant interaction during rumination may be useful in adjusting the feeding procedure.

One medical regimen consists of elevating the child's head and upper body during rest periods and giving small, frequent feedings. Diet management that involves small meals, clear liquids, or no liquids with meals may aggravate weight loss. After a meal, aluminum hydroxide alternating with magnesium hydroxide can be given to decrease esophagitis and improve sphincter pressure in the lower esophagus, thus decreasing reflux. Infants over a year old can be given cimetidine, 20 to 30 mg/kg per day in divided doses, or bethanechol, 8.7 mg per square meter of body surface, in divided doses (Blinder *et al.*, 1989). Oral antiemetic medication is minimally helpful. If severe complications exist after intensive medical management, a Nissen fundoplication may be necessary.

Dietary observations reveal that pureed foods are ruminated at higher rates than normally textured foods (Johnston, 1993). Increasing the amount of chewing decreases rumination, as does participation in after-meal tasks or activities.

Large, high-calorie feedings decrease ruminating after meals in older children (Johnston, 1993; Rast *et al.*, 1985). These satiation diets require that the child consume three to five times the amount of a single-portion feeding. The caloric density is very important because increased calories alone discourage rumination. A full tray is given and refilled as food is eaten. Noncoercive means are used to encourage the child to eat. When the child refuses to eat on three prompts without intervening intake, the meal is over. When the child reaches normal weight, other dietary methods can be considered.

Behavior therapists employ positive reinforcers (e.g., reduced stress and increased attention), satiation, social aversive techniques (e.g., saying "no" when rumination occurs and avoiding contact for five minutes), mouth cleaning or pepper-sauce mouth spray punishment, and other techniques. Behavior therapy is effective when properly done but requires a high degree of sophistication in management and design. The course of therapy often has to be extended. Mild electric shock may be effective, but should be reserved for severe cases in which other therapies have failed. The shock is paired with positive reinforcement for appropriate behavior.

307.59 FEEDING DISORDER OF INFANCY OR EARLY CHILDHOOD

Some 25 to 40% of young children have reportable eating problems. About 30% are "picky eaters." Overeating is rarely a complaint of parents, although 5 to 15% of children under five years of age are obese (Maloney & Ruedisueli, 1993).

Among pediatric admissions, 1 to 5% are for failure to thrive (FTT). Half of these children exhibit no organic explanation for their lack of weight gain (Walsh, 1994). Although FTT is due to inadequate nutrition, that does not always mean that the infant has a feeding disorder. Insecure infant-mother attachment is more common in children who fail to thrive than in other children.

Many parents assume that their young children cannot regulate food intake properly because of erratic eating patterns. Some of these parents use threats or bribes to control eating behavior. In 1928 Clara Davis found that infants who made their own selections from an appropriate diet were healthy and grew well even though eating behavior was erratic at times (Birch *et al.*, 1991). Infants and young children modify their intake in response to the energy content of the diet.

A multidisciplinary team should assess and treat inadequate weight gain in early childhood. If protection from abuse or parental incompetence is a major concern, hospitalization or foster home placement may be necessary. If the etiology of FTT is thought to be functional (i.e., nonorganic), the child should be placed in a controlled environment, and limited laboratory studies (complete blood count, urinalysis, stool examination, and sweat test) carried out. Other studies for etiology may be postponed, since many are affected by malnutrition.

Behavior therapy is often used, along with parent training, support, and attention to the quality of the dyadic relationship. The infant's maladaptive eating behaviors are extinguished and adaptive eating skills supported. Therapy for the mother can be active, practical, and supportive rather than exploratory. If the mother is introspective and motivated, individual psychotherapy may be helpful. Family problems are addressed and most interventions may be home-based. Visiting homemakers, family counseling and education, infant stimulation programs, and assistance with access to support systems may all be helpful.

CHAPTER 34

TIC DISORDERS

307.23 TOURETTE'S DISORDER

It is difficult to tell when Tourette's disorder begins. The most frequent initial symptoms are eye tics; head tics are also common. Throat clearing, sniffing, and coughing are much less commonly seen as initial symptoms, and may be misdiagnosed as upper respiratory tract infections or allergies. Onset is usually between 2 and 15 years of age, with about half of patients presenting their symptoms by the age of seven and 75% by age 11 (Kurlan, 1993). The face, neck, limbs, and torso, in decreasing order, are the most common sites of tics. Additional symptoms may include touching, hitting, jumping, smelling hands or other objects, stomping, squatting, retracing steps, twirling, and doing deep knee bends. When studying the efficacy of treatment, these behaviors must be monitored as well.

Adjustment of the learning disabilities seen in 25 to 50% of child and adolescent Tourette's patients is an important part of treatment. The child needs the freedom to leave the classroom and go to an area where tics or behavioral practice will not be observed. Moderate structure, short work segments, help with directions, support from teachers, and self-pacing can all be useful.

Medication

Medication is used when the tics are interfering significantly with the child's development and when other, less intrusive interventions provide inadequate control. Haloperidol, clonidine, and pimozide are the most commonly used. The goal is to decrease tics by 75% or more while keeping side effects to a minimum. When considering a medication holiday, slowly decreasing the dose is advised; abrupt cessation can produce an exacerbation of symptoms that will last for months.

461

Haloperidol helps up to 80% of patients and is usually considered the medication of choice. About 25% show marked improvement without significant side effects. Pimozide appears to have similar effects and drawbacks, but is better tolerated than haloperidol by many patients. Fluphenazine appears to be clinically effective but has not been adequately studied. Phenothiazines need more study but seem to be less effective than haloperidol and pimozide (Kurlan, 1993).

The efficacy of clonidine has not been clearly established in double-blind studies. Some clinicians use clonidine to avoid the side effects of antipsychotic medications, even though it takes up to three months to produce therapeutic effects.

As many as 50 to 70% of children with Tourette's disorder have some symptoms of ADHD. There is controversy over the use of stimulants in these patients. Up to 50% will develop more tics if stimulants are used (Kurlan, 1993). It is unclear whether or not tricyclic antidepressants increase tics. In open studies of children with both diagnoses, disruptive behavior decreased but imipramine and desipramine had no effect on tics (Ambrosini *et al.*, 1993). Spencer *et al.*, (1993) found significant improvement in both chronic motor tics and ADHD in a small study of nortriptyline. Controlled studies are needed; the lack of major adverse effects makes the response interesting. A retrospective study of bupropion by Spencer, Biederman, Steingard, *et al.* (1993) found exacerbation of tics in four patients with Tourette's and ADHD. Fluoxetine may have beneficial effects in some children with ADHD, but may cause agitation. Clonidine has a positive effect on hyperactivity.

Classroom and behavior management techniques should be tried before considering medication in any motor tic disorder. Even more caution is needed when a child has both ADHD and Tourette's. If all other trials fail, it may be necessary to use a stimulant with a neuroleptic, such as haloperidol or pimozide.

Obsessive-compulsive disorder (OCD) is seen in about half of Tourette's patients, starting around the age of 15 to 18 years and then remaining stable. Fluoxetine decreases OCD symptoms in many of these individuals and has not been reported to increase tics. Patients with OCD with poorly controlled tics may find the addition of clonazepam or neuroleptics helpful. Individual psychotherapy may be needed for the patient's sense of control and integrity. Family counseling or therapy is often required.

Because tics increase with stress, relaxation training can decrease their frequency and severity in stressful situations. Psychotherapy can help the child recognize, understand, and cope with situations that increase symptoms (Schroeder & Gordon, 1991).

Various behavior techniques (self-recording, vicarious learning, response-chain interruption, self-control training, and aversion therapy) are used to treat the self-injurious behavior sometimes seen in Tourette's disorder. There are no controlled studies of medication for SIB in this specific population. It is logical to use medications appropriate for the tic disorder first, then SSRIs, then other medications, if necessary (Towbin *et al.*, 1995).

The natural course of Tourette's disorder makes it difficult to assess treatment methods. In a study of Tourette's patients, 97% had spontaneous changes in the waxing and waning of symptoms, 96% had spontaneous changes in the type of symptoms, and 27% had spontaneous remissions lasting up to seven years. The magnitude of the change is larger than the improvement in many open studies. There is evidence that vocal and motor tics diminish or disappear in adult life. The tic severity decreases in about 30% of adolescent patients and in most adult patients. When treated with placebos, 30% improve, 30% show no effect, and 30% have tics more often.

Information about Tourette's disorder should be given to peers and educational staff members. The Tourette Syndrome Association (42-40 Bell Boulevard, Bayside, NY 11361; 718-224-2999) or a local support group is a useful resource. Books for lay readers, health care personnel, and educational staff are available.

307.22 CHRONIC MOTOR OR VOCAL TIC DISORDER
307.21 TRANSIENT TIC DISORDER
307.20 TIC DISORDER NOS

About one-fourth of school-age children have tics at some time or other. For transient tics, education, reassurance for the child and family, and access to follow-up are usually all that is necessary.

Habit reversal is very effective in chronic motor tic disorders, producing a greater than 90% reduction in tic frequency (Schroeder & Gordon, 1991). The procedure has many specific components, but awareness training and competing-response training are the crucial elements for tic and habit control. Relaxation training and psychotherapy, discussed briefly under Tourette's disorder, can be very helpful. Anxiolytic medication or low doses of major tranquilizers may be helpful.

The patient and family need a full explanation of the disorder. The child can control most tics for a time; families must be aware that loss of tic control is part of the disorder, not necessarily oppositional or defiant behavior.

CHAPTER 35

ELIMINATION DISORDERS

307.7, 787.6 ENCOPRESIS

Bowel training is a more important etiological factor in encopresis than bladder training is in enuresis; however, inadequate potty training alone is not sufficient to cause encopresis. Some children do not have toileting skills (recognizing when they need to go to the bathroom, knowing how to undress and sit on the toilet, etc.). All toileting activity should be focused on the bathroom; for example, one should not place the potty chair in the bedroom or family room.

Diets with little fiber or large amounts of dairy products can increase constipation. Exercise is useful for stimulating elimination. Adult-sized toilets, with which the child's feet do not touch the floor, and fears about going to the bathroom at school or elsewhere may also produce constipation. The parents may wish to check the bathroom facilities at school and make certain that supplies, cleanliness, and privacy are acceptable.

The parents and child must hear a clear, nonjudgmental explanation of encopresis. They must implement the treatment in a neutral fashion. The parents are responsible for checking pants and providing consequences (e.g., return of earned tokens, no star on that day's star chart). The child is responsible for keeping records and maintaining cleanliness. Parents can help younger children maintain a star chart or similar record, or provide a stack of clean pants and require the child to take dirty pants to a parent when soiling occurs. Written details about providing a high-fiber diet and extra fluids should be provided and the child involved in planning the diet.

Most children with encopresis have constipation and overflow incontinence (787.6). Children who are impacted often have poorly functioning anal sphincters and/or sluggish peristalsis in the lower colon. Many children who have developed impaction megacolon do not know they are soiling because rectal sensitivity is decreased.

In severe impaction, bowel evacuation (e.g., with enemas, suppositories, lubricants, or laxatives) must be accomplished before other interventions can work. Parents should be given detailed instructions, with careful follow-up to be certain they have been properly carried out. Some children can retain enema fluid for long periods, possibly producing significant electrolyte problems. Two to five minutes is safe and sufficient when saline is used. An evening oil retention enema with saline wash in the morning may be a safer rectal decompression program. Saline with papain can also be used. Even in safe circumstances, most people wish to avoid enemas; oral laxatives are preferred.

Gleghorn *et al.* (1991) reported a 90% success rate with a program of fecal evacuation (mineral oil, 0.5 to 1.0 ounce per year of age per day, to a maximum of 8 ounces per day); maintenance mineral oil, 15 cc per year of age per day to keep the stool very soft; a high-fiber diet; increased fluid intake; and a toileting program. Parents were reassured that a deficiency of fat-soluble vitamins would not occur (McClung *et al.*, 1993). Three quarters of the children in the study had remission of encopresis; the remainder had decreased frequency. Laxatives were discontinued without relapse.

Other treatment programs for encopresis include behavior modification, biofeedback, medication, hypnosis, relaxation, and psychotherapy. Some compliant children do well with behavior modification alone. Positive reinforcement and mild punishment are better than either alone. Such programs, combined with medication, diet, exercise, enemas, lubricants, and/or laxatives, have been very successful. Walker *et al.* (1989) found that a properly applied combination of behavioral and medical interventions led to remission in almost 100% of patients. Although 15 to 25% relapsed, they usually responded to another course of the same treatment. In the same study, a regimen of behavior modification with laxatives had a clear advantage over behavior modification alone in both remission and relapse rates. Successful treatment also decreased emotional maladjustment. Biofeedback is effective but labor intensive; it is best offered after other approaches have failed. Loening-Baucke (1990) reported that 12 months after therapy, 50% of children who had received biofeedback were still in remission, compared with 16% of those who had experienced conventional therapy.

In most cases, the literature does not support a relationship between emotional disturbance and encopresis; at best, the relationship is unclear (Hersov, 1994; Blum *et al.* 1997). Psychotherapy appears to be of little use (Walker *et al.*, 1989). In the study by McClung *et al.* (1993), less than 5% of the children required psychological interventions.

307.6 ENURESIS (NOT DUE TO A GENERAL MEDICAL CONDITION)

If a young child wets only at night, and is not overly upset by the enuresis, the clinician should encourage parents to delay extensive treatment pending further maturation. There is a high spontaneous-cure rate for bed-wetting. Enuresis occurs in 33% of children at four years of age and 10% at six years of age, and drops about 15% each year after this (Mann, 1991). Eighty percent of patients have primary enuresis (i.e., urinary control has never been firmly established); there is often a strong family history. Secondary enuresis (occurring after months or years of urinary control) is likely to respond to management of the stress that precipitated the episode, if known, as well as to the measures discussed below.

The physician should obtain family histories and educate the family about intervention programs. This may assuage guilt and reduce the potential for child abuse. Reassurance for the parents usually is sufficient for bed-wetting in children under six years of age. For enuretic children over six years old, parent-child education leads to improvement in about 70%. Information is given to the parents and child on the expected decrease in symptoms with maturation, potty training techniques, monitoring for unusual sexual or aggressive stimulation, checking school bathrooms for privacy and adequate facilities, making sure the child knows when to respond to bladder cues and how to remove clothing, and other practical matters. Contrary to some clinical beliefs, nocturnal enuresis is not correlated with depth of sleep as measured by an electroencephalogram (Rapoport, 1993; Shaffer, 1994).

Physicians and families may prefer medication to other treatments, even though the latter are often successful. Star charts seem to be interesting to some children. Restricting fluids before bedtime and waking the child up to go to the bathroom are helpful to very few. Open studies suggest that some forms of hypnosis are effective.

Alarms

An inexpensive and nonintrusive wetness alarm system is effective for many children. The small instrument, similar in appearance to an ordinary pager, is clipped to the underpants and two contacts placed two to three inches from the urethra. A small amount of urine will complete the circuit and sound an alarm, waking the patient. The volume of urine that escapes is usually small, and the alarm is rapidly paired with recognition of bladder or early urination cues. Positive results are seen in a sizable majority of children, with a relapse rate of about one-third (Garfinkel, 1990). A cure rate of 70% for children over eight years old has been reported (Mann, 1991). About two-thirds of the relapsed patients become dry using overlearning (after a dry state has been accomplished, the child drinks extra fluid at bedtime) and an intermittent alarm procedure. Intermittent reinforcement makes the conditioned response more resistant to extinction.

Having the child change (or help the parent change the bed) and clean up is a sufficient behavioral corrective measure; punishment is not indicated. A tactile (vibrating) alarm is now available and is useful for deaf children and for those who do not like noise.

An alarm with arousal training is the treatment of choice for most children 6 to 12 years old. The parents teach the child to turn off the alarm, go to the bathroom, reset the alarm, and return to bed. When the child does this, he gets a token reward (e.g., two stars or stickers). If procedure is not followed, he gives the parents a token. Almost all children become continent with arousal training. A follow-up study by Londen *et al.* (1993) showed a "dry rate" of 92% after two and a half years. Alarm equipment must be kept clean and checked periodically for safety.

Medication

Imipramine is the most commonly used medication for enuresis. Low doses of tricyclic antidepressants are useful if less intensive procedures do not work or if a rapid "cure" is needed for camp or sleepovers. Tricyclics reduce bed-wetting in 80% of children within a week, and a completely dry state occurs in up to 50%. Doses used for enuresis are lower than those for depression, with a maximum of 2.5 mg/kg per day. The mechanism of action is not known. Imipramine is given for three to six months and then tapered over three to six months. There may be side effects, including insomnia, anorexia, anxiety, or, rarely, behavior or personality change.

Demopressin acetate (DDAVP) produces a marked reduction in enuresis. The usual dose is 20 to 40 μg (two to four pump sprays intranasally). The indications for and efficacy of DDAVP are similar to those of imipramine. Neither medication is as effective as an alarm program (Moffatt *et al.*, 1993; Thompson & Rey, 1995). Most children relapse if DDAVP or imipramine is discontinued.

Anticholinergic medications, such as propantheline and oxybutynin, reduce bladder contractions but show conflicting results in enuresis (Miller *et al.*, 1992).

Bladder Capacity and Contractility

In cases that do not respond to conservative therapies, bladder capacity and contractility can be determined and stretching exercises carried out as indicated. For most patients, there is little or no relationship between physical features and enuresis. In the remainder, capacity is less important than contractility. Normal bladder capacity (in ounces) is usually estimated as the child's age plus two, up to 11 years of age. Sphincter practice and bladder stretching produce a cure rate of about 35%.

CHAPTER 36

OTHER DISORDERS OF INFANCY, CHILDHOOD, OR ADOLESCENCE

309.21 SEPARATION ANXIETY DISORDER

Separation anxiety is seen in the normal development of an infant and in a milder form when the child starts school. This episodic anxiety lasts a few days or weeks and then resolves or becomes controllable by the child. It is extremely difficult to make the diagnosis before the age of six years (Klein, 1994), although ICD-10 states that six is the upper age limit. When the child shows persistent severe symptoms, such as school refusal, refusal to sleep alone, or physical complaints, the parents may seek help from a counselor or physician. Children with Tourette's disorder who take haloperidol or pimozide may develop school phobia, also known as neuroleptic separation anxiety syndrome (Linet, 1985).

Separation anxiety has an adaptive function as a signal that the child needs protection. Reactions to separation are abnormal when the child cannot carry out age-appropriate activities. If regular activities resume soon after the child-parent separation, reassurance by the parent is usually sufficient.

Seventy-five percent of children with separation anxiety have school refusal. This form of school refusal is due to the child's being unable to separate from the parent, and not the result of phobia regarding school, situational anxiety, or real (or imagined) parental danger. Livingston (1995) states that the disorder occurs equally in boys and girls, is overrepresented among lower socioeconomic classes, and has a peak incidence at about 11 years of age.

A young child with mild to moderate symptoms of short duration may respond to parental adjustments. The therapist helps the parents understand how the anxiety is generated in the home and why the child needs to experience separation at school time and bedtime. The parents then carry out these separations, even though they may be difficult, and then praise the child for the achievement. Family therapy can be very helpful (Livingston, 1995).

School-phobic children include those with many kinds of anxiety, although separation anxiety usually predominates (Bernstein & Borchart, 1991). School studies are thus not usually limited to separation anxiety *per se*.

In a study of school refusers, Blagg and Yule (1984) found that classical and operant conditioning methods applied for two and a half weeks were very effective, with 83% improvement after one year. Hospitalization averaging 45 days was marginally effective, with 31% improved after a year. Home tutoring and psychotherapy were ineffective; after a mean 72 weeks of treatment, no patients achieved a year of improvement. The patients were not randomly assigned to the groups, which were thus skewed for severity and other factors.

The Children's Manifest Anxiety Scale may not reflect the high level of anxiety these children have, and, therefore, may not be useful in recording changes in the anxiety level (Klein *et al.*, 1992). If severe symptoms persist, hospitalization may be needed to provide an enforced separation. The parents require careful support because this separation is also difficult for them. Failure occurs when the parents do not support the treatment plan.

Separation anxiety is difficult to separate from other childhood anxiety syndromes (Klein *et al.*, 1992). Generic therapy for childhood anxiety may include desensitization, extinction, modeling, counterconditioning, operant conditioning, cognitive-behavioral therapy, and psychotherapy.

Livingston (1991) reports that imipramine is helpful for school-phobic children. In one study, children who did not respond to a short-term behaviorally oriented psychotherapy program were given imipramine or placebo. About half of the children in each group improved. A disinhibiting effect (oppositional behavior) was seen in some children on imipramine (Klein *et al.*, 1992). More data are needed before antidepressants can be fully endorsed for school absenteeism or separation anxiety disorder.

For children who also have attention-deficit/hyperactive disorder, tricyclic antidepressants may be more helpful when stimulants are ineffective or cannot be prescribed (Ambrosini *et al.*, 1993). Double-blind studies have yielded mixed results with benzodiazepines. The side effects are similar to those seen in adults, but behavioral disinhibition is very upsetting to parents. Open trials of buspirone in overanxious children have shown positive results (Livingston, 1995). Thioridazine has been used for anxiety, but there are no good studies to support its use in anxiety disorders of childhood (Livingston, 1991). Although diphenhydramine is sometimes prescribed for anxious children, the literature supporting the use of antihistamines in anxiety is limited. Except for obsessive-compulsive disorders, the effectiveness of treatment for childhood anxiety disorders is uncertain (Klein, 1994; Allen *et al.*, 1995).

313.23 ELECTIVE MUTISM

Four types of elective mutism are described: the symbiotic, submissive-appearing child with a dominant mother and passive father (the largest group); the passive-aggressive child with defiant and often antisocial behaviors; the reactive child, who is depressed and withdrawn, and has parents with similar problems; and the speech-phobic child, who is afraid of his or her own voice. A move to an area in which the local language differs from the primary language of the family is one predisposing factor. Children with elective mutism are a heterogeneous group; a variety of therapeutic modalities may induce the child to talk and address underlying problems.

About one-third of the children with this disorder have a coexisting language disorder. Speech and language therapy is often needed. The *expectation* that the child will talk must be maintained. The parents are taught not to support the child's passivity or to provide any reinforcement, even subtle, for the mute state. Teachers and other adults often are angry with the mute child, even when he or she is functioning well except for talking. Frank punishment should be avoided.

Behavior therapy appears to be more effective than individual or family psychotherapy (Dulcan & Popper, 1991; Krohn *et al.*, 1992). Assertiveness training, paraverbal therapy (in which another patient functions as an assistant therapist), shaping (in which whispering or other near-speech is temporarily rewarded), contingency management, positive reinforcement, response cost (token or other loss for not talking), stimulus fading (gradually increase in the range of people with whom talking is rewarded), and/or desensitization may be employed (Labbe & Williamson, 1984).

A double-blind, placebo-controlled study of fluoxetine by Black and Uhde (1994) reported improvement in both groups, with statistically significant preference for fluoxetine, after 12 weeks. Even with active treatment, the patients remained "very symptomatic." The study was prompted by an earlier case report of the successful treatment of a 12-year-old girl with fluoxetine (Black & Uhde, 1992).

Another case report of severe mutism cited the success of monoamine oxidase inhibitors in adults with social phobia, and the clinical observation that some become very talkative on phenelzine, to justify treating a seven-year-old girl with elective mutism with the drug. At 12 weeks on a mean dose of 52.6 mg/day, she started talking with others outside the home. At week 24, the medication was gradually withdrawn and the mutism did not return. Her father had a panic disorder that responded to phenelzine (Golwyn & Weinstock, 1990). Controlled studies are needed.

After the treatment of 20 children with elective mutism, the Hawthorn Center program reported excellent results in 85% of the children and at least fair results in the remaining 15% (Krohn *et al.*, 1992). The program involved parent education, a child-therapist relationship, firm behavioral expectations, school and family involvement, and careful follow-up. Several levels of intervention were provided at the same time. The findings support the viewpoint that the child is angry about an enmeshed relationship with the mother, and that challenging the anger leads to rapid resolution of the problem behavior. Direct challenge to the symptom did not cause symptom substitution or overwhelming anxiety.

Sometimes the disorder appears to be self-limited. Prognosis is usually good with early detection and intervention. Even with treatment, a few children remain mute and may require hospitalization for more intensive intervention. Specific approaches include behavior therapy, skills training, and family education, as well as speech-language therapy if there is a coexisting language disorder. If the child is still mute after the age of 12, the prognosis is guarded (Baker & Cantwell, 1991).

313.89 REACTIVE ATTACHMENT DISORDER OF INFANCY OR EARLY CHILDHOOD

Parental pathology, life-threatening illness in the infant, multiple caretakers, and other factors may prevent or disrupt the attachment process in the child. The children often present as neglected, abused, nonthriving, or ruminating. Prematurity may require that infants stay in isolettes where life-sustaining care (but limited emotional care) is given. Premature infants without a consistent caring adult may be irritable, fail to thrive, or have increasing organic problems. Some of the consequences of overstimulating the premature infant are known; prevention procedures should be put in place (e.g., avoiding loud noises and bright lights) to enhance development. The attachment needs of the premature infant are not well known, but there is evidence of an interactive system (i.e., response to a caretaker) even in premature infants (Goodfriend, 1993).

State control, alerting, and responsiveness are enhanced in premature infants by having the same person hold the baby for at least two hours each day. Infants who receive massage have more organized behavior than those who do not (Field, 1990). Infants who have skin contact with their mothers cry less than those who do not (Whitelaw *et al.*, 1988). Encouraging parents to have consistent, caring contact with their fragile infants seems to improve outcome. Volunteer baby-holding programs, providing space for parents in neonatal intensive care units, open visiting hours, and assignment of nurse-baby and physician-baby dyads support the attachment needs of the premature infant.

Some prevention programs that focus on potentially inadequate mothers provide trained visitors to work with at-risk mothers from the last trimester of pregnancy through the first postnatal year. Professional consultation is supplied when needed.

If an attachment disorder is severe, with failure to thrive, hospitalization should be seriously considered. (For a discussion of treatment for failure to thrive and rumination, see the section on feeding and eating disorders.) After inpatient assessment, the mother is helped to interact with her baby and provide appropriate stimulation. She may also need individual, group, or family therapy. Group therapy can provide education and guidance in addition to psychotherapy, and may make the mother feel less alone and in need of support. Caring for the mother may allow her to care for her child.

Inpatient interventions for the baby include nutritional habilitation, stimulation, and attention to emotional care. An infant who is responding to treatment increases somatic growth and affective responses. The mother who is improving with treatment feels less alone and more supported and hopeful. If the mother seems able to respond to her infant, care may be provided in the home with careful follow-up by clinic staff and visiting nurses. Family-centered care with counseling in the home may be more effective than office-based care, because of family support issues or avoidance by the mother.

If the infant (or another child) appears to be experiencing significant neglect or possible abuse, legal intervention is necessary and the child must be placed with relatives or in foster care. The possibility of serious risk to the infant is more important than the therapeutic relationship with the mother. Unless it is likely to increase the danger to the child, the therapist should inform the family if a report to a child-protective agency is to be filed.

Transitional objects are soothing to the child in times of stress and can, at times, become more important than the real objects. Bowlby noted that children exhibit unusual attachment to objects when separated from primary caretakers. Preschoolers who show a high attachment to their family homes after leaving them owing due to parental divorce have better behavioral adjustment than do those who move and show low attachment to their former homes. A mother's accepting attitude about her child's references to the family home may allow the child to use the home as an object attachment. Parental education and counseling about the child's needs in this regard are important to later adjustment.

Many (30 to 75%) of these children referred to clinics have peer problems. Because the parent-child relationship is so important to the child's social competence, family (or foster family) intervention should be included when treating the child. When the family begins to function better, the child's social competence improves and peer relationships get better (Schroeder & Gordon, 1991).

307.3 STEREOTYPIC MOVEMENT DISORDER

Stereotypic behavior is both soothing and stimulating to the child. Rhythmic stimulation, such as swinging or rocking in a rocking chair or on a rocking horse, are acceptable nonfunctional behaviors. Normal children exhibit some body rocking at about six months of age, with transient, noninjurious head banging and head rolling at nine months of age. By three years of age, these movements are rare. If there is adequate parenting, padding the crib or making a pallet on the floor to decrease noise is sufficient treatment for most children. If the behavior persists or is severe, as described in DSM-IV criteria, more intensive intervention is needed. Behavior management through overcorrection (waking the child when the behavior occurs, telling the child to assume another position—in which the child typically does not carry out the behavior, holding the position for 15 seconds, and repeating this process 15 to 20 times) is rapidly successful for some infants.

Normal hand, thumb, or finger sucking may begin before birth and by three years of age may become associated with a transitional object. Thumb sucking is not a problem until dentition becomes affected (four to six years of age). Gentle persuasion may be effective, as may removing the transitional object. Habit reversal is very effective. Nail biting appears to reduce tension; habit reversal (through awareness training, competing-response training, and other interventions) is effective in these cases as well.

If it is necessary to treat stereotypies, the first steps are to change the environment and to develop a behavioral program. Functional analysis of the behavior—determining its precursors and the things that influence it—can be used to determine the most appropriate intervention. Enriched visual stimulation, object manipulation (especially toys or playthings), and alternative behavior programs (e.g., interaction with adults or exercise) decrease stereotypy (Crnic & Reid, 1989; Schroeder, 1989).

About one-fourth of blind children exhibit stereotypies. Providing objects with texture and sound helps the blind infant to bring his or her hands together and increases useful hand movement rather than empty fingering.

Overcorrection is effective, but may be associated with an increase in other stereotypies or self-injurious behavior. If the stereotypic behavior results in bodily damage, treatment programs for self-injurious behavior are used. Aversive techniques raise ethical questions when the behavior to be deleted is not particularly harmful to the child (see the section on mental retardation).

Stereotypic behavior often appears to have no external precipitant. When functional analysis does not reveal any motivating factor that perpetuates a nevertheless serious stereotypy, medication may be helpful. Thioridazine (2.5 mg/kg per day) often decreases the behavior(s); thioridazine plus visual screening is slightly more effective. In a study by Singh *et al.* (1993), the best results were obtained by visual screening alone.

Stimulants, antidepressants, and some anticonvulsants (carbamazepine and valproic acid) may increase stereotypic behavior.

References for Part IV

Allen, A. J., Leonard, H., & Swedo, S. (1995): Current knowledge of medications for the treatment of childhood anxiety disorders. *Journal of the American Academy of Child and Adolescent Psychiatry*, 34(8):976–986.

Aman, M. G. (1993): Efficacy of psychotropic drugs for reducing self-injurious behavior in the developmental disabilities. *Annals of Clinical Psychiatry*, 5:171–188.

Aman, M. G., & Rojahn, J. (1992): Pharmacological Intervention. In N. N. Singh, & I. Beale, (Eds.), *Learning Disabilities, Nature, Theory, and Treatment*. New York: Springer-Verlag.

Ambrosini, P. J., Bianchi, M. D., Rabinovich, H., & Elia, J. (1993): Antidepressant treatments in children and adolescents. II: Anxiety, physical, and behavioral disorders. *Journal of the American Academy of Child and Adolescent Psychiatry*, 32(3):483–493.

American Academy of Pediatrics (1993): *Policy Statement on Facilitated Communication*, October 20.

Baker, L., & Cantwell, D. P. (1991): Disorders of language, speech and communication. In M. Lewis, (Ed.), *Child and Adolescent Psychiatry*, Baltimore: Williams & Wilkins.

Barkley, R. A. (1989): Attention deficit-hyperactivity disorder. In E. F. Mash, & R. A. Barkley, (Eds.), *Treatment of Childhood Disorders*. New York: Guilford.

Barness, L. A. (Ed.) (1993): *Pediatric Nutrition Handbook*. (3rd ed.), (pp. 202–208). Elk Grove Village, IL: American Academy of Pediatrics.

Barrickman, L. L., Perry, P. J., Allen, A. J., *et al.* (1995): Bupropion versus methylphenidate in the treatment of attention-deficit hyperactive disorder. *Journal of the American Academy of Child and Adolescent Psychiatry*, 34(5):649–657.

Bernstein, G.A., & Borchardt, C.M. (1991): Anxiety disorders of childhood and adolescence: A critical review. *Journal of the American Academy of Child and Adolescent Psychiatry*, 30(4):519–532.

Bezirganian, S., & Cohen, P. (1992): Sex differences in the interaction between temperament and parenting. *Journal of the American Academy of Child and Adolescent Psychiatry*, 31(5):790–801.

Birch, L. L., Johnson, S. L., Andersen, G., *et al.* (1991): The variability of young children's energy intake. *New England Journal of Medicine*, 324(4):232–235.

Black, B., & Uhde, T.W. (1992): Elective mutism as a variant of social phobia. *Journal of the American Academy of Child and Adolescent Psychiatry*, 31(6):1090–1094.

Black, B., & Uhde, T.W. (1994): Treatment of elective mutism with fluoxetine: A double-blind, placebo-controlled study: *Journal of the American Academy of Child and Adolescent Psychiatry*, 33(7):1000–1006.

Blagg, N. R., & Yule, W. (1984): The behavioral treatment of school refusal: A comparative study. *Behavior Research Therapy,* 22:119–127.

Blinder, B. J., Goodman, S., & Henderson, P. (1989): Pica, rumination. In T. B. Karasu, (Ed.), *Treatments of Psychiatric Disorders.* Washington, DC: American Psychiatric Press.

Bloodstein, O. (1993): *Stuttering.* Needham Heights, MA: Allyn & Bacon.

Blum, N. J., Taubman, B., & Osborne, M. L. (1997): Behavioral characteristics of children with stool toileting refusal. *Pediatrics,* 99(1):50–53.

Buitellar, J. K., Van Engeland, H., DeKogen, K., *et al.* (1992): The adrenocorticotrophic hormone (4–9) analog ORG 2766 benefits autistic children: Report on a second controlled clinical trial. *Journal of the American Academy of Child and Adolescent Psychiatry,* 31(6):1149–1156.

Campbell, M., Anderson, L. T., Small, A. M., *et al.* (1993): Naltrexone in autistic children: Behavioral symptoms and attentional learning. *Journal of the American Academy of Child and Adolescent Psychiatry,* 32(6):1283–1291.

Campbell, M., & Cueva, J. E. (1995): Psychopharmacology in child and adolescent psychiatry: A review of the past seven years. Part I. *Journal of the American Academy of Child and Adolescent Psychiatry,* 34(9):1124–1132.

Crnic, K. A., & Reid, M. (1989): Mental retardation. In E. J. Mash, & R. A. Barkley, (Eds.), *Treatment of Childhood Disorders.* New York: Guilford.

Cueva, J. E., Overall, J. E., Small, A. M., *et al.* (1996): Carbamazepine in aggressive children with conduct disorder: A double-blind, placebo-controlled study. *Journal of the American Academy of Child and Adolescent Psychiatry,* 35(4):480–490.

Dulcan, M. K. (1990): Using psychostimulants to treat behavioral disorders of children and adolescents. *Journal of Child and Adolescent Psychopharmacology,* 1(1):7–20.

Dulcan, M. K., & Popper, C. W. (1991): *Child and Adolescent Psychiatry.* Washington, D.C.: American Psychiatric Press.

Epstein, L. H., Doke, L. A., Sajwaj, T. E., *et al.* (1974): Generality and side effects of over-correction. *Journal of Applied Behavior Analysis,* 7(3):385–390.

Field, T. M. (1990): Neonatal stress and coping in intensive care. *Infant Mental Health Journal,* 2:57–65.

Garfinkel, B. D. (1990): The elimination disorders. In B.D. Garfinkel, G. A. Carlson, & E. B. Weller, (Eds.), *Psychiatric Disorders in Children and Adolescents.* Philadelphia: Saunders.

Gleghorn, E. E., Heyman, M. B., & Rudolph, C.D. (1991): No-enema therapy for idiopathic constipation and encopresis. *Clinical Pediatrics,* 30(12):669–672.

Golwyn, D. H., & Weinstock, R. C. (1990): Phenelzine treatment of elective mutism: A case report. *Journal of Clinical Psychiatry,* 51(9):384–385.

Goodfriend, M. D. (1993): Treatment of attachment disorder of infancy in a neonatal intensive care unit. *Pediatrics,* 91(1):130–142.

Gordon, C. T., State, R. C., Nelson, J. E., *et al.* (1993): A double-blind comparison of clomipramine, desipramine, and placebo in the treatment of autistic disorder. *Archives of General Psychiatry,* 50:441–447.

Green, W. H. (1992): Nonstimulant drugs in the treatment of attention-deficit hyperactivity disorder. *Child and Adolescent Psychiatric Clinics of North America.* 1(2):449–465.

Greenhill, L. L. (1990): Attention-deficit hyperactivity disorder in children. In B. D. Garfinkel, B. A. Carlson, & E. B. Weller (Eds.), *Psychiatric Disorders in Children and Adolescents* (pp. 149–182). Philadelphia: Saunders.

Grizenko, N., Papineau, D. & Sayegh, L. (1993): Effectiveness of a multimodal day treatment program for children with disruptive behavior problems. *Journal of the American Academy of Child and Adolescent Psychiatry,* 32(1):127–134.

Haas, R. H., Rice, M. A., Trauner, D. A. & Merritt, T. S. (1986): Therapeutic effects of a ketogenic diet in Rett syndrome. *American Journal of Medical Genetics,* 24:225–246.

Harris, K. R., Graham, S., & Pressley, M. (1992): Cognitive-behavioral approaches in reading and written language: Developing self-regulated learners. In N. N. Singh, & I. Beale (Eds.), *Learning Disabilities, Nature, Theory, and Treatment* (pp. 415–451). New York: Springer-Verlag.

Hechtman, L. (1992): Long-term outcome in attention-deficit hyperactivity disorder. In G. Weiss (Ed.), *Child and Adolescent Psychiatric Clinics of North America* (pp. 553–565). Philadelphia: Saunders.

Hersov, L. (1994): Faecal soiling. In M. Rutter, E. Taylor, & L. Hersov (Eds.), *Child and Adolescent Psychiatry* (pp. 520–528). Oxford: Blackwell.

Hunt, R. D., Capper, L., & O'Connell, P. (1990): Clonidine in child and adolescent psychiatry. *Journal of Child and Adolescent Psychopharmacology,* 1(1):87–102.

Johnston, J. M. (1993): Phenomenology and treatment of rumination. *Child and Adolescent Psychiatric Clinics of North America.* 2(1):93–107.

Kanner, L. (1957): Rumination. In *Child Psychiatry* (pp. 484–487). Springfield, IL: Charles C Thomas.

Kaplan, H. I., & Sadock, B. J. (1993): *Pocket Handbook of Psychiatric Treatment.* Baltimore: Williams & Wilkins.

Karsh, K. G., & Rapp, A. C. (1992): Computer-assisted instruction: Potential reality. In N. N. Singh & I. Beale (Eds.), *Learning Disabilities, Nature, Theory, and Treatment* (pp. 452–477). New York: Springer-Verlag.

Kernberg, P. F., & Chazan, S. E. (1991): *Children with Conduct Disorders.* New York: Basic Books.

Klein, R. G. (1994): In M. Rutter, E. Taylor, & L. Hersov (Eds.), *Child and Adolescent Psychiatry* (pp. 351–374). Oxford: Blackwell.

Kolmen, B. K., Feldman, H. M., Handen, B. L., & Janowsky, J. E. (1995): Naltrexone in young autistic children: A double-blind, placebo-controlled crossover study. *Journal of the American Academy of Child and Adolescent Psychiatry,* 34(2):223–231.

Krohn, D. D., Weckstein, S. M., & Wright, H. L. (1992): A study of the effectiveness of a specific treatment for elective mutism, *Journal of the American Academy of Child and Adolescent Psychiatry,* 31(4):711–718.

Kurlan, R. (Ed.). (1993): *Handbook of Tourette's Syndrome and Related Tic and Behavioral Disorders.* New York: Marcel Dekker.

Labbe, E. E., & Williamson, D. A. (1984): Behavioral treatment in elective mutism: A review of the literature. *Clinical Psychology Review,* 4:273–292.

Linet, L. S. (1985): Tourette's syndrome, pimozide and school phobia: The neuroleptic separation anxiety syndrome. *American Journal of Psychiatry,* 142:613–615.

Livingston, R. (1991): Anxiety disorders. In M. Lewis (Ed.), *Child and Adolescent Psychiatry* (pp. 673–681). Baltimore: Williams & Wilkins.

Livingston, R. (1995): Anxiety and anxiety disorders. In G. O. Gabbard (Ed.), *Treatment of Psychiatric Disorders* (pp. 229–252). Washington, DC: American Psychiatric Press.

Loening-Baucke, V. (1990): Modulation of abnormal defecation dynamics by biofeedback treatment in chronically constipated children with encopresis. *Journal of Pediatrics*, 116:214–222.

Londen, A. V., Londen-Barentsen, M. W. Mv., Son, M. J. Mv., Mulder, G. A. L. A. (1993): Arousal training for children suffering from nocturnal enuresis: A 2 1/2 year follow-up. *Behavior Research Therapry*, 31(6):613–615.

Lord, R., & Hulme, C. (1987): Perceptual judgements of normal and clumsy children. *Developmental Medicine and Child Neurology*, 29:250–257.

Maloney, M. J., & Ruedisueli, G. (1993): The epidemiology of eating problems in non-referred children and adolescents. *Child and Adolescent Psychiatric Clinics of North America*, 2(1):1–13.

Mann, E. (1991): Nocturnal enuresis. *Western Journal of Medicine*, 155(5):520–521.

McClung, H. J., Boyne, L. J., Linshbeid, T. et al. (1993): Is combination therapy for encopresis nutritionally safe? *Pediatrics*, 91(3):591–594.

McEachin, J. J., Smith, R., & Lovaas, O. I. (1993): Long-term outcome for children with autism who received early intensive behavioral treatment. *American Journal of Mental Retardation*, 97(4):259–272.

McMahon, R. J., & Wells, K. C. (1989): Conduct disorders. In E. J. Mash & R. A. Barkley (Eds.), *Treatment of Childhood Disorders* (pp. 73–132). New York: Guilford.

Miller, K., Atkin, B., & Moody, M. L. (1992): Drug therapy for nocturnal enuresis. *Drugs*, 44(1):47–56.

Moffatt, M. E. K., Harlos, S., Kirshen, A. J., & Burd, L. (1993): Demopressin acetate and nocturnal enuresis: How much do we know? *Pediatrics*, 92(3):420–425.

Newsom, C., & Rincover, A. (1989): Autism. In E. J. Mash, & R. A. Barkley (Eds.), *Treatment of Childhood Disorders* (pp. 286–346). New York: Guilford.

Nielson, J. B., Lou, H. C., Anderson, J. (1990): Biochemical and clinical effects of tyrosine and tryptophan in the Rett syndrome. *Brain Development*, 12(1):143–147.

Pelham, W. E., & Sams, S. E. (1992): Behavior modification. In G. Weiss, (Ed.), *Child and Adolescent Psychiatric Clinics of North America* (pp. 505–518). Philadelphia: Saunders.

Percy, A., Gillberg, C., Hagberg, B., & Witt-Engerstrom, I. (1990): Rett syndrome and the autistic disorders. In *Neurologic Clinics*, 8(3):659–676.

Percy, A., Glaze, D., Schultz, R., *et al.* (1994): Rett syndrome: Controlled study of an oral opiate antagonist, naltrexone. *Annals of Neurology*, 35:464–470.

Perry, A. (1991): Rett syndrome: A comprehensive review of the literature. *American Journal of Mental Retardation*, 96(3):284–285.

Philippart, M. (1986): Clinical recognition of Rett syndrome. *American Journal of Medical Genetics*, 24:111–118.

Popper, C. S., & Frazier, S. H. (Eds.) (1990): *Journal of Child and Adolescent Psychopharmacology*, 1(1):1–102.

Quinn, P. O., & Rappaport, J. L. (1975): One-year follow-up of hyperactive boys treated with imipramine or methylphenidate. *Archives of General Psychiatry*, 132:241–245.

Rappaport, L. (1993): The treatment of nocturnal enuresis—where are we now? *Pediatrics*, 92(3):465–466.

Rast, J. Ellinger-Allen, J. A., & Johnston, J. M. (1985): Dietary management of rumination: Four case studies. *American Journal of Clinical Nutrition,* 42:95–101.

Rojahn, J. & Marshburn, E. (1992): Facial screening and visual occlusion. In J. K. Luiselli, J. L. Matson, & N. N. Singh (Eds.), *Self-Injurious Behavior* (pp. 200–234). New York: Springer-Verlag.

Rozin, P. Poritsky, S. & Sotsky, R. (1970): American children with reading problems can easily learn to read English represented by Chinese characters. *Science,* 30:1264–1267.

Rumsey, J. M. (1992): The biology of developmental dyslexia. *Journal of the American Medical Association,* 268(7):912–915.

Rutter, M. (1985): The treatment of autistic children. *Journal of Child Psychology and Psychiatry,* 26(2):193–214.

Sanchez, L. E., Campbell, M., Small, A. M., *et al.* (1996): A pilot study of clomipramine in young autistic children. *Journal of the American Academy of Child and Adolescent Psychiatry,* 35(4):537–544.

Schroeder, C. S. & Gordon, B. N. (1991): *Assessment and Treatment of Childhood Problems* (pp. 361–371). New York: Guilford.

Schroeder, S. R. (1989): Abnormal stereotyped behaviors. In T. B. Karasu (Ed.), *Treatment of Psychiatric Disorders* (pp. 44–49). Washington, DC: American Psychiatric Association.

Shaffer, D. (1994): Enuresis. In M. Rutter, E. Taylor, & L. Hersov (Eds.), *Child and Adolescent Psychiatry,* (pp. 505–519). Oxford: Blackwell.

Singh, N. N., Landrum, T. J., Ellis, C. R., & Donatelli, L. S. (1993): Effects of thioridazine and visual screening on stereotypy and social behavior in individuals with mental retardation. In *Research in Developmental Disabilities* (pp. 163–177) Tarrytown, NY: Pergamon.

Spencer, T., Biederman, J., Steingard, R. & Wilens, T. (1993): Bupropion exacerbates tics in children with attention-deficit hyperactivity disorder and Tourette's syndrome, *Journal of the American Academy of Child and Adolescent Psychiatry,* 32(1):211–214.

Spencer, T., Biederman, J., Wilens, T., *et al.* (1993): Nortriptyline treatment of children with attention-deficit hyperactivity disorder and tic disorder or Tourette's syndrome, *Journal of the American Academy of Child and Adolescent Psychiatry,* 32(1):205–210.

Stewart, T., Myers, W. C., Burket, R. C., & Lyles, W. B. (1990): A review of the pharmacotherapy of aggression in children and adolescents, *Journal of the American Academy of Child and Adolescent Psychiatry,* 29(2):269–277.

Teicher, M. H., & Glod, C. A. (1990): Neuroleptic drugs: Indications and guidelines for their rational use in children and adolescents. *Journal of Child and Adolescent Psychopharmacology,* 1(1):33–56.

Thompson, D. F., & Thompson, G. D. (1987): Naltrexone in the management of seizures associated with Rett syndrome. *Drug Intelligence and Clinical Pharmacy,* 21:874.

Thompson, S., & Rey, J. M. (1995): Functional enuresis: Is desmopressin the answer? *Journal of the American Academy of Child and Adolescent Psychiatry,* 34:266–271.

Towbin, K. E., Cohen, D. J., & Leckman, J. F., (1995): Tic disorders. In G. O. Gabbard (Ed.), *Treatment of Psychiatric Disorders* (p. 216). Washington, DC: American Psychiatric Press.

Tuten, H., & Miedaner, J., (1989): Effect of hand splints on stereotypic hand behavior of girls with Rett syndrome: A replication study. *Physical Therapy,* 69(11):1099–1103.

Walker, C. E., Kenning, M., & Faust-Campanile, J. (1989): Enuresis and encopresis. In E. J. Mash & R. A. Barkley (Eds.), *Treatment of Childhood Disorders* (pp. 423–448). New York: Guilford.

Walsh, B. T., (Chair, Eating Disorders Work Group), (1994): Feeding disorders of infancy or early development. In *Diagnostic and Statistical Manual of Mental Disorders,* (4th ed.) (pp. 98–100). Washington, DC: American Psychiatric Association.

Wender, P. H. (1990): Attention-deficit hyperactivity disorder in adolescents and adults. In B. D. Garfinkel, G. A. Carlson, & E. G. Weller (Eds.), *Psychiatric Disorders in Children and Adolescents* (pp 183–192). Philadelphia: Saunders.

Whitelaw, A., Heisterkamp, G., Sleath, K., *et al.* (1988): Skin to skin contact for very low birthweight infants and their mothers. *Archives of Diseases of the Child,* 63(11):1377–1381.

Wolf, S. M., & Forsythe, A. (1978): Behavior disturbance, phenobarbital, and febrile seizures. *Pediatrics,* 61:728–731.

Wolraich, M. L., Lindgren, S. D., Stumbo, P. J., *et al.* (1994): Effects of diets high in sucrose or aspartame on the behavior and cognitive performance of children. *New England Journal of Medicine,* 330(5):301–307.

Wynn, K. (1992): Addition and subtraction by human infants. *Nature,* 358:749–750.

Zametkin, A., Rappaport J. L., Murphy, D. L., *et al.* (1985): Treatment of hyperactive children with monoamine oxidase inhibitors. *Archives of General Psychiatry,* 42(10):962–966.

Zappella, M. (1990): A double-blind trial of bromocriptine in the Rett syndrome. *Brain Development,* 12(1):148–150.

APPENDIX A

GENERIC AND TRADE NAMES
OF DRUGS[1]

Note: Many medications have several different clinical indications. A drug's classification in this chart is not necessarily its primary medical use. An asterisk (*) indicates a new drug not available in the United States at the present time. Some older drugs are no longer marketed in the United States.

Generic Name	Brand(s)	Dosage Forms Available[2]
Antipsychotics		
New/Atypical		
clozapine	Clozaril, Leponex	t
olanzapine	Zyprexa	t
quetiapine	Seroquel	*
risperidone	Risperdal	t
sertindole	Serlect, Serdolect	*
ziprasidone	*	*
Butyrophenone		
haloperidol	Haldol, others	t,l,in,dep

[1]Chemical suffixes, such as "HCl" or "maleate," have been omitted unless important for differentiation.

[2]Abbreviations: t = tablet, caplet, or capsule (includes divalproex "sprinkle capsules"); l = oral liquid; in = injection (intramuscular or subcutaneous); dep = depot injection; IV = intravenous

Generic Name	Brand(s)	Dosage Forms Available
Phenothiazines		
acetophenazine	Tindal	t
chlorpromazine	Thorazine, others	t,l,in,suppository
fluphenazine	Prolixin, others	t,l,in,dep
mesoridazine	Serentil	t
perphenazine	Trilafon	t,l,in
prochlorperazine	Compazine	t,l,in,suppository
thioridazine	Mellaril	t,l
trifluoperazine	Stelazine, others	t,l,in
Others		
chlorprothixene	Taractan	t,l,in
loxapine	Loxitane	t
molindone	Moban	t,l
pimozide	Orap	t
thiothixene	Navane	t,l,in

Antiparkinsonians

amantidine	Symmetrel	t,l
benztropine	Cogentin, others	t,in
biperiden	Akineton	t,in
diphenhydramine	Benadryl, others	t,l,in
procyclidine	Kemadrin	t
trihexyphenidyl	Artane	t,l

Antimanics/Mood Stabilizers

carbamazepine	Tegretol, others	t,l
divalproex (sodium valproate + valproic acid)	Depakote	t
lithium carbonate	Eskalith, Lithobid, others	t
lithium citrate		l
valproic acid	Depakene, others	t,c,l

Antidepressants

Selective Serotonin Reuptake Inhibitors

fluoxetine	Prozac	t,l
fluvoxamine	Luvox	t
mirtazapine	Remeron	t
paroxetine	Paxil	t
sertraline	Zoloft	t

Generic Name	Brand(s)	Dosage Forms Available
Other New/Atypical		
brofaromine	*	*
bupropion	Wellbutrin	t
moclobemide	*	*
nefazodone	Serzone	
venlafaxine	Effexor	t
Tricyclic		
amitryptyline	Elavil, others	t,in
clomipramine	Anafranil	t
desipramine	Norpramin, others	t
doxepin	Sinequan, others	t,l
imipramine	Tofranil, others	t
nortriptyline	Pamelor	t,l
protriptyline	Vivactil	t
trimipramine	Surmontil	t
Monoamine Oxidase Inhibitors		
brofaromine	(see "New/Atypical")	*
clorgyline	*	*
isocarboxazid	Marplan	t
moclobemide	(see "New/Atypical")	*
phenelzine	Nardil	t
selegiline, *l*-deprenyl	Eldepryl (Deprenyl)	t
tranylcypromine	Parnate	t
Other		
amoxapine	Asendin	t
maprotiline	Ludiomil	t
trazodone	Desyrel	t

Anxiolytics

(*Note:* Drugs from other classes are often prescribed for anxiety disorders.)

Benzodiazepines

alprazolam	Xanax, others	t
chlordiazepoxide	Librium, others	t,in
clonazepam	Klonopin	t
clorazepate	Tranxene, others	t
diazepam	Valium, others	t,in
halazepam	Paxipam	t
lorazepam	Ativan, others	t,in
oxazepam	Serax, others	t,l
prazepam	Centrax, others	t,l

Generic Name	Brand(s)	Dosage Forms Available
Other		
buspirone	BuSpar	t
clomipramine	Anafranil	t
hydroxyzine	Vistaril, others	t,l

Sedative-Hypnotics

Benzodiazepines		
estazolam	ProSom	t
flurazepam	Dalmane	t
quazepam	Doral	t
temazepam	Restoril	t
triazolam	Halcion	t
New/Atypical		
zolpidem	Ambien	t
zopiclone	*	*
Other		
chloral hydrate		t,l
ethchlorvynol	Placidyl, others	t
glutethimide	Doriden	t
methyprylon	Noludar	t

CNS Stimulants

amphetamine combination	Adderal	t
dextroamphetamine	Dexadrine	t,l
methamphetamine	Desoxyn	t
methylphenidate	Ritalin	t
modafinil	*	*
pemoline	Cylert	t,chewable

Combinations

amitriptyline + chlordiazepoxide	Limbitrol, others	t
perphenazine + amitriptyline	Triavil, others	t

β-Adrenergic Blockers

atenolol	Tenormin	t
metoprolol	Lopressor	t
pindolol	Visken, others	t
propranolol	Inderal, others	t

Generic Name	Brand(s)	Dosage Forms Available
Drugs Used in Substance Abuse		
buprenorphine	Buprenex	in
cyclazocine		
disulfiram	Antabuse	t
levomethadyl (LAAM)	Orlaam	l
methadone	Dolophine, others	t,l
naloxone	Narcan, others	in
naltrexone	Trexan, ReVia	t
Antiandrogens		
cyproterone acetate (CPA)	Androcur	t,dep
medroxy-progesterone acetate (MPA)	Depo-Provera	dep
	Provere	t
Other		
clonidine	Catapres	t
dantrolene	Dantrium	t,in
desmopressin	DDAVP	in, intranasal
dexfenfluramine	Redux	c
donepezil	Aricept	t
ergoloid	Hydergine	t,l
fenfluramine	Pondamin	t
levocarnitine	Carnitor, others	t,l,in
nimodipine	Nimotop	t
tacrine	Cognex	t
yohimbine	Yocon, Yohimex	t

ADULT DOSES OF COMMON PSYCHOACTIVE DRUGS

Note: **Prescribing of any medication must be individualized and based on the clinician's knowledge of the patient, medication, and other factors. This chart represents general dosage ranges, and should not be construed as a recommendation for any specific patient situation, nor should upper limits always be considered the maximum safe dose for patients being appropriately monitored. The ranges given in this chart may not be relevant to some disorders or clinical situations.**

Medication	Emergency or Crisis, Single Dose (mg)[1]	Acute Rx (mg/day)[2]	Maintenance or Chronic Dose (mg/day)[3]
Antipsychotics[4]			
acetophenazine		60–120	40–100

[1]Time between doses and maximum daily dose must also be considered.

[2]Starting doses may be lower. The acute therapeutic dose is often, but not always, less than the maintenance dose. Dosage schedule may be important (e.g., prescribing stimulant drugs early in the day). Note that this is the range for total daily dose, not daily divided dose. Ranges often do not apply to child, elderly, or medically infirm patients.

[3]Maintenance doses are often, but not always, less than the dose for control of early or acute symptoms. Note that this is the range for total dose, not daily divided dose. Ranges often do not apply to child, elderly, or medically infirm patients. Depot doses are given in milligrams every two weeks or milligrams per month.

[4]Although it is common practice to discuss potency of neuroleptics in terms of "chlorpromazine equivalent," we have chosen not to do so. There is no real standard for such comparisons, nor do they effect the variety of currently available antipsychotic drugs.

Medication	Emergency or Crisis, Single Dose (mg)[1]	Acute Rx (mg/day)[2]	Maintenance or Chronic Dose (mg/day)[3]
Antipsychotics (cont'd)			
chlorpromazine			
oral	50–200	200–1,000	200–1,500
injection	25–50		
chlorprothixene		50–600	30–300
clozapine		300–900	300–900

(The patient should not be considered a clozapine "nonresponder" unless the dose is sufficient to maintain plasma level above 350 *nanograms*/ml.)

Medication	Emergency or Crisis, Single Dose (mg)[1]	Acute Rx (mg/day)[2]	Maintenance or Chronic Dose (mg/day)[3]
fluphenazine			
oral		5–30	2–30
decanoate			10–100/2 wks
haloperidol			
oral	2–10	5–50	2–40
injection HCl	2–5		
decanoate			50–200/month
loxapine			
oral	10–20	20–160	10–80
injection	12.5–50		
mesoridazine		100–400	50–400
molindone		40–300	40–300
olanzapine		5–10	5–10
perphenazine		12–64	8–32
pimozide in tic suppression		2–10	2–10
risperidone		4–12	4–12
thiothixene			
oral		10–60	6–40
injection	4–6		
thioridazine	50–200	200–800	100–800
trifluoperazine		8–60	4–40

---

[1]Time between doses and maximum daily dose must also be considered.

[2]Starting doses may be lower. The acute therapeutic dose is often, but not always, less than the maintenance dose. Dosage schedule may be important (e.g., prescribing stimulant drugs early in the day). Note that this is the range for total daily dose, not daily divided dose. Ranges often do not apply to child, elderly, or medically infirm patients.

[3]Maintenance doses are often, but not always, less than the dose for control of early or acute symptoms. Note that this is the range for total dose, not daily divided dose. Ranges often do not apply to child, elderly, or medically infirm patients. Depot doses are given in milligrams every two weeks or milligrams per month.

Medication	Emergency or Crisis, Single Dose (mg)[1]	Acute Rx (mg/day)[2]	Maintenance or Chronic Dose (mg/day)[3]
Antiparkinsonians			
amantidine		100–300	100–300
benztropine			
oral	1–2	1–4	1–4
inject (IM/IV)	1–2		
biperiden	2–4	4–8	4–6
diphenhydramine			
oral	25–50	75–200	75–200
injection	10–100		
procyclidine		5–15	5–15
trihexyphenidyl	2–5	4–15	4–15
Antimanics/Mood Stabilizers			
carbamazepine		400–1,600	400–1,600
(to maintain a plasma level of 6–12 *micrograms*/ml)			
divalproex		750–2,000	750–2,000
(to maintain a plasma level of 45–125 *micrograms*/ml)			
lithium carbonate		900–2100	900–1800
(to maintain a plasma level of 0.6–1.2 mEq/L, slightly higher in acute mania)			
valproic acid		750–2,000	750–2,000
(to maintain a plasma level of 45–125 *micrograms*/ml)			
clozapine		200–600	200–600
(mood stabilizer dose is not clearly established for clozapine but may be less than antipsychotic dose)			
Antidepressants			
amitryptyline		75–300	75–300
amoxapine		100–400	100–400
brofaromine		100–175*	100–175*
bupropion		150–450	150–450
clomipramine		75–300	75–300
desipramine		75–300	75–300

---

*Approximate doses, from limited clinical studies or non-U.S. prescribing experience.

[1]Time between doses and maximum daily dose must also be considered.

[2]Starting doses may be lower. The acute therapeutic dose is often, but not always, less than the maintenance dose. Dosage schedule may be important (e.g., prescribing stimulant drugs early in the day). Note that this is the range for total daily dose, not daily divided dose. Ranges often do not apply to child, elderly, or medically infirm patients.

[3]Maintenance doses are often, but not always, less than the dose for control of early or acute symptoms. Note that this is the range for total dose, not daily divided dose. Ranges often do not apply to child, elderly, or medically infirm patients. Depot doses are given in milligrams every two weeks or milligrams per month.

Medication	Emergency or Crisis, Single Dose (mg)[1]	Acute Rx (mg/day)[2]	Maintenance or Chronic Dose (mg/day)[3]
Antidepressants (cont'd)			
doxepin		75–300	75–300
fluoxetine		20–80	20–80
fluvoxamine		100–300	100–300
imipramine		75–300	75–300
isocarboxazid		10–30	10–20
maprotiline		75–225	75–150
moclobemide		300–600*	300–600*
nefazodone		300–600	300–600
nortriptyline		75–300	75–300
paroxetine		20–50	20–50
phenelzine		60–90	30–60
protriptyline		15–60	15–60
selegiline (l–deprenyl)		10–60*	10–60*
sertraline		50–200	50–200
tranylcypromine		30–60	30–60
trazodone		150–600	150–600
trimipramine		75–300	75–300
venlafaxine		50–350	50–350
Anxiolytics			
alprazolam		1–8	1–8
buspirone		15–60	15–60
chlordiazepoxide	10–25	15–100	15–100
clomipramine in OCD		150–300	150–300
clonazepam		0.5–20	0.5–20
clorazepate	7.5–15	15–60	15–60
diazepam			
oral	5–20	4–40	4–40
injection	2–20		
halazepam		40–160	40–160
hydroxyzine	25–100	100–600	

*Approximate doses, from limited clinical studies or non-U.S. prescribing experience.

[1]Time between doses and maximum daily dose must also be considered.

[2]Starting doses may be lower. The acute therapeutic dose is often, but not always, less than the maintenance dose. Dosage schedule may be important (e.g., prescribing stimulant drugs early in the day). Note that this is the range for total daily dose, not daily divided dose. Ranges often do not apply to child, elderly, or medically infirm patients.

[3]Maintenance doses are often, but not always, less than the dose for control of early or acute symptoms. Note that this is the range for total dose, not daily divided dose. Ranges often do not apply to child, elderly, or medically infirm patients. Depot doses are given in milligrams every two weeks or milligrams per month.

Medication	Emergency or Crisis, Single Dose (mg)[1]	Acute Rx (mg/day)[2]	Maintenance or Chronic Dose (mg/day)[3]
Anxiolytics (cont'd)			
lorazepam		2–10	2–10
oxazepam		20–60	20–60
prazepam		20–60	20–60
Sedative–Hypnotics			
chloral hydrate	500–1,500	500–1,000	
estazolam	1–2	1–2	
ethchlorvynol	500–1,000	500–1,000	
flurazepam	15–30	15–30	
methyprylon	200–400	200–400	
quazepam	7.5–30	7.5–30	
temazepam	15–30	15–30	
triazolam	0.125–0.5	0.125–0.5	
zolpidem	5–10	5–10	
zopiclone	7.5–15	7.5–15	
CNS Stimulants			
dextroamphetamine		5–20	5–20
in narcolepsy		20–60	20–60
methamphetamine		10–40	10–40
in narcolepsy		20–60	20–60
methylphenidate		10–60	10–60
in narcolepsy		20–60	20–60
modafinil in narcolepsy		300–400*	300–400*
pemoline		37.5–75	37.5–75
in narcolepsy		37.5–150	37.5–150

*Approximate doses, from limited clinical studies or non-U.S. prescribing experience.

[1]Time between doses and maximum daily dose must also be considered.

[2]Starting doses may be lower. The acute therapeutic dose is often, but not always, less than the maintenance dose. Dosage schedule may be important (e.g., prescribing stimulant drugs early in the day). Note that this is the range for total daily dose, not daily divided dose. Ranges often do not apply to child, elderly, or medically infirm patients.

[3]Maintenance doses are often, but not always, less than the dose for control of early or acute symptoms. Note that this is the range for total dose, not daily divided dose. Ranges often do not apply to child, elderly, or medically infirm patients. Depot doses are given in milligrams every two weeks or milligrams per month.

Medication	Emergency or Crisis, Single Dose (mg)[1]	Acute Rx (mg/day)[2]	Maintenance or Chronic Dose (mg/day)[3]
Other			
bromocriptine in NMS		10–30	
buprenorphine (sublingual)			
in opioid maintenance		2–16	2–16
clonidine (oral)			
in opiate withdrawal		0.1–2.0[4]	
in tic disorders		0.1–0.25	0.1–0.25
cyproterone acetate (CPA) in paraphilia			
oral		50–200	50–200
depot injection			300–600/1-2wks
dantrolene in neuroleptic malignant syndrome			
oral	400–800	400–800	
IV	50–800		
desmopressin (DDAVP) in enuresis			
oral		20–40 *micrograms*	
nasal spray		10–40 *micrograms*	
disulfiram		125–500	125–500
donepezil		5	5–10
ergoloid		3–4	3–4
fenfluramine for psychiatric indications		60–120	
levocarnitine			2,000–3,000
levomethadyl (LAAM)		20–140 *qd or qod*	20–140 *qd or qod*
medroxy–progesterone acetate (MPA) in paraphilia			
oral		60–80	60–80
depot injection		100–500/wk.	100–500/wk
methadone maintenance		20–100	20–100
naloxone (IV) titrate according to opioid level			
naltrexone (oral)		50	50
tacrine		40–80	40–160
yohimbine		8.1–16.2*	

*Approximate doses, from limited clinical studies or non–U.S. prescribing experience.

[1]Time between doses and maximum daily dose must also be considered.

[2]Starting doses may be lower. The acute therapeutic dose is often, but not always, less than the maintenance dose. Dosage schedule may be important (e.g., prescribing stimulant drugs early in the day). Note that this is the range for total daily dose, not daily divided dose. Ranges often do not apply to child, elderly, or medically infirm patients.

[3]Maintenance doses are often, but not always, less than the dose for control of early or acute symptoms. Note that this is the range for total dose, not daily divided dose. Ranges often do not apply to child, elderly, or medically infirm patients. Depot doses are given in milligrams every two weeks or milligrams per month.

[4]Initial clonidine dose should be very small (0.1–0.3 mg/day); some protocols suggest eventual titration to 0.6–2.0 mg/day.

ADDITIONAL DRUG INFORMATION BIBLIOGRAPHY

Klein, D.F., & Rowland, L.P. (1996): *Current Psychotherapeutic Drugs.* New York: Brunner/Mazel.

Maxmen, J.S., & Ward, N.G. (1995): *Psychotropic Drugs Fast Facts,* (2nd ed.). New York: Norton.

Physicians Desk Reference (1997): 51st edition. Montvale, NJ: Medical Economics.

Name Index

495

Subject Index

XXX